VAT

VETERINARY COLLEGE ADMISSIONS:

A COMPREHENSIVE GUIDE

VAT
VETERINARY
COLLEGE
ADMISSIONS:
A COMPREHENSIVE GUIDE

James W. Morrison
Robert F. Wignall, D.V.M.

ARCO PUBLISHING, INC.
NEW YORK

Published by Arco Publishing, Inc.
215 Park Avenue South, New York, N.Y. 10003

Library of Congress Cataloging in Publication Data

Morrison, James Warner, 1940–
  Veterinary college admissions.

  1. Veterinary colleges—United States—Entrance
examinations—Study guides. 2. Veterinary colleges—
Canada—Entrance examinations—Study guides.
3. Veterinary colleges—Entrance examinations—Study
guides. 4. Veterinary colleges—United States—
Admission. 5. Veterinary colleges—Canada—Admission.
I. Wignall, Robert F.   II. Title.
SF756.35.M67   1985   636.089′076   84-6251
ISBN 0-668-05545-6 (pbk.)

Printed in the United States of America

CONTENTS

ACKNOWLEDGMENTS

The writers gratefully acknowledge the assistance of the American Veterinary Medical Association. Their publications, particularly *Today's Veterinarian*, are important sources of information about the profession. A special note of thanks is due to Dr. Wayne H. Riser, whose *Your Future in Veterinary Medicine* (Arco) brings into focus the difficult issues facing young people who wish to become veterinarians.

In compiling this book, it has been necessary to draw heavily on existing materials in the catalogs, brochures, and information bulletins of American colleges of veterinary medicine. A note of thanks and appreciation is due to these institutions, as well as to institutions offering preveterinary programs, for the use of their announcements.

Acknowledgment is gratefully given to our many colleagues who have provided valuable advice. We would like to thank Mr. Gino Crocetti for permission to use a practice GRE test from his *GRE—Graduate Record Examination General Aptitude Test* (Arco) and Lawrence Solomon, M.D., for permission to use a sample GRE Advanced Biology test from his *Biology: Advanced Test for the GRE* (Arco).

Assistance in many clerical activities was given by Mrs. Blanche Duval and Mrs. Marsha Glance; their many hours of effort are appreciated.

R.F.W., D.V.M.
J.W.M.

PREFACE

It is a difficult task to describe the nature and scope of veterinary medical education in one volume. If, however, you are greatly interested in the profession, this book should encourage your study.

A branch of medicine, veterinary medicine is a separate, self-governing profession with its own system of education, licensure, and code of ethics. The responsibilities of the profession are twofold: to protect animal health and to protect human health. Contributions of the profession to public health include the control of one hundred or so animal diseases that are transmissible to humans (*zoonoses*) and the inspection of foods of animal origin for the protection of consumers. By controlling the diseases of farm animals, veterinarians help to conserve the nation's food supply. Veterinarians are, of course, deeply concerned with relieving suffering among animals.

The activities of veterinarians are highly diversified and include work with all species of animals, wild and domestic. While many of the nation's veterinarians are engaged in private practice, either general or specialized, large numbers are also employed in public health, regulatory, military, industrial, research, and teaching activities.

No matter which professional activity a veterinarian eventually chooses, it takes a lot of hard work to prepare for it. And, like most medical careers, veterinary medicine is a way of life requiring strong vocational motivation and dedication. It is a demanding career but also a rewarding one.

Robert F. Wignall, D.V.M.
James W. Morrison

INTRODUCTION

The purpose of a college of veterinary medicine is to educate young men and women to become practitioners, teachers, and researchers in the science and art of veterinary medicine. Veterinary colleges help to protect the health of livestock, poultry, and companion animals and to support public health programs. They are becoming increasingly important for practicing veterinarians, as well as to the animal-owning public. Their service activities include taking referrals of patients to their clinical departments for diagnostic, medical, or surgical attention; diagnostic laboratory services of serologic, clinical, pathologic, histopathologic, toxicologic, bacteriologic, virologic, and parasitologic nature; and gross autopsy services.

Today, every veterinary college is faced with the task of selecting a small group of students from an overwhelming number of qualified applicants. Only about 25 percent of qualified applicants gain admittance; the vast majority of applicants will not be able to enroll in a professional program in veterinary medicine. Given this competitive situation, it is wise to learn as much as possible about the profession in order to be sure of your interest in and aptitude for it. The following pages give a broad view of veterinary medicine as a profession.

Veterinarians are dedicated to protecting the health and welfare of both animals and people. They are primarily animal doctors, highly educated and skilled in preventing, diagnosing, and treating animal health problems. Because their special knowledge and their training extend to a number of closely related areas, veterinarians are involved in much more than animal medicine. In taking the veterinarian's oath, the veterinary doctor solemnly swears to use his or her scientific knowledge and skills "for the benefit of society, through the protection of animal health, the relief of animal suffering, the conservation of livestock resources, the promotion of public health, and the advancement of medical knowledge."

Veterinarians give animals care similar to that rendered in human medicine. A veterinarian must, accordingly, receive a similar medical education, with a minimum of three years of preveterinary college work and four years of veterinary medicine before a degree of D.V.M., doctor of veterinary medicine. The graduate must then pass the state veterinary medical board examination in order to qualify for a license to practice.

There is no set internship requirement in veterinary medicine at present, but a young doctor usually goes to work for a year or more with an experienced veterinarian before establishing his or her own practice or becoming an associate in practice.

Veterinary medicine, although an ancient calling, has developed more slowly than human medicine; the two fields are benefiting more and more from a growing appreciation of their interdependence. Veterinarians' skills have been refined and greatly enhanced by better scientific education. Today, veterinarians no longer go to the animal to treat it so often as they invite the owner to bring it to their well-equipped hospital or clinic where, with the necessary apparatuses available, they can do a better job of diagnosis and treatment.

The majority of veterinarians are in either large-animal or small-animal private practice, although many do both. The private practitioner may be his or her own boss and can establish his or her own appointment hours, although emergency services and heavy caseloads usually require extra time. Because they are self-employed, most private practitioners can continue to work beyond normal retirement age if they wish. But hours may be long and irregular, particularly for veterinarians who are just starting or who practice alone. The practicing veterinarian also may have to take care of all the bookwork, personnel problems, and other business matters that go along with operating a practice.

Private practice offers a great deal of variety in daily activities. Many different kinds of patients must be treated, and unexpected problems or emergencies can develop at any moment. Work with farm animals usually must be done in a barn or outdoors, often under difficult conditions. Practitioners who treat farm and ranch animals usually spend a great deal of time driving to reach patients who cannot be brought to the clinic or hospital.

Setting up a veterinary practice usually involves purchasing a good deal of expensive equipment and a mobile practice truck or a building. Unlike a community hospital or health clinic, which is financed by tax money, a modern veterinary hospital or clinic must be financed by the owner.

Practicing veterinarians always risk being physically injured or getting one of the many diseases animals can transmit to people. They also have to deal every day with pet and livestock owners, some of whom are not always easy to get along with.

Veterinarians employed by government agencies, laboratories, colleges, and commercial firms usually enjoy fairly regular hours, pleasant surroundings, and a steady income, along with retirement programs and other fringe benefits.

On a college faculty, a veterinarian can find many rewards in teaching both students and graduate veterinarians new knowledge and skills. Veterinarians on college faculties also have opportunities to conduct research, take part in public service programs, and earn advanced academic degrees.

Military veterinarians, too, have opportunities to continue their formal education, usually at government expense. Many retire from the service at a relatively early age and begin a second career in public health or some other area of veterinary medicine.

In order to keep up with the latest scientific developments and new techniques, veterinarians must continue to learn throughout their professional careers by reading, attending scientific meetings, taking additional coursework, and consulting with their colleagues.

Our country still needs more veterinarians than the colleges of veterinary medicine can graduate, although the new graduate probably has somewhat fewer alternatives than were available just a few years ago. The veterinary medical profession offers excellent opportunities for those who have an abiding interest in the diagnosis, treatment, and prevention of animal diseases. The compensation varies greatly, but intelligent and conscientious service is usually rewarded by an adequate income. Those who are genuinely interested in the work will find a veterinary career both challenging and satisfying.

VAT

VETERINARY COLLEGE ADMISSIONS:

A COMPREHENSIVE GUIDE

Part One

GENERAL INFORMATION

THE VETERINARY MEDICAL PROFESSION

A SUMMARY VIEW OF THE PROFESSION

Veterinarians are primarily responsible for the health of farm livestock, poultry, and pet animals. These are the major concerns of most veterinarians in private practice and a large number of those in governmental service. There are also rapidly increasing opportunities available to the graduate veterinarian to use his or her training in a number of other, related areas. These choices include participating in various phases of public health work, such as inspection of production, storage, and distribution of animal food products; being involved in the health care of zoo animals or animals used for biological and medical research; and finding solutions to the health problems of wildlife. Veterinarians are also engaged in research related to animal disease, human medical problems, and basic biological phenomena.

About 76 percent of America's veterinarians are engaged in private practice. Most of these attend the ills of all kinds of animals; a smaller group devotes itself exclusively either to farm animals or to companion animals. The others are involved in a wide variety of careers essential to the support of human health and welfare.

Private practice is a wide field with excellent opportunities. Veterinary practice may be: general, in which the practitioner offers his services in dealing with all species of animals; farm animals, in which the economically important food-producing domestic animals are considered; companion animals, which concerns domestic animals kept as companions or pets; or special, in which only specific conditions or individual species are handled.

Veterinarians are needed both to develop and protect world food supply. Our increasing human population will require more and more food-producing animals. These animals will not only have to be in plentiful supply but will also have to be free from disease so that the meat, eggs, milk, and other dairy products they produce will be wholesome.

The fields of ecology and oceanography also provide unique opportunities for veterinarians. Obviously animals are important elements of our physical environment. Since there are some 100 infectious diseases transmissible between animals and humans, it is essential that companion animals be healthy because they associate so closely with people. It is also extremely important that food-producing animals be free of the residues of drugs and toxic chemicals so that these won't find their way into our food.

Recreational animals, such as riding horses and hunting dogs, are assuming growing importance today. Our shorter work week, earlier retirement, and lengthening life expectancy will doubtless create a need for more pets and recreational animals. There will be a growing demand for more and better veterinary services for these animals.

The veterinary medical profession performs a vital role in research for the benefit of human health. Today's greatest dangers to human health, cancer, heart

3

disease, and the infirmities of old age, are shared by animals, often in almost identical form. In fact, veterinarians have identified more than 250 human diseases and abnormalities that have counterparts in animals. Hence, it is with animals that much of the research on human ailments can be done most productively.

Aside from its human health and humane dimensions, the veterinary profession is of enormous economic importance to the nation. Livestock diseases such as foot-and-mouth disease, contagious pleuropneumonia, and rinderpest— plagues that have repeatedly decimated cattle populations in other parts of the world—have been kept outside the continental limits of the United States through the vigilance of federal and state regulatory veterinarians. Other highly contagious diseases such as tuberculosis, brucellosis, and hog cholera, which caused millions of dollars in annual losses during the first half of this century, have in twenty years been virtually eradicated through a combination of research and preventive medicine. Today, losses to livestock disease are estimated to be in excess of $3 billion annually—and most of this is potentially preventable.

Veterinary care is a necessary adjunct to the economic importance of animals as consumers of agricultural products. The use of grains and grasses by livestock and poultry for conversion to human food products is well-known. Less known is the fact that sales of dog and cat food (also predominately agricultural products) amount to well over a billion dollars annually. Finally, the horse, which declined so rapidly in numbers during the 1940s and 1950s, is now making a remarkable recovery. The capital investment in these animals and their requirements in feed and in health care can be measured in billions of dollars annually.

While most American veterinarians are men, women are entering the profession in increasing numbers. Some 41 percent of the students entering colleges of veterinary medicine are now women. Veterinary medicine also offers unusual opportunities for members of minority groups. The future of the veterinary medical profession seems brighter now than ever before in its long history. The virtual explosion in numbers of small-animal practitioners in the past decade indicates that veterinary medicine today is important in urban as well as in the rural areas of the country. The great increase of veterinarians working in special fields reflects the profession's strength and versatility in new areas such as space exploration and biomedical studies, areas that require the highest degree of specialized knowledge and sophisticated skills.

CAREER OPPORTUNITIES FOR VETERINARIANS

Veterinary Practice

Private practice attracts by far the largest percentage of veterinarians. As the profession has grown, various kinds of practices have evolved. Practices are owned by individuals or groups of veterinarians and range from mixed to highly selective specialty operations.

Large-animal practice is concerned with the nutrition, management, and disease problems of horses, cattle, sheep, and swine. The large-animal veterinarian is in the forefront of the struggle to protect food animals from disease and thus assure an adequate animal protein supply for our nation.

Small-animal veterinarians are concerned with the health, care, and management of dogs, cats, and other small pets. The modern small-animal clinic or hospital is well equipped with surgical units and clinical laboratories necessary for the diagnosis and treatment of the problems of household pets.

Mixed practice is usually concerned with both large and small animals. The practices are often staffed by more than one veterinarian, so that each may concentrate in certain areas.

Specialty practices concentrate their services in one discipline. These include specialties in bovine, equine, avian, and exotic- or zoo-animal medicine, and specialty disciplines such as ophthalmology, radiology, or nutrition.

Laboratory-animal veterinarians direct their efforts towards the management of laboratory animals used for biomedical teaching and research. They are responsible for the health of species varying from pigeons to miniature swine. Others may use animals for drug testing, disease study, or investigating basic biological phenomena.

Space and marine biology veterinarians will become more important as space travel and the use of marine plants and animals for food sources increase.

International Agencies

Veterinarians have helped improve the food supplies in many underdeveloped countries, thus raising the local standards of living. Opportunities for foreign service are based on one- to two-year contracts or appointments. Such positions are available through universities, foundations, or specialized agencies of the United Nations. A few veterinarians also are employed directly by foreign countries, private firms, or individuals on a consultant basis.

Federal Employment

The largest single employer of veterinarians is the U.S. federal government with more than 3200 veterinarians in a variety of duties vital to the health of American citizens. Some federal and state veterinarians are members of teams including physicians and sanitarians who work to safeguard the public health.

The United States Department of Agriculture service employs more veterinarians than any other single agency. Opportunities include meat inspection, animal disease eradication programs, animal disease and parasite research, poultry inspection, livestock inspection, and inspection in biological production plants. The U.S. Department of Agriculture has always needed the services of top-flight veterinarians. USDA veterinarians must be graduates of schools listed by the U.S. Civil Service Commission as accredited veterinary colleges. The U.S. Civil Service Commission conducts examinations for veterinary positions in the government service.

To improve and protect the livestock industry in the United States, the Department of Agriculture performs extensive research on the diseases and parasites of livestock. It is responsible for controlling or eradicating certain animal diseases by the application of suitable measures. These include inspection of animals in the field, at stockyards, and at ports of entry. The protective measures include the control or eradication of animal diseases such as tuberculosis, brucellosis or undulant fever, cattle-tick or splenetic fever, hog cholera, swine erysipelas, sheep and cattle scabies, anthrax, and glanders. It administers a national program to prevent the production, importation, and marketing of any worthless, dangerous or harmful virus, serum, toxin, or analagous product for use in the treatment of domestic animals.

Veterinarians also conduct inspections to assure the wholesomeness, freedom from disease, and cleanliness of meat and meat food products and of poultry and poultry food products shipped in interstate commerce. These activities employ the largest number of veterinarians in the Department.

Listed below are two agencies within the Department of Agriculture that employ veterinarians.

The Animal and Plant Health Inspection Service (APHIS) administers the animal health, veterinary biologics, and meat and poultry inspection programs of the Department of Agriculture. APHIS veterinarians inspect livestock at stockyards or ports of entry into the United States to protect the livestock and poultry industries from disease of foreign origin and prevent the spread of communicable diseases in interstate commerce. Veterinarians also inspect licensed establishments producing veterinary biologics to assure their potency and purity. Many of these veterinarians work in laboratories. Veterinarians are also responsible for the nation's meat and poultry supply to assure its wholesomeness and safety for consumption.

The U.S. Public Health Service and the Food and Drug Administration offers one of the newest and most interesting careers for veterinarians. Communicable-disease control, food sanitation, public health administration, and research in epizootiology and epidemiology represent the major activities of veterinarians employed in these areas.

The Army and the Air Force also have veterinary officers to help protect the health of troops at home and abroad. In addition to safeguarding food and water supplies, Veterinary Corps members carry out research in special military fields such as the effects of space flight on living beings, health of laboratory animals, and human diet development. They also care for animals such as military sentry dogs. Physically qualified graduates of veterinary medical schools who are acceptable to the surgeon generals of the U.S. Army and the U.S. Air Force and who elect to go on active duty are eligible to make application for appointment in grades first lieutenant to colonel, inclusive, the grade being determined by the age, professional experience, and qualifications of the applicant.

State Employment

Each state has a chief livestock sanitary officer, usually identified as "State Veterinarian," whose duty is to enforce the laws, rules, and regulations formulated to suppress diseases of animals within the state and to control the movement of animals through the state. In most states a corps of veterinarians is employed in this regulatory work.

Many state health departments have one or more veterinarians on their staffs engaged in the control of animal diseases transmissible to humans, research, coordination of various state agencies in animal disease control programs, food inspection activities, and numerous other, related functions.

Municipal Government

Most cities and some towns employ veterinarians either full- or part-time as members of their health departments. Such individuals are usually connected with the sanitary control of meat, meat products, milk, and milk products, as well as with the promulgation and enforcement of local disease-control ordinances involving rabies and other diseases transmissible to humans.

Private Industry

Many commercial concerns employ veterinarians on their staffs. Biological and pharmaceutical companies, feed manufacturers, distributors, and dealers have a special need for veterinary services, as do many of the meat-packing companies and some specialized scientific instrument producers.

Academic Positions

Almost every agricultural school in the United States has a veterinary science department where varying numbers of veterinarians are employed in research, teaching, adult education, and other forms of service. There are 27 fully operating schools or colleges of veterinary medicine in the United States, each having from 25 to 100 veterinarians on its staff. In addition, many colleges offer programs in animal technology. Teaching and research opportunities are numerous in these institutions and should be considered seriously by interested and qualified students.

Medical Research and Laboratory Animal Care

A number of veterinarians are employed by medical schools and other institutions to guard the health of laboratory animals and to do cooperative research benefiting humans and animals. Opportunities in this area have been increasing rapidly during recent years.

Other Veterinary Employment Opportunities

By the very nature of the varied patients dealt with and the clientele served, the opportunities available to the veterinarian are numerous. A veterinarian is specially qualified to participate in the solution of problems relating to ecology, food resource management, wildlife preservation, zoo animal care, and space and marine biology. Those individuals interested in local or international service in these areas should consider the opportunities available in the veterinary medical profession.

All these developments forecast an increasing need for veterinarians where shortages already exist. It seems certain, therefore, that veterinarians trained during the next few years will be able to choose from a great variety of challenging and rewarding positions in this essential, growing profession.

VETERINARY MEDICAL EDUCATION

In most colleges of veterinary medicine, the professional program is divided into two phases. During the first phase, preclinical sciences—including anatomy, physiology, pathology, pharmacology and microbiology—are emphasized. Most of the student's time is spent in classroom and laboratory study.

The second phase of professional study is largely clinical. During much of this time, students work with animal patients and deal with owners who use the school's clinical services. The clinical curriculum includes courses on infectious and noninfectious diseases, advanced pathology, applied anatomy, obstetrics, radiology, clinical medicine, and surgery. Students also study public health, preventive medicine, toxicology, nutrition, professional ethics, and business practices.

For most people, veterinary medical study is difficult. Students must learn and remember hundreds of terms and all kinds of facts about many different animals and diseases. They also have to become skilled in surgical techniques and many laboratory and diagnostic procedures. A typical veterinary medical student spends about 5000 hours in classroom, laboratory, and clinical study. And, because the time required for instruction takes up practically all of a student's day, many more hours must be spent at night and on weekends doing lengthy reading assignments, library research, and independent study.

In many ways, a veterinarian's education only begins with a D.V.M. degree. New scientific knowledge and techniques are constantly being developed, and a veterinarian must keep abreast of new information by reading scientific journals and attending professional meetings, short courses, and seminars.

The Doctor of Veterinary Medicine degree can be granted after satisfactory completion of a four-year curriculum. Most institutions require a minimum of six years, including undergraduate courses. The curriculum leading to the D.V.M. includes study of the sciences basic to veterinary medicine and surgery; application of the fundamentals of medicine and surgery; and intensive training in small-animal medicine and surgery, large-animal medicine and surgery, food-animal medicine, equine medicine, public health, exotic and wildlife medicine, and other subspecialties.

Some veterinary colleges have inaugurated an integrated curriculum which compresses a body of knowledge ordinarily presented in a four-year program into a three-year core curriculum to be followed by a one-year track program that delves more intensively into one facet of veterinary medicine. Clinical instruction sometimes begins during the first quarter, correlated with other offerings and carried out through the entire four-year curriculum.

Any student in a D.V.M. program in a school of veterinary medicine who does not hold a baccalaureate degree but has satisfactorily completed the first two years of the professional curriculum and has satisfied the general university requirements is usually eligible to receive a Bachelor of Science (B.S.) degree in veterinary science. A veterinary medicine course of study has at least these goals: to provide a thorough background in both the basic and clinical medical sciences; to offer educational opportunities to observe as well as participate in veterinary medical practice, and to encourage a commitment to scholarship because learning is a

9

lifelong process for the veterinarian. Usually, a substantial portion of the professional education of future veterinarians takes place in the teaching hospital, where they apply knowledge of the basic sciences to solving clinical problems. By working directly with small and large animals and hospital equipment under the supervision of clinical faculty, students gain experience through which they will integrate classroom knowledge with veterinary medical practice.

In the first year of a veterinary medicine program, students commonly examine the structure and function of normal animals. By the second year they usually begin to study pathogenesis of infectious diseases, pathophysiologic concepts, and the principles of therapy. In the last two years of the program, time is spent chiefly in studying prevention, alleviation, and therapy of diseases. Through active involvement with clients and care and management of patients, students learn methods of care, communication, leadership, and administration needed in their later professional practice. Most colleges have a core-elective curriculum sequence; some institutions have more individual courses and offer a broader variety of electives than others. It is not possible to describe in this book all of the professional curricula in colleges of veterinary medicine; the following illustrates in a general way the courses of instruction for the D.V.M. degree.

The subjects of veterinary medical instruction include:

First Year: Gross Anatomy, Developmental Anatomy, Microscopic Anatomy, Introduction to Veterinary Medicine, Introductory Microbiology, Physiology I, Experimental Physiology I, Biochemistry, Neuroscience, Immunology.

Second Year: Animal Production, Poultry Production Methods, Microbiology of Pathogenic Organisms, Physiology II, Experimental Physiology II, Pharmacology, Experimental Pharmacology, Virology, Parasitology, Public Health, General Pathology, Systemic Pathology, The Veterinarian and the Law.

Third Year: Applied Anatomy, Clinical Pathology, Diagnostic Pathology, Radiology, Obstetrics and Reproduction, Correlative Medicine I, Surgery I, Avian Medicine, Food Hygiene, Toxicology.

Fourth Year: Medicine II, Surgery II, Applied Veterinary Medicine (Clinics), Electives.

The following are some of the elective courses that might be available:

Food Animal Clerkship, Equine Clerkship, Studies in Large-animal Clinical Medicine, Studies in Small-animal Clinical Medicine, Small-animal Surgery Clerkship, Small-animal Medicine Clerkship, Clinical Radiology, Radiology Clerkship, Studies in Clinical Anatomy and Radiology, Necropsy Pathology, Advanced Clinical Pathology, Studies in Clinical Veterinary Pathology, Advanced Clinical Microbiology, Diseases of Fishes, Studies in Clinical Medical Microbiology, Laboratory and Exotic Animal Medicine, Clinical Avian Medicine, Diseases of Pet Birds, Studies in Clinical Avian Medicine, Clinical Pharmacology Seminar, Studies in Clinical Physiology and Pharmacology, Studies in Clinical Parasitology.

During the first year, students in veterinary medicine study the gross and microscopic anatomy of food-producing animals, companion animals, and selected laboratory animals. They concurrently study normal functions of cells, tissues, organs, and body systems in physiology and physiologic chemistry. The veterinarian's knowledge of anatomy, physiology, and physiologic chemistry provides the basis for understanding disease processes and the recognition and treatment of animal diseases.

First-year veterinary students study anatomy in laboratory exercises in gross anatomic dissection, microscopic examination of cells and tissues, and study of embryologic and neuroanatomic specimens. Laboratories in physiologic chemistry and physiology provide opportunities for the student to observe and measure the activity of animal organs and tissues.

During the second year, students study pharmacology, which includes actions of drugs and factors influencing the responses of animals to drugs. In the study of toxicology, the student studies disease conditions resulting from poisonous materials including plants, agricultural and industrial chemicals, feed additives, and drugs.

In the clinical years of the professional curriculum, the student is introduced to the art and science of clinical veterinary medicine and surgery. The practical application of the basic principles of medicine to the diagnosis, prevention, and treatment of disease in all species of animals presents a challenge to the mental and physical resources of the student. Proficiency in clinical medicine can be gained by working closely with experienced clinicians in small-animal, large-animal, and ambulatory clinics of teaching hospitals. By the case method of study, professional students are given a considerable amount of responsibility for the total health requirements of animals assigned to their care. Group discussion, formal lectures, and laboratory training guide the progress of the clinical student in systemic medicine and surgery.

Professional courses are also offered, providing instruction in the host response to invading microorganisms, special properties of microorganisms that determine disease-producing potential, and techniques for isolation and identification of microorganisms. Special emphasis is placed on the immunology, transmission, prevention, and control of infectious and parasitic diseases, and on veterinary public health. Lectures, organized laboratory periods, special demonstrations, special projects, and autotutorial programs are offered.

The primary function of the courses in pathology is to teach the morphologic and biochemical changes that occur in animals infected with disease. This is conducted in formal and applied courses in both the professional and graduate programs.

SOME AREAS OF STUDY WITHIN THE VETERINARY CURRICULUM

Following are brief descriptions of areas of study usually offered in a college of veterinary medicine program; students in veterinary medicine take courses in each of these areas. In addition, third- and fourth-year students learn through various field experiences, which are described later under the heading "Clinic Experience" on page 14.

Anatomy. Anatomy includes four related areas: gross anatomy, histology, embryology, and neuroanatomy. In gross anatomy, students first learn the normal structure and function of domestic animals, using the dog as a concept model and dissection subject. Next they study comparative anatomy by dissecting the horse and cow and contrasting them with the pig, sheep, and goat. Clinical anatomy emphasizes gross structures of these animals of special clinical significance. In histology and embryology, students discover normal and abnormal developmental processes as they relate to adult structures; again, both macro- and microfeatures are delineated. Avian morphology is covered during the first year of histology. The focus in neuroanatomy is on identification and definition of structural units. The relationships between these anatomical features and behavior are also studied.

Biochemistry. How biological systems function at the molecular level is the overall question answered in this field. Students learn the ways in which animals digest and absorb nutrients, how they use the absorbed molecules to maintain normal physiological processes, and how the end products, broken down by metabolic processes, are eliminated. Carbohydrates, lipids, proteins, and nucleic acids are explored in depth. After learning about the nature of enzymes, the ways in which they affect biological reactions, and how they are affected by environmental factors, students examine how metabolic processes are regulated. Studying the metabolic role of different tissues in the body and the molecular basis for some metabolic abnormalities provides the foundation needed to understand disease.

Clinical Pathology. Clinical pathology is a broad area of laboratory medicine that crosses several disciplines, including hematology, cytology, surgical pathology, serology, clinical chemistry, and urine analysis. Students evaluate laboratory results and decide when such results may be interpreted with confidence or when they must be applied with reservations. The important aspects of statistical assessment—precision, accuracy, reliability, and interpretability—are presented.

Epidemiology and Public Health. Through epidemiology and public health, veterinary students learn the science of epidemic diseases, food hygiene, environmental health, and zoonoses. These principles are then applied to solve problems encountered in the practice of preventive medicine for all animal species, herd health management for food animals, clinical epidemiology, food protection and hygiene maintenance throughout food production, diseases transmitted from animals to humans, as well as problems related to environmental factors affecting the health of animals and humans.

Microbiology. In microbiology students learn about the taxonomy and metabolic characteristics of bacteria, fungi, and viruses, and their role in both normal and disease processes. Students also study disease-producing microorganisms indigenous to other countries because they pose a possible threat to our susceptible animal population. Mastery of the basic principles of microbiology is essential to the study of infectious diseases, medicine, surgery, pharmacology, and public health—disciplines that comprise the bulk of the last two years of the professional curriculum. Immunology, the study of how animals react to foreign substances, is an important area which is studied concurrently with microbiology and in other courses as well. With the present ease and frequency of long-distance transport of animals, rapid detection, treatment, and control of infectious animal diseases—which require knowledge of microbiology and immunology—take on great economic significance.

Parasitology. Parasitology deals with protozoa, arthropods, and helminths which infest animals. Here students learn about life cycles of parasites, how they affect the health of animals, and their control. Both internal and external parasites are studied. Special attention is given to identifying and classifying parasites, procedures that are commonly used to detect and identify them, and drugs and management procedures that are used for their control.

Pathology. Courses in this field are offered to explain how cells and tissues react to injury, and to relate morphologic changes in them to functional changes. Cell degenerations, cell death, inflammation, immunopathology, and neoplastic and nonneoplastic growth abnormalities are some of the topics taken up. Students are expected to differentiate abnormal from normal cells or tissues at the gross and microscopic levels, identify abnormalities using appropriate terminology, and understand mechanisms (pathogenesis) involved in the development of the abnormalities.

Pharmacology. The goals for students in this discipline are twofold: to understand the general principles underlying drug action and use, thus building the conceptual framework within which to integrate subsequent training in veterinary therapeutics, and to acquire adequate knowledge of drugs used therapeutically by considering prototypes from major drug groups. The following topics concerning drugs in general are examined: chemical nature, the relationship between the structure of the drug and its biological activity, the ways in which drugs are absorbed and distributed in the body, how drug action is terminated and how the drug is eliminated from the body, biological variability in response of animals to drugs, dose-response and time-response relationships, drug interactions, toxicity and abuse, and regulation of drugs.

Physiology. Physiology is closely related to both anatomy and biochemistry, focusing on the function of all the major body organs and organ systems: circulatory, digestive, renal, reproductive, respiratory, etc. Since clinical problems frequently involve digestion and reproduction, these areas are emphasized. The endocrine organs are studied in endocrinology. The structure of hormones, their principal effects and target organs, and their regulation are presented, with emphasis on reproductive endocrinology. Students also learn about interrelationships among hormones and the consequences of the secretion of abnormal quantities of hormones.

Anesthesiology. Anesthesiology covers the pharmacology of anesthetic agents, cardiopulmonary physiology, and the use of anesthetic agents and equipment for various kinds of patients and surgical procedures. Students also learn to deal with shock, the traumatized or critically ill patient, and various methods of monitoring the surgical patient. Techniques are usually practiced in special anesthesiology laboratories, the surgery teaching laboratory, and on patients in a veterinary teaching hospital.

Large-animal Medicine. This field includes work with food- and fiber-producing animals, horses, and zoo animals. Students learn how to approach a clinical case, do a thorough physical examination, reach a diagnosis, carry out a course of therapy, give a prognosis, and recommend methods of control and prevention of a disease. Field investigations of disease problems are a valuable part of the learning experience. Students also participate in establishing and conducting herd health programs and in handling diseases in herds of animals. Zoo-animal medicine is approached in lectures and by experience at a local zoo or with zoo animals brought to a veterinary teaching hospital. Externships enable fourth-year students to work with animal health problems by participating in veterinary medical practices throughout the country.

Small-animal Medicine.   Students are prepared for this specialty by providing them with current information on all aspects of diseases of pet animals. Techniques and procedures used in the diagnosis, therapy, and management of such diseases are demonstrated and practiced. Courses in diagnostic and therapeutic techniques and physical diagnosis prepare students for active participation in small-animal clinical care. In clinics, students integrate and use information obtained in both basic science and clinical courses to solve pet-animal health problems.

Radiology.   Radiology concentrates on the properties and production of X rays; their use in diagnosis and therapy; their safe use, including the major regulations concerning the subject; and understanding and controlling film processing. Interpreting radiograms and basic principles of radiation therapy and nuclear medicine are highlighted.

Large-animal Surgery.   Theories and techniques of veterinary surgery, as applied to large animals, are covered in this disciplinary area. Additional important areas of study are the etiology and pathophysiology of diseases that require surgical intervention. Students learn to correlate information from preclinical and clinical courses in making decisions about surgery and in managing the surgical patient. Course work includes basic principles of veterinary surgery, surgical diagnosis, therapeutic techniques, and aftercare of specific disease entities. Surgery laboratory courses afford firsthand experience in certain surgical procedures— casting, splinting, and bandaging techniques; patient care; and experience in large-animal anesthesia.

Small-animal Surgery.   The small-animal surgery program provides students with a broad basic education in principles, theories, and techniques of veterinary surgery and anesthesiology. The program includes study of the etiology and pathophysiology of diseases that require surgical intervention. Knowledge of the other clinical sciences as well as the basic sciences is brought to bear in developing sound programs for the management and therapy of surgical patients.

Theriogenology.   In theriogenology students learn the parameters of normal fertility and reproductive efficiency for most species of domestic animals. The roles of environment, nutrition, genetics, management, and other factors influencing normal body functions are studied, as well as the relationship between these factors and anatomic abnormalities, physiologic alterations, or diseases that ultimately result in lower fertility. Students develop the skill to recognize clinical signs that may indicate lower reproductive efficiency, and they make clinical examinations. Training is provided in laboratories, on hospital cases, and on farms served by ambulatory clinics.

Clinic Experience.   Direct experience with veterinary medical problems and patients forms an important part of the fourth-year curriculum. Field, clinic, and laboratory assignments last from one to six weeks, are offered both on and off campus, and accompany corresponding course work. They include assignments to the clinical areas described above as well as externships, ambulatory clinics, and preventive veterinary medicine programs.

In externships students are typically placed off campus for two weeks to work with practicing veterinarians not associated with the college, although selected by it. The location and kind of animal cared for cover a broad range.

Ambulatory clinics are mobile units dispatched on demand to deliver on-site veterinary medical care to animals on university farms and on farms within a reasonable distance from the campus.

In preventive medicine, production animals and their farm environments are examined and tested on a regularly scheduled basis by students and staff of the college. Herd health programs are provided for beef cattle, dairy cattle, horses, poultry, and swine.

VETERINARY COLLEGE ADMISSIONS

The competition for admission to veterinary medical college is intense because of the limited number of openings for first-year students. Only about one of every four qualified applicants is accepted. It is important, therefore, to know what is taken into consideration in the admissions process, so that you can prepare yourself as thoroughly as possible. You should also give some thought to alternative career plans, in the event that you are not accepted into a program of veterinary medical study.

Most veterinary medical colleges evaluate applicants according to both objective and subjective critera. Examples of objective critera that may be used are undergraduate grade point average, undergraduate grades in specific prerequisite science and/or mathematics courses, and scores on standardized examinations such as the Veterinary Aptitude Test VAT, Medical College Admission Test MCAT, Graduate Record Examination GRE, or GRE Advanced Biology Test. Subjective criteria that may be considered include personal interviews, letters of recommendation, contact and experience with animals, and an applicant's motivation, maturity, leadership abilities, and extracurricular activities. Often the objective criteria carry more weight in the admission decision than do the subjective criteria.

Each school of veterinary medicine sets its own entrance policies and requirements. Most admissions committees try to select those well-qualified applicants who, in their judgment, are best able to complete the veterinary medical studies successfully and who have the potential to become competent, responsible veterinarians dedicated to a lifetime of productive community service and continued learning. Admissions requirements vary from one veterinary college to another. Many schools have state residency requirements or preferences. Write to the particular school or schools that interest you to find out exactly when the deadline for application is and what specific requirements must be met.

VETERINARY MEDICAL COLLEGES ACCREDITED BY THE AMERICAN VETERINARY MEDICAL ASSOCIATION

Alabama

School of Veterinary Medicine
Auburn University
Auburn, AL 36849

School of Veterinary Medicine
Tuskegee Institute
Tuskegee, AL 36088

California

School of Veterinary Medicine
University of California
Davis, CA 95616

Colorado

College of Veterinary Medicine
and Biomedical Sciences
Colorado State University
Ft. Collins, CO 80523

Florida

College of Veterinary Medicine
University of Florida
Gainesville, FL 32601

Georgia

College of Veterinary Medicine
University of Georgia
Athens, GA 30601

Illinois

College of Veterinary Medicine
University of Illinois
Urbana, IL 61801

Indiana

School of Veterinary Medicine
Purdue University
West Lafayette, IN 47907

Iowa

College of Veterinary Medicine
Iowa State University
Ames, IA 50011

Kansas

College of Veterinary Medicine
Kansas State University
Manhattan, KS 66502

Louisiana

College of Veterinary Medicine
Louisiana State University
Baton Rouge, LA 70803

Massachusetts

School of Veterinary Medicine
Tufts University
Boston, MA 02111

Michigan

College of Veterinary Medicine
Michigan State University
East Lansing, MI 48824

Minnesota

College of Veterinary Medicine
University of Minnesota
St. Paul, MN 55108

Mississippi

College of Veterinary Medicine
Mississippi State University
Mississippi State, MS 39762

Missouri

College of Veterinary Medicine
University of Missouri
Columbia, MO 65201

New York

New York State College of
Veterinary Medicine
Cornell University
Ithaca, NY 14853

North Carolina

School of Veterinary Medicine
North Carolina State University
Raleigh, NC 27607

Ohio

College of Veterinary Medicine
Ohio State University
Columbus, OH 43210

Oklahoma

College of Veterinary Medicine
Oklahoma State University
Stillwater, OK 74074

Texas

College of Veterinary Medicine
Texas A&M University
College Station, TX 77843

Oregon

School of Veterinary Medicine
Oregon State University
Corvallis, OR 97331

Virginia

Virginia-Maryland Regional
    College of Veterinary Medicine
Virginia Polytechnic Institute
Blacksburg, VA 24061

Pennsylvania

School of Veterinary Medicine
University of Pennsylvania
Philadelphia, PA 19104

Washington

College of Veterinary Medicine
Washington State University
Pullman, WA 99163

Tennessee

College of Veterinary Medicine
University of Tennessee
Knoxville, TN 37901

Wisconsin

School of Veterinary Medicine
University of Wisconsin
Madison, WI 53706

REQUIREMENTS AND PRIORITIES FOR VETERINARY MEDICAL COLLEGES

College	Admissions Priorities	Test Requirements
Auburn University Auburn, Alabama	Alabama, Kentucky, and North Carolina residents	none
Colorado State University Ft. Collins, Colorado	Colorado residents or residents of Western Interstate Commission for Higher Education (WICHE) states—currently, Alaska, Arizona, Hawaii, Montana, Nevada, New Mexico, Utah, Wyoming	GRE Aptitude Test

College	Admissions Priorities	Test Requirements
Cornell University Ithaca, New York	none given	GRE Aptitude Test
Iowa State University Ames, Iowa	Iowa residents and approved residents of states having contracts with I.S.U. for educating veterinary medical students	VAT
Kansas State University Manhattan, Kansas	1. Kansas residents 2. residents of contract states—Arizona, Arkansas, New Mexico, North Dakota, Puerto Rico, South Dakota, Utah, Wyoming	none
Louisiana State University Baton Rouge, Louisiana	Louisiana, Arkansas, and West Virginia residents	MCAT
Michigan State University East Lansing, Michigan	1. Michigan residents 2. residents of states other than Michigan, including U.S. Territories and Trust Possessions 3. all others	MCAT
Mississippi State University Mississippi State, Mississippi	Mississippi residents only	MCAT
North Carolina State University Raleigh, North Carolina	1. North Carolina residents 2. residents of other states, including U.S. Territories and Trust Possessions 3. all others	VAT
Ohio State University Columbus, Ohio	residents of Ohio, Maryland, Nevada, New Hampshire, New Jersey, Puerto Rico, West Virginia	VAT

College	Admissions Priorities	Test Requirements
Oklahoma State University Stillwater, Oklahoma	Oklahoma residents	GRE Aptitude Test; SCAT (School & College Ability Test)
Purdue University West Lafayette, Indiana	1. Indiana residents 2. residents of other states without colleges of veterinary medicine	VAT
Texas A&M University College Station, Texas	1. Texas residents who are either U.S. citizens or in the United States on a visa permitting permanent residence 2. residents of other states without colleges of veterinary medicine permitting permanent residence 3. residents of states with colleges of veterinary medicine and foreign students	GRE Aptitude Test
Tufts University Boston, Massachusetts	residents of Massachusetts, Connecticut, Rhode Island, Maine, and New Mexico	GRE Aptitude Test
Tuskegee Institute School of Veterinary Medicine Tuskegee, Alabama	1. residents of Alabama, South Carolina, Mississippi, West Virginia, Georgia, Arkansas, Kentucky, New Jersey, Puerto Rico, Guyana, Jamaica, Barbados 2. all others	VAT

College	Admissions Priorities	Test Requirements
University of California Davis, California	1. California residents only, with rare exceptions 2. when an exception is made, priority is given to residents of states participating in the Western Interstate Commission for Higher Education (WICHE)	GRE Aptitude Test; GRE Advanced Biology Test
University of Florida Gainesville, Florida	1. Florida residents 2. limited number of non-Florida residents with outstanding academic qualifications and/or unique personal backgrounds	GRE Aptitude Test
University of Georgia Athens, Georgia	Georgia, South Carolina, and West Virginia residents	VAT; GRE Aptitude Test; GRE Advanced Biology Test
University of Illinois Urbana, Illinois	1. Illinois residents 2. limited number of applicants with superior qualifications, usually from states that have no veterinary college or that have no contractual agreement with a veterinary college in another state	VAT
University of Minnesota St. Paul, Minnesota	1. Minnesota residents; minority applicants, regardless of state of residence; contracting states—Nebraska, North Dakota, Wisconsin 2. residents of other states that do not have an accredited veterinary college 3. all others	GRE Aptitude Test; VAT

College	Admissions Priorities	Test Requirements
University of Missouri Columbia, Missouri	1. Missouri residents 2. residents of states without colleges of veterinary medicine 3. all others	VAT
University of Pennsylvania Philadelphia, Pennsylvania	special preference is given to children and close relatives of alumni, faculty and staff of the university and to children of other veterinarians	GRE Aptitude Test
University of Tennessee Knoxville, Tennessee	Tennessee residents and residents of those states under a contractual agreement with the Southern Regional education Board	VAT
Virginia Polytechnic Institute Blacksburg, Virginia	Virginia and Maryland residents	GRE Aptitude Test; GRE Advanced Biology Test
*Washington–Oregon–Idaho Program	Washington, Idaho and Oregon residents and residents of WICHE states—Alaska, Arizona, Hawaii, Montana, New Mexico, Utah, Wyoming	GRE Aptitude Test
University of Wisconsin Madison, Wisconsin	Wisconsin residents and residents of contracting states	GRE Aptitude Test; GRE Advanced Biology Test

*This is a regional program in which the University of Idaho, Oregon State University, and Washington State University participate.

ADMISSIONS EXAMINATIONS·

Most veterinary medical colleges require applicants to take one or more of the following examinations: Veterinary Aptitude Test (VAT), Medical College Admission Test (MCAT), Graduate Record Examination (GRE), or GRE Advanced Biology Test. An applicant's scores on these tests will comprise an important part of the objective criteria used to evaluate the prospective veterinary student's abilities.

It is your responsibility to find out which of these exams are required by the veterinary school(s) to which you are applying and what the school's deadline is for receiving your test results. You must then register for and take the tests. General information about and registration forms for these exams are available from the organizations that administer them, at the following addresses.

Veterinary Aptitude Test
The Psychological Corporation
7500 Old Oak Blvd.
Cleveland, OH 44130
(216) 234-5300

Medical College Admission Test
The American College Testing Program
P.O. Box 414
Iowa City, IA 52243
(319) 337-1276

Graduate Record Examinations
Educational Testing Service
Box 955
Princeton, NJ 08541
New Jersey telephone: (609) 771-7670
California telephone: (415) 849-0950

Note: Use the same address for both the GRE and the GRE Advanced Biology Test.

Read carefully the information you receive for registration deadlines, testing fees, and test dates. Be sure that you register to take the necessary tests early enough to ensure that the school(s) to which you are applying will receive your scores before the admissions application deadline.

Once you have decided to take any of these standardized examinations, begin to prepare for it as soon as possible. None of the standardized tests given on this level of study are tests for which you can cram. Systematic study is the only approach likely to improve your performance considerably, although practice with the types of questions you'll encounter on the examination will keep unfamiliarity with the forms of the questions from hurting your score. Moreover, in the course of preparing for these examinations with practice examinations like those that follow, you'll learn what your strengths and weaknesses are. The direction this knowledge will give to your study is likely to result in an improved score.

This section contains four practice examinations—one VAT, one MCAT, one GRE, and one GRE Advanced Biology Test—to help you prepare for the test or tests you need to take. These practice tests are designed to simulate the actual exams as closely as possible in length, content, number and kind of questions, and level of difficulty. An answer key and explanatory answers to the questions are given immediately following each exam.

TAKING THE PRACTICE EXAMINATIONS

To get the most out of these practice tests, you should take them under conditions similar to those you will encounter during the actual exams. Assemble all the necessary materials (pencils, answer sheet, clock or watch, and this book) in a quiet room with a desk or other writing surface and a chair. Plan to take the tests at a time when you will be least likely to be interrupted by telephone calls or other distractions. Some of these tests take several hours to complete; if you cannot arrange to take a test in one large block of time, you can take it in several shorter sessions—just make sure that you adhere to the time limits specified for each section of the test. Mark your answers on the answer sheets provided.

In order to pace yourself, you may find it helpful to calculate the approximate amount of time you have available to answer each question in a test section. To do this, convert the number of minutes allotted to complete the section into seconds, then divide the total number of seconds by the number of questions in the section. This will give you the number of seconds allotted per question. Check your clock or watch at regular intervals to see how fast you are working. Keep in mind, however, that this is only a guideline for pacing yourself—not everyone is expected to complete every question in every section of these tests.

When you finish a practice test, check your answers with the answer key and the explanatory answers. You may find that you are weak in one or two particular subject areas. You may decide to review these areas in appropriate textbooks and then retake the practice test sections that gave you trouble. You may want to retake the entire exam as a review and to familiarize yourself more thoroughly with the test's format.

Even if the veterinary school(s) to which you are applying requires only one of these exams, you may find it helpful, as an additional review of subject matter, to take one or more of the other practice tests.

Note: More detailed information about the MCAT, the GRE, and the GRE Advanced Test in Biology as well as more practice examinations can be found in Arco's preparation books for these examinations:

Medical College Admissions Test (MCAT) (Bramson and Solomon); *Graduate Record Examination General (Aptitude) Test* (GRE) (Crocetti); *Graduate Record Examination Biology; Advanced Test* (Miller and Solomon) Fourth Edition.

Part Two

VETERINARY APTITUDE TEST
(VAT)

VETERINARY APTITUDE TEST (VAT)

The Veterinary Aptitude Test is designed to measure an applicant's preparation in the elementary natural sciences and his or her reading comprehension and quantitative reasoning abilities. The examination is composed of five subtests: Reading Comprehension; Biology; Chemistry; Quantitative Ability; and Study–Reading.

VAT ANALYSIS AND TIMETABLE		
Subtest	*Number of Questions*	*Testing Time*
Reading Comprehension	60	40 minutes
Biology	45	25 minutes
Chemistry	45	25 minutes
Quantitative Ability	50	45 minutes
Study–Reading	50	40 minutes
TOTALS	250 questions	175 minutes (2 hours 55 minutes)

Each VAT subtest is scored separately; the total of these five scores is also reported as your combined score. Because your VAT scores are based only on the number of correct answers, it is to your advantage to answer every question. Guess even if you are not sure of an answer—no points are deducted from your scores for wrong answers.

When you take this practice exam, read and follow all directions for each subtest. Record your answers on the answer sheet provided.

ANSWER SHEET FOR THE VAT PRACTICE EXAMINATION

Reading Comprehension

1 ① ② ③ ④	13 ① ② ③ ④	25 ① ② ③ ④	37 ① ② ③ ④	49 ① ② ③ ④
2 ① ② ③ ④	14 ① ② ③ ④	26 ① ② ③ ④	38 ① ② ③ ④	50 ① ② ③ ④
3 ① ② ③ ④	15 ① ② ③ ④	27 ① ② ③ ④	39 ① ② ③ ④	51 ① ② ③ ④
4 ① ② ③ ④	16 ① ② ③ ④	28 ① ② ③ ④	40 ① ② ③ ④	52 ① ② ③ ④
5 ① ② ③ ④	17 ① ② ③ ④	29 ① ② ③ ④	41 ① ② ③ ④	53 ① ② ③ ④
6 ① ② ③ ④	18 ① ② ③ ④	30 ① ② ③ ④	42 ① ② ③ ④	54 ① ② ③ ④
7 ① ② ③ ④	19 ① ② ③ ④	31 ① ② ③ ④	43 ① ② ③ ④	55 ① ② ③ ④
8 ① ② ③ ④	20 ① ② ③ ④	32 ① ② ③ ④	44 ① ② ③ ④	56 ① ② ③ ④
9 ① ② ③ ④	21 ① ② ③ ④	33 ① ② ③ ④	45 ① ② ③ ④	57 ① ② ③ ④
10 ① ② ③ ④	22 ① ② ③ ④	34 ① ② ③ ④	46 ① ② ③ ④	58 ① ② ③ ④
11 ① ② ③ ④	23 ① ② ③ ④	35 ① ② ③ ④	47 ① ② ③ ④	59 ① ② ③ ④
12 ① ② ③ ④	24 ① ② ③ ④	36 ① ② ③ ④	48 ① ② ③ ④	60 ① ② ③ ④

Biology

1 ① ② ③ ④	10 ① ② ③ ④	19 ① ② ③ ④	28 ① ② ③ ④	37 ① ② ③ ④
2 ① ② ③ ④	11 ① ② ③ ④	20 ① ② ③ ④	29 ① ② ③ ④	38 ① ② ③ ④
3 ① ② ③ ④	12 ① ② ③ ④	21 ① ② ③ ④	30 ① ② ③ ④	39 ① ② ③ ④
4 ① ② ③ ④	13 ① ② ③ ④	22 ① ② ③ ④	31 ① ② ③ ④	40 ① ② ③ ④
5 ① ② ③ ④	14 ① ② ③ ④	23 ① ② ③ ④	32 ① ② ③ ④	41 ① ② ③ ④
6 ① ② ③ ④	15 ① ② ③ ④	24 ① ② ③ ④	33 ① ② ③ ④	42 ① ② ③ ④
7 ① ② ③ ④	16 ① ② ③ ④	25 ① ② ③ ④	34 ① ② ③ ④	43 ① ② ③ ④
8 ① ② ③ ④	17 ① ② ③ ④	26 ① ② ③ ④	35 ① ② ③ ④	44 ① ② ③ ④
9 ① ② ③ ④	18 ① ② ③ ④	27 ① ② ③ ④	36 ① ② ③ ④	45 ① ② ③ ④

Chemistry

1 ① ② ③ ④   9 ① ② ③ ④   17 ① ② ③ ④   25 ① ② ③ ④   38 ① ② ③ ④   41 ① ② ③ ④
2 ① ② ③ ④   10 ① ② ③ ④   18 ① ② ③ ④   26 ① ② ③ ④   32 ① ② ③ ④   42 ① ② ③ ④
3 ① ② ③ ④   11 ① ② ③ ④   19 ① ② ③ ④   27 ① ② ③ ④   33 ① ② ③ ④   43 ① ② ③ ④
4 ① ② ③ ④   12 ① ② ③ ④   20 ① ② ③ ④   28 ① ② ③ ④   34 ① ② ③ ④   44 ① ② ③ ④
5 ① ② ③ ④   13 ① ② ③ ④   21 ① ② ③ ④   29 ① ② ③ ④   35 ① ② ③ ④   45 ① ② ③ ④
6 ① ② ③ ④   14 ① ② ③ ④   22 ① ② ③ ④   30 ① ② ③ ④   36 ① ② ③ ④
7 ① ② ③ ④   15 ① ② ③ ④   23 ① ② ③ ④   31 ① ② ③ ④   39 ① ② ③ ④
8 ① ② ③ ④   16 ① ② ③ ④   24 ① ② ③ ④   37 ① ② ③ ④   40 ① ② ③ ④

Quantitative Ability

1 ① ② ③ ④   10 ① ② ③ ④   19 ① ② ③ ④   28 ① ② ③ ④   37 ① ② ③ ④   46 ① ② ③ ④
2 ① ② ③ ④   11 ① ② ③ ④   20 ① ② ③ ④   29 ① ② ③ ④   38 ① ② ③ ④   47 ① ② ③ ④
3 ① ② ③ ④   12 ① ② ③ ④   21 ① ② ③ ④   30 ① ② ③ ④   39 ① ② ③ ④   48 ① ② ③ ④
4 ① ② ③ ④   13 ① ② ③ ④   22 ① ② ③ ④   31 ① ② ③ ④   40 ① ② ③ ④   49 ① ② ③ ④
5 ① ② ③ ④   14 ① ② ③ ④   23 ① ② ③ ④   32 ① ② ③ ④   41 ① ② ③ ④   50 ① ② ③ ④
6 ① ② ③ ④   15 ① ② ③ ④   24 ① ② ③ ④   33 ① ② ③ ④   42 ① ② ③ ④
7 ① ② ③ ④   16 ① ② ③ ④   25 ① ② ③ ④   34 ① ② ③ ④   43 ① ② ③ ④
8 ① ② ③ ④   17 ① ② ③ ④   26 ① ② ③ ④   35 ① ② ③ ④   44 ① ② ③ ④
9 ① ② ③ ④   18 ① ② ③ ④   27 ① ② ③ ④   36 ① ② ③ ④   45 ① ② ③ ④

Study-Reading

1 ① ② ③ ④   10 ① ② ③ ④   19 ① ② ③ ④   28 ① ② ③ ④   37 ① ② ③ ④   46 ① ② ③ ④
2 ① ② ③ ④   11 ① ② ③ ④   20 ① ② ③ ④   29 ① ② ③ ④   38 ① ② ③ ④   47 ① ② ③ ④
3 ① ② ③ ④   12 ① ② ③ ④   21 ① ② ③ ④   30 ① ② ③ ④   39 ① ② ③ ④   48 ① ② ③ ④
4 ① ② ③ ④   13 ① ② ③ ④   22 ① ② ③ ④   31 ① ② ③ ④   40 ① ② ③ ④   49 ① ② ③ ④
5 ① ② ③ ④   14 ① ② ③ ④   23 ① ② ③ ④   32 ① ② ③ ④   41 ① ② ③ ④   50 ① ② ③ ④
6 ① ② ③ ④   15 ① ② ③ ④   24 ① ② ③ ④   33 ① ② ③ ④   42 ① ② ③ ④
7 ① ② ③ ④   16 ① ② ③ ④   25 ① ② ③ ④   34 ① ② ③ ④   43 ① ② ③ ④
8 ① ② ③ ④   17 ① ② ③ ④   26 ① ② ③ ④   35 ① ② ③ ④   44 ① ② ③ ④
9 ① ② ③ ④   18 ① ② ③ ④   27 ① ② ③ ④   36 ① ② ③ ④   45 ① ② ③ ④

VAT PRACTICE EXAMINATION

READING COMPREHENSION

Time: **40 minutes**
60 questions

Directions: You will find questions following each of the reading passages in this subtest. Select the one best answer from the numbered choices that follow each question.

The quantitative breeding practices of commercial poultry breeders have changed very little over the last thirty years. Highly heritable traits, such as growth rate, body conformation, and egg weight, are perpetuated by mass selection because little advantage is gained from hybrid vigor. Low heritable traits (egg production, fertility, and disease resistance) are perpetuated by crossbreeding and identified through progeny and family testing.

The goals of the industry are to increase egg production of the layers—both in quality and quantity—and, with broilers and turkeys, to improve growth rate, feed efficiency, and yield, as well as to reduce body fat and the incidence of defects.

The technologies of artificial insemination (AI) and semen preservation have accelerated the advances made through quantitative breeding technology. AI is widely used in commercial turkey breeding because of the inability of modern strains to mate. It makes breeding tests more efficient, steps up selection pressure on the male line, reduces the number of necessary breeder males, and increases the number of females that may be mated to one male. Semen diluents were introduced to the turkey industry about ten years ago to lower the cost of AI. Currently, a little over half of the turkeys are inseminated with diluted semen.

Preservation of poultry semen by freezing is now practiced by several primary breeders. Although freezing chicken semen causes it to lose some potency, the practice allows increased genetic advancement and the distribution of genetic material worldwide.

The amount of genetic variation available for breeding stock is not expected to diminish in the near future. Ceilings for certain traits will eventually be reached, but certainly not in the 1980s. Advances in breeding laying chickens will be less dramatic than in the past, but efforts will continue to develop new genetic lines and to improve reserve lines and crosses to meet future needs.

The growth rate of broilers will continue to increase at four percent a year, which suggests that birds will be reaching 4.4 pounds in five weeks by the 1990s. Breeding for stress resistance will be increasingly important, not only because of the increased use of intensive production systems, but also to meet the physiological stresses resulting from faster growth and greater weight.

AI will assume increasing importance. Recent advances in procedures for long-term freezing of chicken semen will allow breeders to extend the use of outstanding sires. The sale of frozen semen may eventually substitute, in part, for the sale of breeder males.

Dwarf broiler breeders will also assume increasing importance over the next few years. The dwarf breeder female is approximately twenty-five percent smaller than the standard female, and even though the dwarf's egg is smaller and the progeny's growth rate slightly less than that of the standard broiler, the lower cost of producing broiler chicks from the dwarf breeder more than offsets the slight loss in their growth rate. Dwarf layers and the dwarf breeder hens could reduce production costs by twenty percent and two percent, respectively.

There is some interest among poultry breeders in cloning, gene transfer, and sex control, but progress toward successful technologies is slow.

1. Which of the following is not listed as resulting from the use of AI in commercial turkey breeding?
   (1) It makes breeding tests more efficient.
   (2) It reduces the number of breeder males necessary.
   (3) It increases the number of females that may be mated to one male.
   (4) It decreases the ability of modern strains to mate.

2. Of what use are semen diluents to the turkey industry?
   (1) They make breeding tests more efficient.
   (2) They lower the cost of AI.
   (3) They increase the number of breeder males.
   (4) They improve the growth rate of offspring.

3. Approximately what percentage of turkeys are presently inseminated with diluted semen?
   (1) 25 percent
   (2) 50 percent
   (3) 75 percent
   (4) 100 percent

4. Which of the following is listed as an advantage of freezing poultry semen?
   (1) It allows the worldwide distribution of genetic material.
   (2) It increases semen potency.
   (3) It makes breeding tests more efficient.
   (4) It reduces the incubation period.

5. When are the ceilings for genetic traits in poultry breeding expected to be reached?
   (1) the 1980s
   (2) the 1990s
   (3) by the early twenty-first century
   (4) The specific date is not stated in the passage.

6. Which of the following technologies has thus far enjoyed the greatest success?
   (1) gene transfer
   (2) cloning
   (3) artificial insemination
   (4) sex control

7. Which of the following is not listed as a goal of commercial poultry breeders as regards broilers and turkeys?
   (1) to reduce body fat
   (2) to improve feed efficiency
   (3) to improve the growth rate
   (4) none of the above

As for the relation between man and other forms, we study not only paleontological evidence but the similarities in structure and functioning of the living representations of related types. Such a demonstration as has been given by Gregory in tracing the bones of the face, item by item, from the fish, through intermediate types, to man, shows how widespread are these resemblances. Many similarities between man and his closest primate relations, the great apes, have been described. That none of these forms has a tail, that they alone have the vermiform appendix, that they have similar blood-types, have almost the same structure of uterus and placenta, are omnivorous, having the dental equipment to chew either meat or herbivorous foods, have stereoscopic vision, and possess the opposable thumb, indicate how numerous are these resemblances. Most important is the fact that only man and the anthropoid apes share the tendency to upright posture and bipedal locomotion. Though man is the only true biped, and the apes employ their arms to assist them in walking, yet only man and the great apes have posterior extremities that can be put to such use.

The attainment of upright posture was fundamental in bringing about the changes that made of man the erect, speaking, tool-using, culture-building creature he has become. We cannot here debate the question whether or not the forms that preceded man began the march toward erect posture by coming out of the trees to lead a terrestrial rather than an arboreal life. The play of cause and effect is much too obscure, much too complex to permit any conclusive answer. It is quite possible, however, that a period of arboreal life did encourage the development of upright posture by shifting the axis of support to a line between the great toe and the rest of the foot. What is important here is to trace the consequences that followed when man's anterior extremities came exclusively to function as grasping organs, and his legs and feet came to be his only means of support and locomotion.

8. The relationship between man and other animals is shown by
   (1) a period of arboreal life
   (2) man's upright posture
   (3) paleontological and physiological evidence
   (4) stereoscopic vision

9. These paragraphs would most probably be found in a book on
   (1) comparative zoology
   (2) paleontology
   (3) physiology
   (4) ontogeny

10. "Upright posture was a primary causal factor in the development of the intellectual skills of man." This statement
    (1) is contrary to the information in the section
    (2) may be inferred from the section
    (3) is foreign to the subject matter of the section
    (4) is true for all stages of evolution

11. On the basis of the section, one should conclude that in studies of evolutionary phenomena,
    (1) cause and effect are quite clear
    (2) observations of structure and function offer basic data
    (3) the best explanations are teleological
    (4) the best observations are often misinterpreted

12. Which of the following is not listed as one of the similarities between man and the great ape?
    (1) Both are able to chew meat and herbivorous food.
    (2) Both have the vermiform appendix.
    (3) They have similar blood types.
    (4) none of the above

13. Which of the following is suggested by the author as the reason that a period of arboreal life may have encouraged the development of upright posture?

(1) Arboreal life effected a shift in the axis of support.
(2) Primitive forms were forced to hold on to branches to balance themselves.
(3) To climb trees, it was necessary to stand erect and reach to the higher limbs.
(4) none of the above

A staminate cone consists of a central axis and a series of spirally arranged *sporophylls*. Each sporophyll bears two pollen-sacs, or microsporangia, on its lower surface. Each microsporangium contains numerous cells called microspore mother cells, which divide by reduction division to form microspores, or pollen grains, four from each microspore mother cell. The large cell of the pollen grain divides to form two, known as the generative and tube cells. On the upper surface of each scale of the ovulate cone are two ovules. The greater part of each ovule is a mass of cells called the nucellus or megasporangium. As the ovule develops, one (or sometimes more) of the cells in the nucellus becomes distinct from the other cells because of its larger size and denser protoplasm. This is the megaspore mother cell. It divides by reduction division to form a row of three or four cells, one of which becomes the megaspore, the others degenerating. The single megaspore divides into many cells, which form the female gametophyte or megagametophyte. At the end of the megagametophyte nearest the micropyle several *archegonia* develop. Each archegonium contains a single very large egg cell.

The pollen grain, carried by the wind, comes in contact with a small drop of fluid that has been secreted by cells in the region of the micropyle to the surface of the nucellus. There the pollen grain puts out a pollen tube that grows through the nucellus tissue until it reaches the tip of the megagametophyte. During this development a final division of the generative nucleus has occurred, and two male gametes or sperm nuclei are formed. When the top of the tube reaches an archegonium, these nuclei are discharged into the egg. One of the nuclei passes to the egg nucleus and fuses with it; the other disintegrates.

The nucleus of the fertilized egg passes to the basal end, dividing twice, and forms a rosette of four nuclei. Each of these divides again, forming two tiers of four nuclei. Walls then begin to form, separating the apical tier from the other. Subsequent nuclear divisions increase the number of tiers to four, each composed of four cells. The apical tier presently divides and forms the embryo; the second tier, called the suspensor, elongates greatly, shoving the embryo down into the gametophyte tissue. There the embryo absorbs food substances from the tissues around it and matures.

14. A staminate cone is to a sporophyll as an ovulate cone is to
    (1) a megaspore mother cell
    (2) a megagametophyte
    (3) an ovule
    (4) a sporophyte

15. The staminate derivative analogous to the egg is the
    (1) nucellus
    (2) sperm nucleus
    (3) gametophyte
    (4) pollen grain

16. How many sperm nuclei may arise from one megaspore cell?
    (1) 0
    (2) 1
    (3) 3 or 4
    (4) an infinite number

17. A nonembryonic structure derived from the fused nuclei is the
    (1) apical layer
    (2) archegonium
    (3) gametophyte tissues
    (4) suspensor

18. The staminate process analogous to the reduction division of the megaspore mother cell takes place in the
    (1) apical layer
    (2) archegonium
    (3) pollen grain
    (4) microsporangium

19. The structure analogous to the archegonium in terms of function is the
    (1) megasporangium
    (2) microspore
    (3) nucellus
    (4) microgametophyte

20. How many sperm nuclei may arise from a single microspore mother cell?
    (1) 1
    (2) 4
    (3) 3
    (4) 8

21. How many gametophytes may arise from the ovule?
    (1) 1
    (2) 3
    (3) 4
    (4) an indeterminate number

An action of apparent social significance among animals is that of migration. But several different factors are at work causing such migrations. These may be concerned with food-getting, with temperature, salinity, pressure, and light changes, with the action of sex hormones, and probably other combinations of these factors.

The great aggregations of small crustaceans, such as copepods found at the surface of the ocean, swarms of insects about a light, or the masses of unicellular organisms making up a part of the plankton in the lakes and oceans, are all examples of nonsocial aggregations of organisms brought together because of the presence or absence of certain factors in their environment, such as air currents, water currents, food or the lack of it, oxygen or carbon dioxide, or some other contributing causes.

Insects make long migrations, most of which seem due to the urge for food. The migrations of the locust, both in this country and elsewhere, are well known. While some fish, such as salmon, return to the same stream where they grew up, such return migrations are rare in insects, the only known instance being in the monarch butterfly. This is apparently due to the fact that it is long-lived and has the power of strong flight. The mass migrations of the Rocky Mountain and the African species of locust seem attributable to the need for food. Locusts live, eat, sun themselves, and migrate in groups. It has been suggested that their social life is in response to the two fundamental instincts, aggregation and imitation.

Migrations of fish have been studied carefully by many investigators. Typically the migrations are from deep to shallow waters, as in the herring, mackerel and many other marine fish. Freshwater fish in general exhibit this type of migration in the spawning season. Spawning habits of many fish show a change in habitat from salt to fresh water. Among these are the shad, salmon and alewife. In the North American and European eels, long migrations take place at the breeding season. All these migrations are obviously not brought about by a quest for food, for the salmon and many other fish feed only sparingly during the spawning season, but are undoubtedly brought about by metabolic changes in the animal initiated by the interaction of sex hormones. If this thesis holds, then here is the beginning of social life.

Bird migrations have long been a matter of study. The reasons for the migration of the golden plover from the Arctic regions to the tip of South America and return in a single year are not fully explainable. Several theories have been advanced, although none have been fully proved. The reproductive "instinct," food scarcity, temperature and light changes, the metabolic changes brought about by the activity of the sex hormones and the length of the day, have all been suggested, and ultimately several may prove to be factors. Aside from other findings, it is interesting to note that bird migrations take place year after year on about the same dates. Recent studies in biochemistry of metabolism, showing that there is a seasonal cycle in the blood sugar that has a definite relation to activity and food, seem to be among the most promising leads.

In mammals the seasonal migrations that take place, such as those of the deer, which travel from the high mountains in summer to the valleys in winter, or the migration of the caribou in the northern areas of Canada, are based on the factor of temperature that regulates the food supply. Another mystery is the migration of the lemming, a small, ratlike animal found in Scandinavia and Canada. The lemming population varies greatly from year to year, and, at times when it greatly increases, a migration occurs in which hordes of lemmings march across the country, swimming rivers and even plunging into the ocean if it bars their way. This again cannot be a purely social association of animals. The horde is usually made up entirely of males, as the females seldom migrate.

22. The migration of the lemmings cannot be considered one of social association since
    (1) only males migrate
    (2) migrations occur only with population increases
    (3) it is probably due to the absence of some factor in the environment
    (4) the migrants do not return

23. Animals which apparently migrate in quest for food are the
    (1) fish
    (2) birds
    (3) mammals
    (4) insects

24. A characteristic of migration is the return of the migrants to their former home areas. This is, however, not true of the
    (1) birds
    (2) insects
    (3) mammals
    (4) fish

25. The reproductive instinct is probably not a factor in the actual migration of the
    (1) shad
    (2) lemming
    (3) golden plover
    (4) monarch butterfly

26. Return migrations are usually associated with animals that
    (1) make long migrations
    (2) are long-lived
    (3) migrate to spawn
    (4) make short migrations

27. The author indicates that careful investigation has shown that fish migration is probably concerned with
    (1) spawning habits
    (2) feeding habits
    (3) neither spawning nor feeding
    (4) both spawning and feeding

28. Which is not mentioned as likely to bring about migration?
    (1) changes in temperature
    (2) lack of available food

(3) longing to experience new environments
(4) the action of sex hormones

The function of the heart is to discharge, with adequate force, an amount of blood sufficient for the metabolic needs of the body. The amount discharged in a unit of time is determined by the stroke volume and rate of heartbeat. As the demand for blood by the body varies from moment to moment, it is evident that the rate, force, and systolic output of the heart must be governed in accordance. This control is both neural and humoral.

The origin of the heartbeat is not dependent upon the central nervous system. But it is a fact, proved by everyday observation, that the state of mind or body can modify the action of the heart. The heart is connected with the central nervous system by means of two nerves, the vagus and the cervical sympathetic. From the brain there issue twelve pairs of cranial nerves; of these the vagus, or pneumogastric nerve, forms the tenth pair. The vagus springs from the lowest division of the brain, known as the medulla oblongata, which may be looked upon as the connection between the brain and the spinal cord. This nerve is very widely distributed, sending branches to the heart, lungs, trachea, esophagus, stomach, pancreas, gall bladder, intestines, etc.; it is, therefore, one of the most important nerves in the body. To the heart the vagus nerve sends both afferent and efferent fibers; the latter fibers belong to the autonomic nervous system. The efferent vagal fibers end in a peripheral ganglion lying in the heart; from this ganglion the impulses are carried by very short postganglionic fibers to the sino-auricular and the auriculo-ventricular nodes and the bundle of His.

In an animal the vagus nerve may be exposed without any great difficulty. Under the influence of an anesthetic the skin in the neck, a little to either side of the larynx, is slit open; the structures immediately below the skin are pushed aside, and the carotid artery is brought to view. Alongside this vessel lies a large nerve trunk, the vagus. When the vagus on one side is cut, there is usually little or no result, but when both vagi are severed, there is a marked cardiac acceleration. Stimulation of the vagus nerve may cause a decrease in the rate, or it may diminish the force without affecting the rate, or it may cause a complete cessation of the heartbeat in diastole. This slowing or stoppage of the heart, cardiac inhibition, is the result of a reduction in the irritability of the sino-auricular node and a decrease in the conductivity of the auriculo-ventricular bundle; upon the ventricular musculature the vagus is said to have no direct influence.

29. The statement that the vagus nerve is connected with involuntary action is
    (1) made in the paragraphs
    (2) neither made nor implied in the paragraphs
    (3) definitely stated by the author
    (4) not made, but implied in the paragraphs

30. Which of the following is *least* true of the vagus nerve?
    (1) It belongs to the autonomic system.
    (2) It comes from the medulla oblongata.
    (3) It is one of the tenth pair of cranial nerves.
    (4) It serves the heart through both efferent and afferent fibers.

31. Which of the following is true of the vagus nerve?
    (1) It completely controls heart action.
    (2) It controls blood temperature.
    (3) Either branch of the vagus nerve can take over the functions of the other.
    (4) It only accelerates the heart rate.

32. Choose the phrase that makes the following most nearly true: The rate, force and systolic output of the heart are controlled by
    (1) neural connections
    (2) the central nervous system
    (3) the sino-auricular node
    (4) the vagus and cervical sympathetic systems

33. That the state of mind can modify heart action is
    (1) shown to operate through control from the brain
    (2) shown by cardiac inhibition
    (3) shown by cardiac stimulation
    (4) stated but its mode of operation is not shown

34. The statement "This control is both neural and humoral" means
    (1) both neural pathways and the mood control heartbeat
    (2) heartbeat is controlled by both efferent and afferent nerves
    (3) substances in the blood may affect heartbeat as well as the stimulation via neural pathways
    (4) both postganglionic fibers and the bundle of His are necessary to control the heartbeat

Chemical investigations show that during muscle contraction the store of organic phosphates in the muscle fibers is altered as energy is released. In doing so, the organic phosphates (chiefly adenosine triphosphate and phospho-creatine) are transformed anaerobically to organic compounds plus phosphates. As soon as the organic phosphates begin to break down in muscle contraction, the glycogen in the muscle fibers also transforms into lactic acid plus free energy. This energy the muscle fiber uses to return the organic compounds plus phosphates into high-energy organic phosphates ready for another contraction. In the presence of oxygen, the lactic acid from the glycogen decomposition is changed also. About one-fifth of it is oxidized to form water and carbon dioxide and to yield another supply of energy. This time the energy is used to transform the remaining four-fifths of the lactic acid into glycogen again.

35. The energy for muscle contraction comes directly from the
    (1) breakdown of the organic phosphates
    (2) resynthesis of adenosine triphosphate
    (3) breakdown of glycogen into lactic acid
    (4) oxidation of lactic acid

36. Lactic acid does not accumulate in a muscle that
    (1) is in a state of lacking oxygen
    (2) has an ample supply of oxygen
    (3) is in a state of fatigue
    (4) is repeatedly being stimulated

37. The energy for the resynthesis of adenosine triphosphate and phospho-creatine comes from the

    (1) synthesis of organic phosphates
    (2) oxidation of lactic acid
    (3) change from glycogen to lactic acid
    (4) resynthesis of glycogen

38. The energy for the resynthesis of glycogen comes from the
    (1) breakdown of organic phosphates
    (2) resynthesis of organic phosphates
    (3) change occurring in one-fifth of the lactic acid
    (4) change occurring in four-fifths of the lactic acid

39. The breakdown of the organic phosphates into organic compounds plus phosphates is an
    (1) anabolic reaction
    (2) aerobic reaction
    (3) endothermic reaction
    (4) anaerobic reaction

The first representatives of the Osteichthyes appeared in the middle Devonian, soon after the earliest sharks. As the fossils are known, these bony fishes are separated at the outset into the three types of lobe-finned fishes, ray-finned fishes, and lung-fishes, which means that their differentiation from a common ancestry was well advanced. The lobe-fins in turn can be identified as including forms that were forerunners of the first land vertebrates.

Surprising as it may seem, a lung or lungs appear to have been present in many, if not all, of these early bony fishes, perhaps as an adaptation to life in stagnant pools that may have been formed recurrently in the watercourses under the climatic conditions of the Devonian. Apparently the swim bladder of modern bony fishes, which is homologous with the lungs of tetrapod vertebrates, is not the organ from which lungs arose but a modification of the primitive lung in the early ancestors of these fishes. After making a beginning of air-breathing, it seems that one line, the lobe-finned fishes, gave rise to the Amphibia and so to the land vertebrates...., while another line, the ray-finned fishes, gave rise to the bony fishes of the present day, in which the primitive lung was transformed into a hydrostatic organ, the swim bladder.

It is significant in this connection that in the most primitive of existing ray-finned fishes, such as the "bichir" of the Nile, *Polypterus*, the lung still persists in its original function; another and independent survival of the primitive lung appears in the three genera of lung-fishes (Dipnoi), *Ceratodus*, *Protopterus*, and *Lepidosiren*. In North America the sturgeon, *Acipenser*, the paddle fish, *Polyodon*, the gar pike, *Lepisosteus*, and the bow-fin, *Amia*, are ray-fins of primitive type, although they do not have lungs as does the more primitive *Polypterus*. The more specialized ray-fins include all the most familiar fishes of fresh and salt water, such as the trout, salmon, carp, bass, perch, catfish, cod, herring, mackerel, and many others.

40. The word *homologous* as used in the section means
    (1) compatible
    (2) having the same function
    (3) having the same origin
    (4) having the same structure

41. Which one of the following belongs to the most primitive type?
    (1) catfish
    (2) frog
    (3) sturgeon
    (4) codfish

42. The mammals are derived from
    (1) fish with swim bladders
    (2) the lobe-fins
    (3) the ray-fins
    (4) fish without lobe-fins

43. The Devonian is a
    (1) climatic region
    (2) geological period
    (3) oceanic drift area
    (4) sunken continent

44. The *Osteichthyes* are
    (1) algae
    (2) bony fish
    (3) amphibians
    (4) sharks

45. The gar pike, found in the midwestern U.S.A., is a
    (1) lobe-finned fish
    (2) lung-fish

(3) ray-finned fish
(4) amphibian

Much improvement can be made in the germ-plasm of all major farm animal species using existing technology. The expanded use of artificial insemination (AI) with stored frozen sperm, especially in beef cattle, would benefit both producers and consumers. New techniques for synchronizing estrus should encourage the wider use of AI. Various manipulations of embryos will find limited use in producing breeding stocks, and sex selection and twinning techniques should be available for limited application within the next ten to twenty years.

The most important technology in reproductive physiology will continue to be AI. Due in part to genetic improvement, the average milk yield of cows in the United States has more than doubled in the past thirty years, while the total number of milk cows has been reduced by more than half. AI, along with improved management and the availability and use of accurate progeny records of breeding stock, has caused this great increase.

The improvement lags behind what is theoretically possible. In practice, the observed increase is about 100 pounds of milk per cow per year, while a hypothetical breeding program using AI would result in a yearly gain of 220 pounds of milk per cow. The biological limits to this rate of gain are not known.

In comparison with the dairy cattle industry, the beef cattle industry has not applied AI technology widely. Only three to five percent of U.S. beef is artificially inseminated, compared to fifty percent of the dairy herd. This low rate for beef cattle can be explained by several factors, including management techniques (range versus confined housing) and the conflicting objectives of individual breeders, ranchers, breed associations, and commercial farmers.

The national calf crop—calves alive at weaning as a fraction of the total number of cows exposed to breeding each year—is only 65 to 81 percent. An improvement of only a few percentage points through AI would result in savings of hundreds of millions of dollars to producers and consumers.

Coupled with a technology for estrus cycle regulation, the use of AI could be expanded for both dairy and beef breeding. Embryo transfer technology, already well-developed but still costly, can be used to produce valuable breeding stock. Sexing technology, which is not yet perfected, would be of enormous benefit to the beef industry because bulls grow faster than heifers.

46. The most important technology in reproductive physiology is
    (1) sex selection
    (2) twinning techniques
    (3) embryo manipultion
    (4) artificial insemination

47. Which of the following is not listed as having contributed to the great increase in the milk yield of cows in the United States in the last thirty years?
    (1) improved management
    (2) artificial insemination
    (3) twinning techniques
    (4) use of progeny records on breeding stock

48. Which of the following technologies is most useful in light of the fact that bulls grow faster than heifers?
    (1) artificial insemination
    (2) twinning techniques
    (3) embryo manipulation
    (4) none of the above

49. Which of the statements below is contradicted by the passage?
    (1) Using AI, it is possible to gain 220 pounds of milk per cow per year.
    (2) In the last thirty years, the number of milk cows has been reduced by half.
    (3) In the last thirty years, the milk yield per cow has increased four-fold.
    (4) none of the above

50. The author treats recent advances in reproductive biology with
    (1) enthusiasm
    (2) chagrin
    (3) subjectivity
    (4) servility

51. AI technology has been applied by the dairy cattle industry approximately how much more frequently than by the beef cattle industry?

    (1) 12 to 20 times
    (2) 10 to 30 times
    (3) 18 to 30 times
    (4) 15 to 20 times

52. The author cites which of the following as the major problem with embryo transfer technology?
    (1) It is costly.
    (2) It is undeveloped.
    (3) It cannot be made to conform with Food and Drug Administration regulations.
    (4) none of the above

As the world's population grows, the part played by man in influencing plant life becomes more and more important. In old and densely populated countries, as in western Europe, man determines almost wholly what shall grow and what shall not grow. In such regions, the influence of man on plant life is in large measure a beneficial one. Laws, often centuries old, protect plants of economic value and preserve soil fertility. In newly settled countries, the situation is unfortunately quite the reverse. The pioneer's life is too strenuous for him to think of posterity.

Some years ago, Mt. Mitchell, the highest summit east of the Mississippi, was covered with a magnificent forest. A lumber company was given full rights to fell the trees. Those not cut down were crushed. The mountain was left a waste area where fire would rage and erosion would complete the destruction. There was no stopping the devastating foresting of the company, for the contract had been given. Under a more enlightened civilization, this could not have happened. The denuding of Mt. Mitchell is a minor chapter in the destruction of lands in the United States; and this country is by no means the only or chief sufferer. China, India, Egypt, and East Africa all have their thousands of square miles of waste land, the result of man's indifference to the future.

Deforestation, grazing, and poor farming techniques are the chief causes of the destruction of land fertility. Wasteful cutting of timber is the first step. Grazing then follows lumbering, often bringing about ruin. The Caribbean slopes of northern Venezuela are barren wastes, owing first to ruthless cutting of forests and then to destructive grazing. Hordes of goats roamed these slopes until only a few thorny acacias and cacti remained. Erosion completed the devastation. What is illustrated there on a small scale is the story of vast areas in China and India, countries where famines are of regular occurrence.

Man is not wholly to blame, for nature is often merciless. In parts of India and China, plant life, when left undisturbed by man, cannot cope with either the disastrous floods of wet seasons or the destructive winds of the dry season. Man has learned much; prudent land management has been the policy of the Chinese people since 2700 BC, but even they have not learned enough.

When the American forestry service was in its infancy, it met with much opposition from legislators who loudly claimed that the protected land would in one season yield a crop of cabbages of more value than all the timber on it. Herein lay the fallacy, that one season's crop is all that need to be thought of. Nature, through the years, adjusts crops to the soil and to the climate. Forests usually occur where precipitation exceeds evaporation. If the reverse is true, grasslands are found; and where evaporation is still greater, desert or scrub vegetation alone survives. The phytogeographic map of a country is very similar to the climatic map based on rainfall, evaporation, and temperature. Man ignores this natural adjustment of crops and strives for one "bumper" crop in a single season; he may produce it, but "year in and year out, the yield of the grassland is certain, that of the planted fields, never."

Man is learning; he sprays his trees with insecticides and fungicides; he imports ladybugs to destroy aphids; he irrigates, fertilizes, and rotates his crops; but he is still indifferent to many of the consequences of his shortsighted policies.

In spite of the evidence from the experience of this country, the people of other countries still in the pioneer stage farm as wastefully as did our own pioneers. In the interiors of Central and South America, natives fell superb forest trees and leave them to rot in order to obtain virgin soil for cultivation. Where the land is hillside, the soil readily washes away, and after one or two seasons the land is unfit for crops. So the frontier farmer pushes back into the primeval forest, moving his hut as he goes, and fells more monarchs to lay bare another patch of ground for his plantings to support his family. Valuable timber that will require a century to replace is destroyed and the land laid waste to produce what could be supplied for a pittance.

How badly man can err in his handling of land is shown by the draining of extensive swamp areas, which to the uninformed would seem to be a very good thing to do. One of the first effects of the drainage is the lowering of the water-table, which may bring about the death of the dominant species and leave to another species the possession of the soil, even when the difference in water level is little more than an inch. Frequently, bog country will yield marketable crops of cranberries and blueberries but, if drained, neither these nor any other economic plant will grow on the fallow soil. Swamps and marshes have their drawbacks but also their virtues. When drained they may leave wasteland, the surface of which rapidly erodes, then to be blown away in dust blizzards disastrous to both man and wild beasts.

53. The best title for this passage is
  (1) How to Increase Soil Productivity
  (2) Conservation of Natural Resources
  (3) Man's Effect on Soil
  (4) Soil Conditions and Plant Growth

54. A policy of good management is sometimes upset by
  (1) the indifference of man
  (2) centuries-old laws
  (3) floods and winds
  (4) grazing animals

55. Areas in which the total amounts of rain and snow falling on the ground are greater than that which is evaporated will support
  (1) forests
  (2) grasslands
  (3) scrub vegetation
  (4) no plants

56. Phytogeographic maps are those that show
  (1) areas of grassland
  (2) areas of bumper crops
  (3) areas of similar climate
  (4) areas of similar plants

57. The basic cause of frequent famines in China and India, according to the passage, is probably
  (1) allowing animals to roam wild

(2) drainage of swamps
(3) overpopulations
(4) destruction of forests

58. What is meant by "the yield of the grassland is certain; that of the planted field, never" is that
    (1) it is impossible to get more than one bumper crop from any one cultivated area
    (2) crops, planted in former grassland, will not give good yields
    (3) through the indifference of man, dust blizzards have occurred in former grasslands
    (4) if man does not interfere, plants will grow in the most suitable environment

59. The first act of prudent land management might be to
    (1) prohibit drainage of swamps
    (2) use irrigation and crop rotation in planted areas
    (3) increase use of fertilizers
    (4) prohibit excessive forest lumbering

60. The results of good land management may usually be found in
    (1) heavily populated areas
    (2) areas not given over to grazing
    (3) underdeveloped areas
    (4) ancient civilizations

STOP

END OF READING COMPREHENSION QUESTIONS

BIOLOGY

Time: **25 minutes**
45 questions

Directions: Select the one best answer from the numbered choices that follow each question.

1. If the pancreatic duct is tied, which of the following functions of the pancreas is inhibited?
   (1) endocrine functions only
   (2) exocrine functions only
   (3) both endocrine and exocrine functions
   (4) neither endocrine nor exocrine functions

2. For approximately 10 hours after birth, a newly hatched duckling will adopt as its mother the first moving object that it encounters. This is an example of
   (1) instinct
   (2) habituation
   (3) taxis
   (4) imprinting

3. The stage in embryology at which the primitive gut is well formed is called the
   (1) blastula
   (2) gastrula
   (3) hollow ball stage
   (4) morula

4. Which of the following is a ductless gland?
   (1) thyroid
   (2) liver
   (3) spleen
   (4) salivary gland

5. Blood is carried to the heart by the
   (1) auricles
   (2) ventricles
   (3) veins
   (4) arteries

6. Of the following hormones, the one that is most directly associated with the maintenance of pregnancy is
   (1) insulin
   (2) progestin
   (3) secretin
   (4) somatotrophin

7. Pictured below is a schematic diagram of an animal cell. Which structure is primarily concerned with the release of energy from nutrients?
   (1) 4
   (2) 2
   (3) 1
   (4) 3

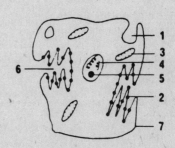

8. The correct sequence of digestive structures is
   (1) esophagus, liver, large intestine, small intestine
   (2) stomach, spleen, liver, large intestine
   (3) esophagus, stomach, large intestine, small intestine
   (4) esophagus, stomach, small intestine, large intestine

9. What is the probable order of evolution among the following phyla?

1. protozoa 4. birds 7. fish
2. sponges 5. arthropods 8. amphibians
3. mammals 6. worms 9. reptiles
(1) 1, 5, 6, 4, 7, 6
(2) 1, 2, 7, 9, 8, 3
(3) 2, 9, 7, 8, 3, 4
(4) 1, 2, 8, 9, 4, 3

10. A dolphin's flipper, and a horse's foreleg have similar embryological and anatomical relationships and are therefore
(1) genetic isolates
(2) analogous structures
(3) homologous structures
(4) evolved from one common ancestor

11. Cells are broadly divided into eucaryotes and procaryotes according to whether
(1) their genes are enclosed by a nuclear membrane
(2) the nuclear membrane is permeable
(3) they have ribosomes
(4) they are plant or animal

12. Which one of the following compounds stores energy that is immediately available for active muscle cells?
(1) creatine phosphate
(2) glycogen
(3) glucose
(4) glycine

Base your answers to 13 and 14 on the chart that follows.

	0.7B	0.3b
0.7B	0.49	0.21
0.3b	0.21	0.09

13. As indicated, the homozygous dominant individuals constitute what proportion of the population?
(1) 42%
(2) 16%
(3) 49%
(4) 65%

14. The proportion of offspring that contain the gene b is
(1) 40%
(2) 51%
(3) 52%
(4) 16%

15. Place the following in increasing order of complexity.
 I. proteins
 II. CH_4 and NH_3
 III. amino acids
 IV. C, H, O, N

(1) I, II, III, IV
(2) II, IV, I, III
(3) IV, I, II, III
(4) IV, II, III, I

16. In which of the following kinds of symbiosis do both species benefit from the association?
(1) commensalism
(2) parasitism
(3) mutualism
(4) none of the above

17. Which of the following is true of enzyme catalysis but not true of inorganic catalysis?
(1) Enzyme catalysis speeds up the reaction.
(2) The inorganic catalyst itself undergoes no change in the reaction.
(3) Enzyme catalysis is subject to cellular controls.
(4) Only a small amount of the inorganic catalyst is necessary.

18. An albino corn plant lacks chlorophyll and therefore cannot carry on photosynthesis. Continuation of this genetic trait in corn plants occurs because
(1) albino plants become green in the sunlight
(2) self-pollination occurs in albino plants
(3) green plants may carry the albino gene
(4) albino plants mutate to green plants

19. Unicellular organisms ingest large molecules into their cytoplasm from the external environment without previously digesting them.

This process is called
(1) pinocytosis
(2) plasmolysis
(3) osmosis
(4) transpiration

20. Which environmental change is most likely to increase the rate of photosynthesis in a bean plant?
    (1) an increase in the intensity of green light
    (2) a rise in the oxygen concentration in the air
    (3) a rise in the carbon dioxide concentration in the air
    (4) an increase in plant fertilization

21. According to recent studies, a bacteriophage consists essentially of an internal metabolic mechanism that contains nucleic acid and an external coat of
    (1) keratin
    (2) phosphide
    (3) polysaccharide
    (4) protein

22. An organism that can reproduce successfully without utilizing the process of meiosis is the
    (1) fruit fly
    (2) dog
    (3) ameba
    (4) grasshopper

For questions 23–26, match the smaller structures listed below with the larger structures named in each question.

(1) cristae
(2) ribosomes
(3) grana
(4) microtubules

23. Chloroplast

24. Mitochondria

25. Endoplasmic reticulum

26. Cilia

27. The center for temperature regulation in the human is the

(1) skin
(2) thalamus
(3) medulla
(4) cerebellum

28. Select the cross in which all offspring will be hybrids.
    (1) RRYY X rryy
    (2) RrYy X RrYy
    (3) RrYy X rryy
    (4) rryy X rryy

Choose the numbered term that is most closely related to the statements in questions numbered 29–32 below.

(1) morula
(2) blastula
(3) gastrula
(4) mesoderm formation

29. Shows the presence of the blastocoele.

30. Is the end result of cleavage.

31. In amphibians, this stage results from the process of gastrulation.

32. The next structure to develop directly from the zygote, in mammals.

33. Consider the knee-jerk reflex. The pathway of this reflex involves
    (1) 2 neurons: 1 from knee to spinal cord; 1 from spinal cord to leg muscle
    (2) 3 neurons: 1 from knee to spinal cord; 1 from 1st to 3rd within spinal cord; 1 from spinal cord to leg muscle
    (3) 4 neurons: the three from (B); 1 along the leg muscle
    (4) 5 neurons: 1 from knee to spinal cord; 1 from spinal cord to brain; 1 within brain (affected by other stimuli); 1 from brain to spinal cord; 1 from spinal cord to muscle

34. Bile is used in digesting
    (1) sugars
    (2) proteins
    (3) amino acids
    (4) fats

35. The human embryo goes through various states resembling lower forms of animals. Which of the following structures has a similar structure appearing sometime during the development of the human embryo?
    I. gills
    II. tail
    III. spiracles

    (1) I
    (2) II
    (3) III
    (4) I and II

36. Which of the following kind of bond is formed between the strands of a DNA molecule?
    (1) disulfide
    (2) hydrogen
    (3) hydrophobic
    (4) covalent

37. In which of the following cell functions is the lysosome involved?
    (1) protein synthesis
    (2) protein packaging
    (3) digestion
    (4) photosynthesis

38. Facultative anaerobes
    (1) are found only among the green plants
    (2) require oxygen to live
    (3) may make use of oxidative phosphorylation
    (4) die from exposure to oxygen

39. The arms of a human and the forelimbs of a dog are
    (1) analogous structures
    (2) homologous structures
    (3) both analogous and homologous structures
    (4) neither analogous nor homologous structures

40. Which of the following structures arises from the embryonic cell layer known as the *mesoderm*?
    (1) heart
    (2) bone
    (3) muscle
    (4) all of the above

41. If it is known that in a certain DNA molecule 10% of the bases are guanine, it can be concluded that
    (1) 40% are thymine
    (2) 80% are cytosine
    (3) 45% are adenine
    (4) 90% are adenine

42. External fertilization is most likely to be carried on by organisms that live in
    (1) meadows
    (2) forests
    (3) tundra
    (4) ponds

43. With a genotype AaBb, the fraction of gametes that will be ab is
    (1) $\frac{1}{16}$
    (2) $\frac{1}{4}$
    (3) $\frac{1}{2}$
    (4) $\frac{1}{8}$

44. The dark reaction of photosynthesis *cannot* occur in the absence of
    (1) CO_2
    (2) O_2
    (3) chlorophyll
    (4) nitrogen

45. The DNA code is directly dependent upon the
    (1) relative abundance of the adenine–thymine guanine–cytosine pairs
    (2) number of deoxyribose molecules
    (3) arrangement of purine–pyrimidine pairs
    (4) position of the phosphate groups

STOP

END OF BIOLOGY QUESTIONS

PERIODIC TABLE OF THE ELEMENTS

1a	2a	3b	4b	5b	6b	7b	8	8	8	1b	2b	3a	4a	5a	6a	7a	0
1 H 1.0097																	2 He 4.0026
3 Li 6.939	4 Be 9.0122											5 B 10.811	6 C 12.01115	7 N 14.0067	8 O 15.9994	9 F 18.9984	10 Ne 20.183
11 Na 22.9898	12 Mg 24.312											13 Al 26.9815	14 Si 28.086	15 P 30.9738	16 S 32.064	17 Cl 35.453	18 Ar 39.948
19 K 39.102	20 Ca 40.08	21 Sc 44.956	22 Ti 47.90	23 V 50.942	24 Cr 51.996	25 Mn 54.9380	26 Fe 55.847	27 Co 58.9332	28 Ni 58.71	29 Cu 63.546	30 Zn 63.37	31 Ga 69.72	32 Ge 72.59	33 As 74.9216	34 Se 78.96	35 Br 79.904	36 Kr 83.80
37 Rb 85.47	38 Sr 87.62	39 Y 88.905	40 Zr 91.22	41 Nb 92.906	42 Mo 95.94	43 Tc (97)	44 Ru 101.07	45 Rh 102.905	46 Pd 106.4	47 Ag 107.868	48 Cd 112.40	49 In 114.82	50 Sn 118.69	51 Sb 121.75	52 Te 127.60	53 I 126.9044	54 Xe 131.30
55 Cs 132.905	56 Ba 137.34	57* La 138.91	72 Hf 178.49	73 Ta 180.948	74 W 183.85	75 Re 186.2	76 Os 190.2	77 Ir 192.2	78 Pt 195.09	79 Au 196.967	80 Hg 200.59	81 Tl 204.37	82 Pb 207.19	83 Bi 208.980	84 Po (209)	85 At (210)	86 Rn (222)
87 Fr (223)	88 Ra (236)	89** Ac (227)														104 –	

Transition Elements — Group 8

*Lanthanides	58 Ce 140.12	59 Pr 140.907	60 Nd 144.24	61 Pm (145)	62 Sm 150.35	63 Eu 151.96	64 Gd 157.25	65 Tb 158.924	66 Dy 162.50	67 Ho 164.930	68 Er 167.26	69 Tm 168.934	70 Yb 173.04	71 Lu 174.97
**Actinides	90 Th (232)	91 Pa (231)	92 U (238)	93 Np (237)	94 Pu (244)	95 Am (243)	96 Cm (247)	97 Bk (247)	98 Cf (251)	99 Es (254)	100 Fm (257)	101 Md (256)	102 No (254)	103 Lw (254)

Numbers in parentheses are mass numbers of most stable isotope of that element.

CHEMISTRY

Time: 25 minutes
45 questions

Directions: Select the one best answer from the numbered choices that follow each question. The Periodic Table of the Elements appears on page 49.

1. Given the reaction below, which of the following will not increase the amount of NH_3 produced?

$$\Delta H = -80 \text{ Kcal}$$
$$2NH_3 \rightleftharpoons N_2 + 3H_2$$
$$\Delta H = +80 \text{ Kcal}$$

   (1) increasing the temperature
   (2) increasing the pressure
   (3) adding NH_3
   (4) none of the above

2. Which of the following cannot result from the oxidation of a primary alcohol?
   (1) a ketone
   (2) an aldehyde
   (3) a carboxylic acid
   (4) none of the above

3. A compound having a molecular weight of 58 is shown by analysis to consist of 5/29 hydrogen and the remainder carbon by weight. The number of carbon atoms in one molecule of the compound is
   (1) 5
   (2) 4
   (3) 8
   (4) 10

4. The maximum number of electrons that may be found in the "L" shell of an atom is
   (1) 6
   (2) 8
   (3) 18
   (4) 10

5. Which of the following statements best describes the action of catalysts?
   (1) They alter the ratio of products.
   (2) They change the rate of reactions.
   (3) They change the ratio of products and the rate of reaction.
   (4) They alter the equilibrium of the reaction.

6. The acid in the reaction $NH_3 + H_2O \rightarrow NH_4^+ + OH^-$ is
   (1) NH_3
   (2) H^+
   (3) H_2O
   (4) NH_2^-

7. Rutherford's bombardment of gold foil with alpha particles helped to establish the electron theory by
   (1) determining the mass of the atom
   (2) determining the number of particles in a mole
   (3) determining the charge on a single electron
   (4) demonstrating that the atom is largely empty space with a concentrated positive charge

8. The mass of material deposited on the cathode of an electrolytic cell, other things being equal, is proportional to the
   (1) area of the cathode surface
   (2) quantity of charge passing through the cell
   (3) concentration of electrolyte in solution
   (4) degree of metallic character of the cathode

9. As we go from left to right in period two of the Periodic Table, the gram atomic volume of the elements

(1) will change indefinitely
(2) increases at a constant rate
(3) first increases, then decreases
(4) decreases

10. Chemical analysis of a gas shows that it contains one atom of carbon for each two atoms of hydrogen. If its density is 1.25 g per liter at standard temperature and pressure, its formula is (Atomic weights: C = 12; H = 1)
    (1) CH_2
    (2) C_2H_4
    (3) C_4H_8
    (4) C_3H_6

11. The volume of 0.25 molar H_3PO_4 necessary to neutralize 25 ml of 0.30 molar $Ca(OH)_2$ is
    (1) 8.3 ml
    (2) 20 ml
    (3) 50 ml
    (4) 40 ml

12. Naphthalene, $C_{10}H_8$, is most soluble in
    (1) water
    (2) alcohol
    (3) benzene
    (4) acetic acid

13. Which of the following is a balanced chemical equation?
    (1) $H_2 + Br_2 \rightarrow HBr$
    (2) $P_4 + O_2 \rightarrow P_4O_{10}$
    (3) $C_3H_8 + 5O_2 \rightarrow 3CO_2 + 4H_2O$
    (4) $H_2 + O_2 \rightarrow 2H_2O$

14. Element 102, with a mass number of 253, was synthesized by bombarding $_{96}Cm^{240}$ with a single nuclear particle, which it captured. The particle used was
    (1) $_6X^{13}$
    (2) $_{13}X^6$
    (3) $_6X^{12}$
    (4) $_9X^{17}$

15. In beta emission from the nucleus, an atom
    (1) increases by one in atomic weight
    (2) decreases by one in atomic weight
    (3) decreases by four in atomic weight
    (4) increases by one in atomic number

16. The weight in grams of nitrogen in 11.2 liters (S.T.P.) of ammonia is (Atomic weight of nitrogen = 14)
    (1) 7
    (2) 8.5
    (3) 14
    (4) 3.5

17. Gamma rays have
    (1) unit mass and minus charge
    (2) unit mass and zero charge
    (3) zero mass and zero charge
    (4) zero mass and minus charge

18. Which of the following statements best distinguishes electrolytes from nonelectrolytes?
    (1) Electrolytes are always ionic compounds, while nonelectrolytes are always covalent compounds.
    (2) Electrolytes are usually covalent compounds, while nonelectrolytes are usually ionic compounds
    (3) Nonelectrolytes are usually insoluble in water, while electrolytes are usually soluble.
    (4) Electrolytes can be covalent or ionic compounds but must be ionic in solution.

19. Of the following gases, the lightest is
    (1) carbon monoxide
    (2) sulfur dioxide
    (3) hydrogen sulfide
    (4) fluorine

20. When small particles are added to a liquid, they can often be seen to be undergoing very rapid motion on the surface of the liquid. The explanation for this motion is best described by which of the following?
    (1) the electrical interactions between the liquid and the suspended particles
    (2) the molecular vibrations of the liquid causing collisions with the suspended particles
    (3) eddy currents in the surface of the liquid
    (4) thermal induction at the surface of the liquid

21. A radioisotope has a half-life of twenty days; after forty days the fraction of pure radioisotope that remains is

(1) ½
(2) ¼
(3) ⅙
(4) ⅛

22. The reaction $3O_2 \rightleftharpoons 2O_3 - 69,000$ calories is aided in the forward direction by
    (1) higher temperature and lower pressure
    (2) higher temperature and higher pressure
    (3) lower temperature and lower pressure
    (4) lower temperature and higher pressure

23. An element that forms amphoteric compounds is
    (1) Zn
    (2) La
    (3) F
    (4) Cl

24. What is the efficiency of a reversible Carnot cycle having a mass of steel as working substance?
    (1) 10%
    (2) 50%
    (3) 80%
    (4) 100%

25. According to the Bronsted definition of acids and bases,
    (1) any acid can yield a base by gaining a proton
    (2) a base cannot be a cation
    (3) a base may be an electrically neutral substance
    (4) a base cannot be an anion

26. Compounds in which electrovalent bonds predominate have liquid forms characterized by
    (1) low freezing point and slight electrical conductivity
    (2) low freezing point and good electrical conductivity
    (3) high freezing point and good electrical conductivity
    (4) high freezing point and slight electrical conductivity

27. Different compounds with the same crystalline form are said to be
    (1) isogonic
    (2) isomorphic
    (3) isotropic
    (4) isotopic

28. Properties which depend upon the number rather than the nature of the dissolved particles in a solution are called
    (1) colligative
    (2) isotropic
    (3) isotonic
    (4) isoelectronic

29. In a chemical reaction, equilibrium has been established when the
    (1) concentrations of the reactants and the products are equal
    (2) reaction ceases to generate heat
    (3) order of the reaction is larger than two
    (4) velocity of the opposing reaction is the same as that of the forward reaction

30. Which one of the following is a product of the reaction between copper and hot concentrated sulfuric acid?
    (1) hydrogen
    (2) sulfur dioxide
    (3) sulfur trioxide
    (4) cuprous ions

31. The process $_1H^2 + {}_1H^3 \rightarrow {}_2H^4 + {}_0n^1$ represents the type of reaction known as
    (1) fission
    (2) chemical
    (3) autocatalytic
    (4) fusion

32. If a surface film behaves as an ideal two-dimensional gas, its equation of state becomes (f = force, A = area)
    (1) $PV = RT$
    (2) $fV = PT$
    (3) $fA = kT$
    (4) $AR = PT$

33. Of the following metals, the two whose oxides are often reduced with hydrogen are
    (1) iron and nickel
    (2) titanium and zirconium
    (3) vanadium and chromium
    (4) tungsten and molybdenum

34. The number of elements in each of the *long* periods in the Periodic Table is
    (1) 8
    (2) 18
    (3) 36
    (4) 10

35. The relative abundance of two rubidium isotopes of atomic weights 85 and 87 is 75% and 25%, respectively. The average atomic weight of rubidium is
    (1) 75.5
    (2) 85.5
    (3) 87.5
    (4) 86.5

36. In the series of active metals (Na, K, Rb, Cs) cesium is the most active because it (its)
    (1) incomplete shell is closest to the nucleus
    (2) exerts the greatest attractive force on valence electrons
    (3) has the largest number of valence electrons
    (4) valence electron has a larger orbit than the orbit of the valence electron of any of the others

37. A certain metal will liberate hydrogen from dilute acids. It will react with water to form hydrogen only when the metal is heated, and the water is in the form of steam. The metal is probably
    (1) Fe
    (2) Cu
    (3) K
    (4) Hg

38. 500 ml of a 0.1N solution of $AgNO_3$ are added to 500 ml of a 0.1N solution of KCl. The concentration of nitrate ion in the resulting mixture is
    (1) 0.05N
    (2) 0.01N
    (3) 0.1N
    (4) 0.2N

39. A 0.3M HCl solution contains the following ions:
    $$Hg^{++}, Cd^{++}, Sr^{++}, Fe^{++}, Cu^{++}$$

The addition of H_2S to the above solution will precipitate
    (1) Cd, Fe, and Sr
    (2) Hg, Cu, and Fe
    (3) Cu, Sr, and Fe
    (4) Cd, Cu, and Hg

40. In the ion Cu $(NH_3)_4{}^{++}$, the valence and coordination number of the copper are respectively
    (1) + 4 and 12
    (2) + 2 and 8
    (3) + 2 and 4
    (4) + 2 and 12

41. The conjugate base of $NH_4{}^+$ is
    (1) NH_3
    (2) NH_4OH
    (3) OH^-
    (4) NH_2

42. The reaction $H_2O + C_{12}H_{22}O_{11} \rightarrow 4CO_2 + 4C_2H_5OH$ is an example of
    (1) fermentation
    (2) esterification
    (3) polymerization
    (4) photolysis

43. An example of a polar covalent compound is
    (1) NaCl
    (2) CCl_4
    (3) HCl
    (4) CH_4

44. The valence of ruthenium in the compound $K_2Ru(OH)Cl_5$ is
    (1) plus 2
    (2) minus 2
    (3) plus 3
    (4) plus 4

45. A solution contains the following ions: $Ag^+, Hg^+, Al^{+++}, Cd^{++}, Sr^{++}$. The addition of dilute HCl will precipitate
    (1) Al and Cd
    (2) Ag, Cd and Sr
    (3) Al and Sr
    (4) Ag and Hg

STOP

END OF CHEMISTRY QUESTIONS

QUANTITATIVE ABILITY

Time: 45 minutes
50 questions

Directions: Select the one best answer from the numbered choices that follow each question.

1. The length of each side of the square below is $\frac{2x}{3} + 1$. The perimeter of the square is

   (1) $\frac{8x + 4}{3}$

   (2) $\frac{8x + 12}{3}$

   (3) $\frac{2x}{3} + 4$

   (4) $\frac{2x}{3} + 16$

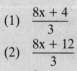

2. To find the radius of a circle whose circumference is 60 inches,
   (1) multiply 60 by π
   (2) divide 60 by 2 π
   (3) divide 30 by 2 π
   (3) divide 60 by 3 π

3. If the outer diameter of a metal pipe is 2.84 inches and the inner diameter is 1.94 inches, the thickness of the metal is
   (1) .45 of an inch
   (2) .90 of an inch
   (3) 1.94 inches
   (4) 1.42 inches

4. The ratio of the sides of 2 cubes is 3:4. The difference of their volumes is 296. The side of the smaller cube is
   (1) 8
   (2) 3
   (3) 4
   (4) 6

5. From a piece of tin in the shape of a square 6 inches on a side, the largest possible circle is cut out. Of the following, the ratio of the area of the circle to the area of the original square is closest in value to
   (1) $\frac{4}{5}$
   (2) $\frac{2}{3}$
   (3) $\frac{3}{5}$
   (4) $\frac{3}{4}$

6. A motorist travels 120 miles to his destination at an average speed of 60 miles per hour and returns to the starting point at an average speed of 40 miles per hour. His average speed for the entire trip is
   (1) 50 miles per hour
   (2) 48 miles per hour
   (3) 45 miles per hour
   (4) 52 miles per hour

7. As shown in the diagram, AB is a straight line and angle BOC=20°. If the number of degrees in angle DOC is 6 more than the number of degrees in angle x, find the number of degrees in angle x.
   (1) 77
   (2) 75
   (3) 78
   (4) 87

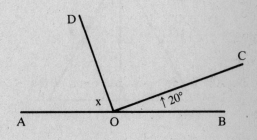

8. As shown in the figure, a cylindrical oil tank is $\frac{1}{3}$ full. If 3 more gallons are added, the

51

tank will be half full. What is the capacity, in gallons, of the tank?

(1) 16
(2) 17
(3) 18
(4) 19

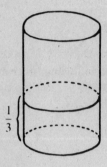

9. A boy receives grades of 91, 88, 86, and 78 in four of his major subjects. What must he receive in his fifth major subject in order to average 85?
   (1) 85
   (2) 84
   (3) 83
   (4) 82

10. In the figure, PS is perpendicular to QR. If PQ=PR=26 and PS=24, then QR=
    (1) 16
    (2) 18
    (3) 20
    (4) 22

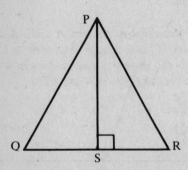

11. If p pencils cost $2D$ dollars, how many pencils can be bought for c cents?

(1) $\dfrac{pc}{2D}$

(2) $\dfrac{pc}{200D}$

(3) $\dfrac{50pc}{D}$

(3) $\dfrac{2Dp}{c}$

12. If a man walks ⅖ mile in 5 minutes, what is his average rate of walking in miles per hours?
    (1) 4
    (2) 4½
    (3) 4⅘
    (4) 5⅕

13. One end of a dam has the shape of a trapezoid with the dimensions indicated. What is the dam's area in square feet?
    (1) 1000
    (2) 1200
    (3) 1500
    (4) 1800

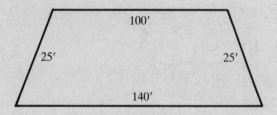

14. If $1 + \dfrac{1}{t} = \dfrac{t+1}{t}$, what does t equal?
    (1) $+2$ or -2 only
    (2) $+2$ or -1 only
    (3) -2 or $+1$ only
    (4) none of the above

15. Point A is 3 inches from line b as shown in the diagram. In the plane that contains point A and line b, what is the total number of points which are 6 inches from A and also 1 inch from b?
    (1) 1
    (2) 2
    (3) 3
    (4) 4

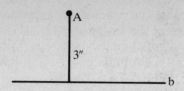

16. If R and S are different integers, both divisible by 5, then which of the following is *not necessarily* true?
    (1) R − S is divisible by 5
    (2) RS is divisible by 25
    (3) R + S is divisible by 5
    (4) R + S is divisible by 10

17. If a triangle of base 7 is equal in area to a circle of radius 7, what is the altitude of the triangle?
    (1) 14π
    (2) 10π
    (3) 12π
    (4) 8π

18. The coordinates of the vertices of quadrilateral PQRS are P(0,0), Q(9,0), R(10,3), and S(1,3), respectively. The area of PQRS is
    (1) 9√10
    (2) ½√10
    (3) 27
    (4) 27½

19. In the circle shown, AB is a diameter. If secant AP=8 and tangent CP=4, find the number of units in the diameter of the circle.
    (1) 6
    (2) 6½
    (3) 8
    (4) 3√2

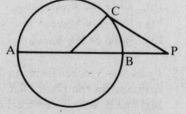

20. A certain type of siding for a house costs $10.50 per square yard. What does it cost for the siding for a wall 4 yards wide and 60 feet long?
    (1) $800
    (2) $840
    (3) $2520
    (4) $3240

21. A circle whose radius is 7 has its center at the origin. Which of the following points are outside the circle?
    I. (4, 4)
    II. (5, 5)
    III. (4, 5)
    IV. (4, 6)

    (1) II and III only
    (2) II, III, and IV only
    (3) II and IV only
    (4) III and IV only

22. A merchant sells a radio for $80, thereby making a profit of 25% of the cost. What is the ratio of cost to selling price?
    (1) ⅘
    (2) ¾
    (3) ⅚
    (4) ⅔

23. How many degrees are there between the hands of a clock at 3:40?
    (1) 140°
    (2) 130°
    (3) 125°
    (4) 120°

24. Two fences in a field meet at 120°. A cow is tethered at their intersection with a 15-foot rope, as shown in the figure. Over how many square feet may the cow graze?
    (1) 75π
    (2) 80π
    (3) 85π
    (4) 90π

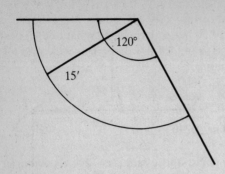

25. In the figure below, r, s, and t are straight lines meeting at point p, with angles formed as indicated; then y =
    (1) 120°
    (2) 3x
    (3) 180 − x
    (4) 180 − 3x

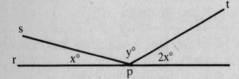

26. $^{18}\!/_{33} = \dfrac{\sqrt{36}}{\sqrt{?}}$

    (1) 121
    (2) 66
    (3) 144
    (4) 1089

27. If we write all the whole numbers from 200 to 400, how many of these contain the digit 7 once and only once?
    (1) 34
    (2) 35
    (3) 36
    (4) 38

28. $(r + s)^2 − r^2 − s^2 =$
    (1) 2rs
    (2) rs
    (3) rs^2
    (4) $2r^2 + 2s^2$

29. In the figure, angle S is obtuse, PR = 9,

PS = 6, and Q is any point on RS. Which of the following inequalities expresses possible values of the length of PQ?
    (1) $9 \geq PQ \geq 6$
    (2) $9 \geq 6 \geq PQ$
    (3) $PQ \geq 9 \geq 6$
    (4) $9 \leq PQ \leq 6$

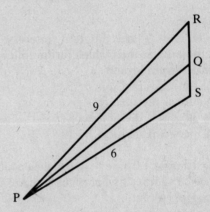

30. If a man buys several articles for K cents per dozen and sells them for $\dfrac{K}{8}$ cents per article, what is his profit, in cents, per article?

    (1) $\dfrac{K}{48}$ (3) $\dfrac{K}{18}$

    (2) $\dfrac{K}{12}$ (4) $\dfrac{K}{24}$

31. If all P are S and no S are Q, it necessarily follows that
    (1) all Q are S
    (2) all Q are P
    (3) no P are Q
    (4) some Q are P

32. The average of four numbers is 45. If one of the numbers is increased by 6, the average will remain unchanged if each of the other three numbers is reduced by
    (1) 1
    (2) 2
    (3) ¾
    (4) ⁴⁄₃

33. A set of papers is arranged and numbered from 1 to 40. If the paper numbered 4 is drawn first and every seventh paper thereafter is drawn, what will be the number of the last paper drawn?
    (1) 37
    (2) 38
    (3) 39
    (4) 40

34. If the angles of a triangle are in the ratio of 2:3:5, the triangle is
    (1) obtuse
    (2) isosceles
    (3) right
    (4) equilateral

35. In the figure, a rectangular piece of cardboard 18 inches by 24 inches is made into an open box by cutting a 5-inch square from each corner and building up the sides. What is the volume of the box in cubic inches?
    (1) 560
    (2) 1233
    (3) 1560
    (4) 2160

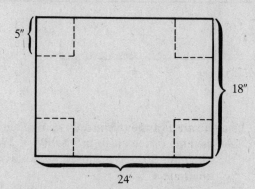

36. The figure that follows represents the back of a house. Find, in feet, the length of one of the equal rafters PQ or QR, if PV and TR are each 12 inches long.
    (1) 19
    (2) 21
    (3) 23
    (4) 25

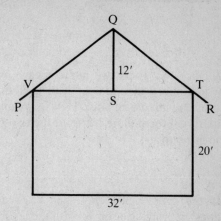

37. The scale of a certain map is ¾ inch = 9 miles. Find in square miles the actual area of a park represented on the map by a square whose side is ⅞ inch.
    (1) 10½
    (2) 110¼
    (3) 121
    (4) 125⅔

38. A relationship that holds for all waves is expressed by the formula $V = fL$, where V is the velocity, f is the frequency, and L the wavelength. Express the wavelength L in terms of V and f.

    (1) $L = \dfrac{V}{f}$

    (2) $L = Vf$

    (3) $L = V + f$

    (4) $L = \dfrac{f}{V}$

39. If t represents the ten's digit and u the unit's digit of a two-digit number, then the number is represented by
    (1) $t + u$
    (2) tu
    (3) $10u + t$
    (4) $10t + u$

40. The pages of a typewritten report are numbered from 1 to 100 by hand. How many times will it be necessary to write the number 5?

(1) 10
(2) 12
(3) 19
(4) 20

41. A clock that gains two minutes each hour is synchronized at midnight with a clock that loses one minute an hour. How many minutes apart will the minute hands of the two clocks be at noon?
    (1) 30
    (2) 24
    (3) 14
    (4) 12

42. Instead of walking along two adjacent edges of a square lot, a boy walks along the diagonal. About what percent did he save?
    (1) 29
    (2) 33
    (3) 24
    (4) 22

43. The figure represents a wooden block, 3 inches on an edge, all of whose faces are painted black. If the block is cut up along the dotted lines, 27 blocks result, each 1 cubic inch in volume. Of these, how many will have no painted faces?
    (1) 1
    (2) 3
    (3) 4
    (4) 5

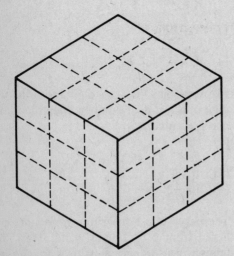

44. The number 6 is called a *perfect* number because it is the sum of all its integral divisors except itself. Another perfect number is
    (1) 36
    (2) 28
    (3) 24
    (4) 16

45. The morning classes in a school begin at 9 A.M. and end at 11:51 A.M. There are 4 class periods with 5 minutes between classes. How many minutes are there in each class period?
    (1) 37¾
    (2) 38½
    (3) 39
    (4) 40

46. A man plans to build a fenced-in enclosure along a riverbank, as shown in the figure. He has 90 feet of fencing available for the three sides of the rectangular enclosure. All of the following statements are true *except*

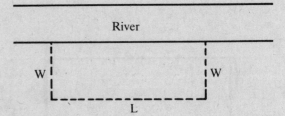

    (1) the area of the enclosure is LW
    (2) the area of the enclosure is $90W - 2W^2$
    (3) when W=20, the enclosed area is 1000 square feet
    (4) the enclosed area is greatest when L=W

47. A desk was listed at $90.00 and was bought for $75.00. What was the rate of discount?
    (1) 15%
    (2) 16⅔%
    (3) 18%
    (4) 20%

48. In the figure that follows, a running track goes around a football field in the shape of a rectangle with semicircles at each end, with

dimensions as indicated on the figure. The distance around the track in yards is

(1) $100 + 60\pi$
(2) $200 + 30\pi$
(3) $200 + 60\pi$
(4) $100 + 30\pi$

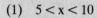

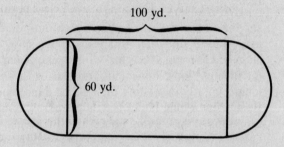

100 yd.

60 yd.

49. How many feet does an auto travel in 1 second if it is moving at the rate of 45 miles per hour? There are 5280 feet in one mile.

(1)   44
(2)   66
(3)   88
(4)   112

50. In the figure below, $\triangle$ PQR is isosceles with the legs each equal to 5. If angle P may take on values between 90° and 180°, which inequality best expresses the possible values of the base x?

(1) $5 < x < 10$
(2) $5\sqrt{3} < x < 10$
(3) $7 < x < 10$
(4) $5\sqrt{2} < x < 10$

P

5   5

Q   R

x

STOP

END OF QUANTITATIVE ABILITY QUESTIONS

STUDY–READING

Time: **20 minutes to read the passage;**
20 minutes to answer the 50 questions

Directions: You will be given 20 minutes to read the following passage. Later in the examination, you will be given 20 additional minutes to answer 50 questions based on the passage. Study the passage carefully for the entire 20 minutes. You will not be permitted to refer to it after this time is expired.

(*Note*: The study–reading passage and the questions may be separated by a completely unrelated test section.)

Strictly speaking, the skeletal system consists of the bones and related cartilages of the body. More broadly, it also includes the *articulations* (joints). The study of bones is called *osteology*, while the study of joints is called *arthrology*. Bone is the major support tissue in the vertebrates. The human skeletal system consists of 206 specific bones that can be subdivided into two major groups, the *axial* and *appendicular skeletons*. The axial skeleton contains 80 bones, including those of the skull, vertebral column and thorax, while the appendicular skeleton contains 126 bones, including those of the pectoral and pelvic girdles and the upper and lower limbs. Each subdivision is further arranged as follows:

Axial Skeleton (80 bones):
  Skull (29)
  Vertebral column (26)
  Thorax (sternum and ribs) (25)

Appendicular Skeleton (126 bones):
  Pectoral girdle (4)
  Upper limbs (60)
  Pelvic girdle (2)
  Lower limbs (60)

The four major functions of human bones are: (1) support for soft body tissue; (2) protection for vital body organs; (3) to serve as centers for hematopoeisis (blood cell formation); and (4) passive involvement in movement, with the bones serving as lever systems upon which muscles can act. Based on their shapes, bones may be classified as long, short, flat, or irregular. Characteristically, long bones are tubular with their length greatly exceeding their other dimensions. Examples of long bones are the humerus, femur, tibia, and fibula. Short bones may be tubular or cuboidal with no one dimension significantly exceeding any other. Examples of short bones are the *carpals* (wrist bones) and *tarsals* (ankle bones). Flat bones are generally quite broad and thin. Examples of flat bones are ribs and skull bones that form the brain case. Each bone has a specific set of relationships with other tissues and organs of the body. These relationships are suggested by a variety of surface features, which range from irregularly roughened areas and ridges to well-defined knobs and processes. No less than 18 special terms are assigned to these surface features. These terms are an important part of the vocabulary necessary to describe bones.

On the basis of development, there are two kinds of bones: (1) *intramembranous* bone, which develops directly from *mesenchymal tissue*, and (2) *endochordral* bone, which develops from hyaline cartilage. In both cases, the specialized *osteoblasts* (immature bone cells) lay down a homogenous matrix of amorphous ground substance composed of mucopolysaccharides, and protein fibers composed primarily of collagen. This is followed by the deposition of lime salts in the matrix. As the matrix solidifies, it imprisons osteoblasts and blood vessels in *lacunae* (chambers) and canaliculi, haversian canals, and Volkmann's canals. The entire process is called *calcification*. Calcification is dependent on an adequate supply of calcium, phosphorus, vitamin D, *parathormone* (parathyroid hormone) and specific enzymes known as *phosphatases*.

The human skull is composed of 8 cranial bones (which surround the brain), 14 facial bones (which support and protect the eyes and the respiratory and digestive system entryways), 6 middle ear bones, and 1 *hyoid bone* (which is found in the base of the tongue). The teeth of the oral cavity are set in three of the facial bones: the mandible (which forms the lower jaw) and two maxillae (which form the upper jaw). The mandible forms a horseshoe-shaped body with two perpendicular rami (branches). It also contains 16 *mandibular alveoli* (tooth sockets). The remaining 16 alveoli are distributed equally in the two maxillae. *Foramina* (openings) in all three bones provide passageways for blood vessels and nerves. The opening on each side, the *mandibular foramen*, provides the innervation for the lower teeth on each side of the lower jaw. This single innervation on each side provides the dentist with a single injection site for an anesthetic, which then renders half the lower jaw insensitive. There is no corresponding arrangement in either of the maxillae.

Histologically speaking, the teeth and *gingivae* (gums) are considered to be part of the digestive system. The gingivae are composed of dense, fibrous connective tissue that is attached to the neck of each tooth and to the margins of maxillae and mandible. On the outside, the gingiva is covered by a mucus membrane that is continuous with the mucus membrane of the lips and cheek. On the other side, the gingiva reflects into each alveolus, where it is continuous with the *periodontal membrane* (a special type of dense connective tissue). The fibers of the periodontal membrane penetrate the cementum layer binding each tooth to the alveolar wall, permitting only limited movement of the tooth in its alveolus. The fibers, composed of the protein *collagen*, are so arranged as to respond best to the pressures of *mastication* (chewing) and thereby transmit mastication pressures in such a way as to avoid direct influence on the bone. If these pressures were allowed to act directly on the bone, the response would be the localized resorption of bone tissue, resulting in alveolar enlargement and the ultimate loosening of the tooth in its socket.

Teeth serve two purposes in humans. First, they are the organs of mastication, being specialized for cutting, tearing, or grinding. Second, they are an integral part of articulate speech. As seen in the illustration, teeth are embedded in alveoli of the mandible and maxillae. This arrangement thereby forms the *superior* and *inferior dental arches* of the oral cavity. Irrespective of function, all teeth are composed of a *crown* (exposed portion), a *neck* (slightly constricted region at the gum line), and a *root* (region embedded in the bony alveolus). The *apical foramen* serves as the entryway for nerves and blood vessels that enter and leave the *pulp cavity*. The channel that leads from the apical foramen to the pulp cavity is called the *root canal*. The pulp cavity contains *pulp*, which consists mainly of a loose kind of connective tissue with both thin collagenous and reticular fibers arranged in no particular pattern, plus amorphous ground substance containing mucopolysaccharides.

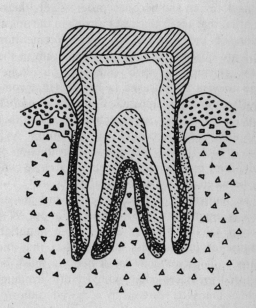

▨ Crown Enamel	▱ Peridontal Membrane
▨ Dentin	▨ Alveolar Bone
▭ Pulp Cavity & Root Canal	▨ Gingiva Connective Tissue
▬ Cementum	▨ Gingiva Epithelium

The three mineralized layers of the tooth are the: (1) *enamel*, (2) *dentin*, and (3) *cementum*. With the exception of root canal openings, the dentin completely surrounds the pulp cavity and root canals, and the dentin itself is surrounded by cementum in the alveolar region and by enamel in the crown region. Dentin is a calcified tissue similar to bone, only harder due to its high content of calcium, as much as 80% of the tooth's dry weight. The remaining 20% is composed of collagenous fibers and the mucopolysaccharides *chondroitin sulfate* or *hyaluronic acid*. *Odontoblasts*, specialized bonelike cells that line the internal surface of the tooth, are responsible for synthesizing the organic matrix of dentin. Dentin is quite sensitive to heat, cold, acids, trauma, and other forms of stimuli. Although the pulp is richly innervated and the dentin is not, impulses appear to be readily transmitted from the point of stimulation outside of the dentin to the pulp nerves inside the dentin layer. It is not known exactly how this phenomenon occurs.

Cementum is another calcified tissue similar to bone, although it lacks the haversian canals and blood vessels commonly found in bones. Cementum starts out as a thin covering over the dentin in the neck region and becomes progressively thicker until it reaches its thickest layering in the apical region of the root. *Cementocytes* (cementum cells) are observed only in the cementum in the apical region. As with osteocytes in bone, cementocytes are encased in lacunae that communicate through canaliculi. Cementum is *labile* (sensitive) and reacts to respective stress by either resorption or production of new cementum. As a tooth grows, there is a continuous production of cementum, maintaining the necessary close contact between the root and the alveolus.

The hardest known substance in the human body is enamel. It is composed of about 97% calcium salts and about 3% organic material. Because of its hardness and the fact that the matrix collapses when decalcified, it must be prepared for microscopic study by dry grinding. Enamel matrix is secreted by cells called *ameloblasts*. When the enamel is fully calcified, the ameloblasts first become cuboid cells, then gradually atrophy and disappear once the *enamel cuticle* forms on the external surface of the enamel. Mature enamel is composed of elongated *enamel prisms* (hexagonal rods in the shape of prisms) bound together by *interprismatic substance*. The prisms run through the entire thickness of the enamel and are arranged to provide the greatest degree of strength to the outer layer of the crown.

The alveolar bone is an immature bone in direct contact with the periodontal membrane. Its collagen fibers are not arranged in the lamellar pattern typical of adult bone. Collagenous fibers of the periodontal membrane penetrate both the cementum and alveolar bone, thereby bridging these structures.

Human teeth are varied in form. The front *incisors* (chisel-shaped) are for cutting; on either side are the pointed *canines* for tearing, followed by the *premolars* (bicuspids) and *molars*, which are for grinding and crushing. We all start life with a set of 20 deciduous (milk, temporary) teeth. The first of these generally show up with the eruption of the central incisors between the first 6–8 months of life. The general pattern continues as follows: lateral incisors (7–12 months), canines (16–20 months), first molars (12–16 months), and finally the second molars (20–30 months). Deciduous teeth are usually shed between the ages of 6–13 years. As deciduous teeth are shed, they are replaced by the permanent teeth. As with the deciduous teeth, the first permanent teeth to appear are the central incisors (7–8 years). These are followed by the lateral incisors (7–10 years), canines (9–14 years), first premolars (9–13 years), second premolars (10–14 years), first molars (5–8 years), second molars (10–14 years), and the third molars or wisdom teeth (17–24 years). A full set of permanent teeth consists of 32 units: 8 incisors, 4 canines, 8 premolars, and 12 molars.

It is interesting to note that both deciduous and permanent teeth begin their development during embryonic and fetal life. Deciduous teeth begin forming around the sixth week after conception, while the permanent teeth initiate development around the fourth month after conception. Deciduous tooth calcification occurs partially during intrauterine life and partially after birth. Permanent tooth calcification occurs during infancy and childhood. Deciduous tooth calcium is initially derived from the mother's blood, which contains calcium from her diet and some withdrawn from her bones. After birth, calcium is derived from the child's diet. It should be noted that phosphorus and vitamin D are also necessary to ensure good tooth development.

The most common tooth problem is the appearance of *dental caries*. There is no question that the single factor that favors bacterial growth leading to the formation of dental caries is a high carbohydrate diet. Frequent monitoring of the teeth is important to ensure early recognition of dental caries and periodontal disease, as well as other potentially serious tooth-related problems. Early intervention often avoids undue pain, suffering, and expense.

STUDY–READING QUESTIONS

Directions: You will have 20 minutes to answer the following questions. You may *not* refer to the passage when answering these questions. Select the one best answer from the numbered choices following each question.

1. The axial skeleton consists of all the bones of the
   (1) skull, vertebrae, and upper limbs
   (2) upper limbs, lower limbs, and girdle
   (3) pectoral girdle, skull, and thorax
   (4) skull, vertebrae, and thorax

2. An arthrologist would be a person who works specifically with
   (1) the teeth of children and adults
   (2) bone physiology and embryonic development
   (3) skeletal joints and joint-related diseases
   (4) the skull degenerative diseases

3. The human skeleton is composed of
   (1) 80 bones
   (2) 126 bones
   (3) 206 bones
   (4) 116 bones

4. One body system that can be directly influenced by changes in the skeletal system is the
   (1) circulatory system
   (2) digestive system
   (3) reproductive system
   (4) endocrine system

5. One important function of the skeletal system is to
   (1) reduce the amount of gravitational pull on the brain
   (2) augment the muscle system during movement activities
   (3) secrete the hormones that feed back to the pituitary gland
   (4) display the visceral organs of the body

6. The largest number of bones in the axial skeleton are located in the
   (1) thorax
   (2) skull
   (3) vertebral columm
   (4) upper limbs

7. One way a bone can be identified is by
   (1) preparing a piece for microscopic examination
   (2) performing a nitric acid test
   (3) observing color change in ultraviolet light
   (4) looking for surface features unique to each type of bone

8. Mesenchymal tissue plays an important role in the
   (1) destruction of bone in the root canal
   (2) impulse transmission in the pulp nerves
   (3) calcification of the tooth crown
   (4) formation of intramembranous bone

9. Both mesenchymal and endochordral bone formation depend on adequate supplies of
   (1) milk, eggs, and celery
   (2) vitamin C, thyroxin, and glucose
   (3) vitamin D, phosphorus, calcium, and parathyroid hormone
   (4) cementocytes, osteocytes, ameloblasts, and erythrocytes

10. The most important element in any calcified tissue is
    (1) iron
    (2) magnesium
    (3) potassium
    (4) calcium

11. Of the 29 skull bones,
    (1) only 3 play a role in mastication
    (2) 9 form the cranial vault
    (3) 6 form the support for the base of the tongue

(4) only 2 hold deciduous teeth

12. The mandible, maxillae, and hyoid bone
    (1) all possess rami and cementocytes
    (2) belong to the appendicular skeleton
    (3) belong to the axial skeleton
    (4) are all covered by a gingiva

13. Dense fibrous connective tissue is characteristic of
    (1) dental pulp
    (2) the gingivae
    (3) bone matrix
    (4) the mandibular foramen

14. It would be safe to assume that an infectious organism that causes destruction of the periodontal membrane would
    (1) cause decay in the crown
    (2) be ultimately responsible for loosening of the tooth in the alveolus
    (3) digest only the collagen fibers
    (4) cause excessive hardening of the enamel

15. There is a continuity between the
    (1) enamel and the periodontal membrane
    (2) periodontal membrane and the gingiva
    (3) gingiva and the dentin
    (4) dentin and the alveolar bone

16. One maxilla in the adult possesses
    (1) 10 dental alveoli
    (2) 20 dental alveoli
    (3) 8 dental alveoli
    (4) 32 dental alveoli

17. It would be accurate to say that
    (1) cementocytes respond only to cold
    (2) the arrangement of collagen in the periodontal membrane is specific
    (3) vertebrae are all long bones
    (4) calcium is found in greater combinations in soft tissues than in hard tissues

18. One important role for the teeth in humans is to
    (1) serve a repository for calcium in the body
    (2) participate in the digestive process
    (3) influence the development of the cranial vault during embryogenesis

(4) assure all endochordral bone development

19. Innervations for the dental pulp enter the tooth through the
    (1) apical foramen
    (2) inferior dental arch
    (3) tibia
    (4) gingivae

20. The root of a typical tooth is composed of
    (1) gingiva and alveolar bone
    (2) alveolar bone and periodontal membrane
    (3) periodontal membrane and cementum
    (4) cementum and dentin

21. It would be accurate to say that
    (1) all teeth have two roots, each with its own canal
    (2) the inferior dental arch holds 10 deciduous teeth in a child
    (3) fibrous connective tissue is the major component of enamel
    (4) innervation in the enamel makes it insensitive to cold

22. The three mineralized portions of the tooth are the
    (1) enamel, alveolar bone, and periodontal membrane
    (2) enamel, gingiva, and cementum
    (3) gingiva, dentin, and enamel
    (4) enamel, cementum, and dentin

23. The composition of pulp includes
    (1) cementocytes and calcium salts
    (2) enamel, nervous tissue, and blood vessels
    (3) mainly a loose connective tissue with collagenous and reticular fibers in no particular arrangement
    (4) mucopolysaccharides, ameloblasts, and osteoblasts

24. The most richly innervated part of the tooth is the
    (1) cementum
    (2) pulp cavity
    (3) dentin
    (4) periodontal membrane

25. The organic matrix of dentin is synthesized by
    (1) erythrocytes
    (2) chondrocytes
    (3) odontoblasts
    (4) phosphatases

26. Cementocytes are commonly found in the
    (1) cementum in the apical region
    (2) cementum and dentin both
    (3) entire cementum region
    (4) cementum and periodontal membrane

27. Most calcified tissue cells are encased in
    (1) foramina
    (2) canals
    (3) lacunae
    (4) alveolar bone

28. The amount of calcium salts in a tooth weighing 100 milligrams is about
    (1) 50 milligrams
    (2) 80 milligrams
    (3) 100 milligrams
    (4) 97 milligrams

29. The best way to prepare enamel tissue for microscopic study is to
    (1) decalcify and section it
    (2) dry grind it until it is thin enough
    (3) fix it in formalin
    (4) digest the calcium with phosphatases

30. Enamel matrix is secreted by
    (1) osteoblasts
    (2) cementocytes
    (3) ameloblasts
    (4) cementocytes

31. A typical structure found in enamel formation is the
    (1) enamel prism
    (2) enamel odontoblast
    (3) enamel formina
    (4) alveola arch

32. It would be accurate to say that the inferior dental arch
    (1) develops from the bones of the cranial vault
    (2) houses six molars in the adult
    (3) houses four canines in the adult
    (4) is composed of two maxillae

33. The teeth that are structurally designed for cutting are the
    (1) premolars and molars
    (2) bicuspids, canines, and molars
    (3) canines
    (4) incisors

34. By the age of 18 months one would normally expect a child to have
    (1) a full set of deciduous teeth
    (2) all permanent incisors
    (3) a full set of deciduous teeth minus the second molars
    (4) only the central incisor and first molars to be present

35. First molars normally appear in the child between
    (1) 6–8 months of life
    (2) 7–12 months of life
    (3) 12–16 months of life
    (4) 16–20 months of life

36. A permanent set of teeth in the inferior dental arch would consist of
    (1) 8 incisors, 4 canines, 8 premolars, and 12 molars
    (2) 4 incisors, 2 canines, 4 premolars, and 6 molars
    (3) 2 incisors, 2 canines, 4 premolars, and 5 molars
    (4) 4 incisors, 4 canines, 8 premolars, 6 molars, and 4 wisdom teeth

37. It would be accurate to say that
    (1) deciduous and permanent tooth development begin simultaneously in the fetus
    (2) deciduous tooth calcification is complete at the time of birth
    (3) dentin is harder than enamel because it is supported by alveolar bone
    (4) permanent tooth development is initiated in the second trimester (4–6th month) of pregnancy

38. Normally, if a mother's diet is moderately deficient in calcium, it is safe to say that

(1) fetus tooth development would be inhibited

(2) calcium would be withdrawn from the mother's bone to supply the needed calcium

(3) vitamin D would replace the needed calcium, resulting in good tooth development

(4) the teeth would grow well without the needed calcium

39. The single most important factor in the actual production of dental caries is
    (1) a deterioration of the gingivae
    (2) bacterial growth encouraged by a rich carbohydrate diet
    (3) a deficiency of calcium in the diet
    (4) simultaneous destruction of the dental pulp and alveolar bone by bacteria

40. It would be safe to assume that *if* a tooth were a bone of the body, it would most probably be classified as
    (1) long
    (2) short
    (3) flat
    (4) irregular

41. Both the upper and lower limbs of the appendicular skeleton contain 60 bones, and yet
    (1) all of the bones would be expected to be alike
    (2) one would expect many more small bones in the lower limbs
    (3) one would expect differences related to functional differences
    (4) the girdle bones would be expected to be greater in total weight

42. The gland that would play the most influential role in bone calcification is the
    (1) pituitary gland
    (2) thyroid gland
    (3) thymus gland
    (4) parathyroid gland

43. The gradual transition between enamel and cementum occurs in the region of the
    (1) crown
    (2) neck
    (3) apical foramen
    (4) mandibular foramen

44. Once encased in the lacunae, the cementocytes
    (1) are isolated from one another
    (2) derive nourishment from the alveolar bone
    (3) communicate with one another through canaliculi
    (4) mature into odontoblasts

45. The major histological difference between bone and tooth is the
    (1) time of embryonic development
    (2) amount of calcium salts in the matrix
    (3) total length of the pulp cavity
    (4) type of calcium isotope absorbed during matrix mineralization

46. One inference to be made from this passage is that the
    (1) pattern of tooth development in humans is fairly precise
    (2) skull is the most important part of the skeletal system
    (3) blood analysis is important in assessing the condition of teeth
    (4) proportion of bone to muscle in humans determines bone shape

47. During the course of the passage, light is shed on all of the following except
    (1) the relationship between diet and potential tooth problems
    (2) the formal similarities of tooth types vis-à-vis their functional differences
    (3) a system that is presently utilized to classify bones based on their shape
    (4) the detrimental effects of periodontal decay

48. The initial section of this passage may best be entitled
    (1) The Structure and Function of the Teeth
    (2) The General Structure and Function of the Skeletal System
    (3) A List of the Bones of the Body
    (4) How Bones Develop

49. The closing section of this passage may best be entitled
    (1) The Form and Development of Teeth
    (2) The Structure and Function of a Particular Tooth
    (3) Deciduous Teeth
    (4) The Tooth and Diet

50. The most appropriate title for the entire passage is
    (1) The Control, Cure, and Prevention of Dental Caries
    (2) The Functions of the Skeletal System
    (3) Some Aspects of the Skeletal System and Related Structures
    (4) The Biology of Teeth

STOP

END OF TEST

ANSWER KEY FOR THE VAT PRACTICE EXAMINATION

Reading Comprehension

1.	4	16.	1	31.	2	46.	4
2.	2	17.	4	32.	4	47.	3
3.	2	18.	4	33.	4	48.	4
4.	1	19.	2	34.	3	49.	4
5.	4	20.	4	35.	1	50.	1
6.	3	21.	1	36.	2	51.	1
7.	4	22.	1	37.	3	52.	1
8.	3	23.	4	38.	3	53.	3
9.	1	24.	2	39.	4	54.	3
10.	2	25.	2	40.	3	55.	1
11.	2	26.	3	41.	3	56.	4
12.	4	27.	1	42.	2	57.	4
13.	1	28.	3	43.	2	58.	4
14.	3	29.	4	44.	2	59.	4
15.	2	30.	1	45.	3	60.	1

Biology

1.	2	11.	1	21.	4	31.	3	41.	1
2.	4	12.	1	22.	3	32.	1	42.	4
3.	2	13.	3	23.	3	33.	1	43.	2
4.	1	14.	2	24.	1	34.	4	44.	1
5.	3	15.	4	25.	2	35.	4	45.	3
6.	2	16.	3	26.	4	36.	2		
7.	4	17.	3	27.	2	37.	3		
8.	4	18.	3	28.	1	38.	3		
9.	4	19.	1	29.	2	39.	2		
10.	3	20.	3	30.	1	40.	4		

Chemistry

1.	3	11.	2	21.	2	31.	4	41.	1
2.	1	12.	3	22.	2	32.	3	42.	1
3.	2	13.	3	23.	1	33.	4	43.	3
4.	2	14.	1	24.	4	34.	2	44.	4
5.	2	15.	4	25.	3	35.	2	45.	4
6.	3	16.	1	26.	3	36.	4		
7.	4	17.	3	27.	2	37.	1		
8.	2	18.	4	28.	1	38.	1		
9.	4	19.	1	29.	4	39.	4		
10.	2	20.	2	30.	2	40.	3		

Quantitative Ability

1.	2	11.	2	21.	3	31.	3	41.	2
2.	2	12.	3	22.	1	32.	2	42.	1
3.	1	13.	4	23.	2	33.	3	43.	1
4.	4	14.	4	24.	1	34.	3	44.	2
5.	1	15.	4	25.	4	35.	1	45.	3
6.	2	16.	4	26.	1	36.	2	46.	4
7.	1	17.	1	27.	3	37.	2	47.	2
8.	3	18.	3	28.	1	38.	1	48.	3
9.	4	19.	1	29.	1	39.	4	49.	2
10.	3	20.	2	30.	4	40.	4	50.	4

Study–Reading

1.	4	11.	1	21.	2	31.	1	41.	3
2.	3	12.	3	22.	4	32.	2	42.	4
3.	3	13.	2	23.	3	33.	4	43.	2
4.	1	14.	2	24.	2	34.	3	44.	3
5.	2	15.	2	25.	3	35.	3	45.	2
6.	2	16.	3	26.	1	36.	2	46.	1
7.	4	17.	2	27.	3	37.	4	47.	4
8.	4	18.	2	28.	2	38.	2	48.	2
9.	3	19.	1	29.	2	39.	2	49.	1
10.	4	20.	4	30.	3	40.	2	50.	3

EXPLANATORY ANSWERS FOR THE
VAT PRACTICE EXAMINATION

Reading Comprehension

1. **(4)** (1), (2), and (3) are presented in the third paragraph. Only (4) is not listed anywhere in the passage.

2. **(2)** This is stated explicitly in paragraph three.

3. **(2)** The last sentence of paragraph three gives this percentage.

4. **(1)** This is stated in paragraph four.

5. **(4)** Paragraph five states only that ceilings would begin to be reached following the 1980s.

6. **(3)** (1), (2), and (3) are listed in the final paragraph only as having aroused some interest among poultry breeders, while AI is already widely used.

7. **(4)** (1), (2), and (3) are all stated explicitly in paragraph two.

8. **(3)** The first sentence of the passage states that the relationship between man and other animals is shown by paleontological evidence and the similarities in structure and functioning of the organic internal structures (physiological evidence).

9. **(1)** Numerous comparisons are made between various animal groups. The study of the anatomy and development of different animal phyla is known as comparative zoology.

10. **(2)** The entire second paragraph discusses the attainment of upright posture as being fundamental in bringing about intelligent behavior and accomplishments. It is stated midway in this paragraph that "the play of cause and effect is much too obscure, much too complex to permit any conclusive answer." However, the statement posed is definitely inferred from this reading.

11. **(2)** Numerous examples of physical composition are correlated with different evolutionary attainments in the section. Observations of structure and function are traced from simple vertebrates to primates.

12. **(4)** (1), (2), and (3) are all similarities noted in the first paragraph.

13. **(1)** The author suggests this hypothesis in paragraph two.

14. **(3)** The fifth sentence states that two ovules are located on the upper surface of each scale of the ovulate cone.

15. **(2)** In plants, the pollen is the male sex cell, corresponding to the sperm of animals. The staminate part of the plant bears the male reproductive structures that are responsible for producing the pollen. The sperm nucleus is contained within the pollen grain, analogous to the egg (ovule) of the female.

16. **(1)** At the end of the first paragraph, the fate of the megaspore mother cell is described. The eventual resulting single megaspore divides to form the female gametophyte. No pollen grains, and hence no sperm nucleus, are found within the female gametophyte or megagametophyte.

17. **(4)** The final paragraph discusses the fused nuclei and the embryology of the fertilized egg. The second tier, called the suspensor, pushes the embryo down into the gametophyte tissue.

18. **(4)** As stated before, the megaspore mother cell undergoes meiosis to produce eventually one megaspore cell which forms the female gametophyte. The corresponding process occurs in the microsporangium, where microspore mother cells divide by meiosis to form microspores. In turn, the microspores form the pollen grains, or male gametophytes.

19. **(2)** The archegonium contains a rather large ovule, or female gametophyte. The microspores are really pollen grains, or male gametophytes.

20. **(4)** The microspore mother cell undergoes reduction division to form four microspores. The third sentence in the second paragraph states that two male gametes, or sperm nuclei, are formed within

each pollen grain. Therefore, if there are four pollen grains, each containing two sperm nuclei, the total would be eight.

21. **(1)** Toward the end of the first paragraph, we learn that the megaspore mother cell eventually produces the female gametophyte. The archegonium is found on this megagametophyte and contains only one large egg cell. Therefore, only one gametophyte results from one ovule.

22. **(1)** The reason why migration cannot be purely social association is given in the last sentence of the passage.

23. **(4)** This is stated in the first sentence of the third paragraph.

24. **(2)** Paragraph three discusses insect migration. The monarch butterfly is cited as the only known example of return migration in insects. The search for food is given as the primary reason for insect migration.

25. **(2)** Lemmings migrate when their population increases greatly, as explained in the final paragraph.

26. **(3)** This can be deduced by reading paragraph four with the information given about salmon in paragraph three in mind: salmon return to the stream in which they grew up when they are ready to spawn.

27. **(1)** This is implied in paragraph four.

28. **(3)** Changes in environment, lack of food supply, and the action of sex hormones are all suggested in the first paragraph as reasons for migration.

29. **(4)** The author states (midway in the second paragraph) that the vagus nerve sends branches to specifically named organs. These organs, upon analysis by the reader, are all concerned with vital involuntary functions. Therefore, it is suggested or implied that the vagus nerve would be similarly concerned with involuntary regulation.

30. **(1)** All of the other choices are directly true of the vagus nerve and are stated in the passage. However, only the efferent fibers of the vagus nerve belong to the autonomic nervous system. This is verified near the end of the second paragraph.

31. **(2)** The vagus nerve regulates the rate of the heartbeat. When the heart beats faster, more blood reaches the muscles, causing them to expend more energy. Any increase in muscular activity is accompanied by a corresponding increase in temperature.

32. **(4)** The second paragraph states that the heart is connected with the central nervous system by means of two nerves, the vagus and the cervical sympathetic. The last sentence in the first paragraph summarizes that the rate, force and systolic output of the heart is controlled by nerves and by chemicals that nerve endings or other structures produce.

33. **(4)** This statement is made in the second sentence of the second paragraph, but not elaborated upon any further.

34. **(3)** Neural control refers directly to nerves; humoral control refers to chemicals secreted into the bloodstream (hormones, etc.) by various glands, structures, or organs.

35. **(1)** This is stated in the third sentence: "As soon as the organic phosphates begin to break down in muscle contraction...."

36. **(2)** The third sentence from the end of the passage states that lactic acid undergoes change in an oxygen environment.

37. **(3)** Organic phosphates are composed chiefly of ATP and phospho-creatine, which begin to break down in muscle contraction only to be reformed after glycogen is changed to lactic acid. This sequence is described in the middle of the passage.

38. **(3)** The last sentence clearly states that "the energy is used to transform the remaining four-fifths of the lactic acid into glycogen again."

39. **(4)** The second sentence states that the organic phosphates are transformed anaerobically to organic compounds plus phosphates.

40. **(3)** The meaning of *homologous* is clearly stated in the second sentence of the second paragraph; in effect, the swim bladder and lungs arose from a modification of the primitive lung found in a common ancestor.

41. **(3)** The sturgeon is an elasmobranch possessing plates on its body, similar to those of armor-plated fish which are long extinct.

42. (2) See latter part of second paragraph: "...the lobe-finned fishes gave rise to the Amphibia and so to the land vertebrates," in which the mammals are included.

43. (2) The Devonian was one of six periods of the Paleozoic era in which fossils of the first amphibians are found.

44. (2) The definition of Osteichthyes is stated in the second sentence of the first paragraph: "...these bony fishes are separated...."

45. (3) This is stated in the next to last sentence of the passage: "...the gar pike...are rayfins of primitive type...."

46. (4) The first sentence of paragraph two states this explicitly.

47. (3) (1), (2), and (4) are cited in paragraph two as having contributed to the great increase.

48. (4) As indicated in the final sentence of the passage, sexing technology (not listed among the choices) is useful in this respect.

49. (4) All of the other choices are either mentioned specifically or may be deduced from paragraphs two and three.

50. (1) Choices (2) and (4) make no sense. (3) is incorrect because the passage is written objectively.

51. (1) Three to five percent of U.S. beef cattle are artificially inseminated. Sixty percent of U.S. dairy cattle are artificially inseminated.

$$60 : 5 :: 12 : 1$$
$$60 : 3 :: 20 : 1$$

Therefore, the dairy cattle industry uses AI technology 12 to 20 times as frequently as the beef cattle industry.

52. (1) This is stated explicitly in the final paragraph.

53. (3) The variables that affect soil (and over which man has control) are discussed throughout the passage.

54. (3) This is stated in paragraph four.

55. (1) According to paragraph five, forests usually occur where precipitation exceeds evaporation.

56. (4) There is a direct relation between climate and plant life. Paragraph five mentions that the phytogeographic map is similar to the climatic map based on rainfall, evaporation, and temperature.

57. (4) Deforestation is given as a chief cause of the destruction of land fertility.

58. (4) In paragraph five, this quotation is introduced to give credence to the danger of man's being ignorant of the natural adjustment of crops.

59. (4) Again, deforestation is given as one of the chief causes of the destruction of land fertility.

60. (1) The author asserts this in the first paragraph of the passage.

Biology

1. (2) Endocrine functions are not affected because the bloodstream is used to transport hormones to the various target sites throughout the body. Enzymes secreted by the pancreas, however, travel through the pancreatic duct and would be trapped if it were tied.

2. (4) This is the classic example of a behavior that is learned by imprinting.

3. (2) The primitive gut differentiates into the alimentary canal during the gastrula stage of embryology. In the horse, this process starts on the eighteenth day. It is during gastrulation that the cells of the primary germ layers start differentiating into the various organs and organ systems of the embryo. The prefix "gastr-" indicates "stomach" (*Gastēr, Gr.—belly*).

4. (1) The thyroid is a ductless gland. Ductless glands secrete directly into the bloodstream and therefore are endocrine glands.

5. (3) The veins carry blood toward the heart.

6. (2) Progestin (progesterone) is produced by the corpus luteum, and is vital to the establishment and development of pregnancy. It makes possible implantation of the zygote in the uterine wall, and causes development of the mammary glands during late pregnancy.

7. (4) Structure three is a mitochondrion. It is concerned with extracting the energy that resides in the bonds of organic molecules.

8. **(4)** The mouth-to-anus digestive tube is specialized along its length into a number of structures, including the esophagus, stomach, small intestine, and large intestine.

9. **(4)** One-celled animals, followed by simple multicelled animals, followed by amphibians (living in water and on land), followed by reptiles (living on land only), followed by birds, followed by mammals, perhaps the newest comer of all.

10. **(3)** Homologous structures are inherited from a common ancestor, while analogous structures are similar in function and often in superficial structure but have different evolutionary origins. The animals mentioned in this question are mammals and are fairly closely related, having a common ancestry.

11. **(1)** This question is elementary to cell biology. Cells are divided into eucaryotes and procaryotes according to whether their genes are enclosed by a nuclear membrane. The only cytoplasmic inclusions always found in procaryotes are the ribosomes and a nuclear body, whereas eucaryotes have all the features of procaryotes and more.

12. **(1)** Creatine phosphate participates in muscle metabolism after exhaustion of the immediately available ATP reserve by virtue of the freely reversible reaction with ATP:

$$creatine + ATP \rightarrow ADP + creatine\ phosphate$$

The phosphoamide structure of this compound is highly reactive with respect to phosphate group transfer.

13. **(3)** In a monohybrid cross only one of the four boxes represents the homozygous dominant when the parents are heterozygous. In this case, BB is the box representing 0.49, or 49%.

14. **(2)** Three out of four offspring will contain the b gene: the two heterozygotes and the homozygous recessive. $0.21 + 0.21 + 0.09 = 51\%$

15. **(4)** Proteins are composed of amino acids; amino acids can be formed from such molecules as CH_4 and NH_3; and these in turn are composed of C, H, N, or O; therefore, the correct sequence is IV, II, III, I.

16. **(3)** Both species benefit in *mutualism*. One benefits while the other is unharmed in *commensalism*. But in *parasitism* one species benefits while the other is harmed.

17. **(3)** Enzyme catalysis takes place in living systems and therefore is subject to cellular controls. This is not true of inorganic catalysis.

18. **(3)** Albinism is a recessive trait and can manifest itself only when two such genes meet. However, phenotypically "normal" photosynthetic plants can transmit this gene via their heterozygous genetic makeup. The plants possessing this hybrid condition are completely normal as far as ability to manufacture food is concerned.

19. **(1)** Large molecules adhere to the surface of the cell membrane, which then infolds or invaginates. Eventually, the sides of the pocket meet, trapping the large molecules within the cytoplasm. Special digestive structures within the cytoplasm convert these large insoluble molecules into a soluble form. Pinocytosis literally means "cell-drinking process" (*pinein*, to drink; *cyto*, cell; *osis*, process).

20. **(3)** An increase in the number of carbon dioxide molecules will cause more of these to accept hydrogen atoms stored in the plant. Powered by APT, the excess hydrogen atoms being transported by molecules of carbon dioxide will form a highly reactive compound, PGA (phosphoglyceric acid). These molecules combine to form sugar. The more PGA molecules, the more sugar produced. All of these sequences stem from an original increase in carbon dioxide availability.

21. **(4)** The head of a typical bacteriophage virus consists of DNA surrounded by a protein coat. Using the tail portion as an inoculation needle, the phage penetrates the bacteria by injecting its DNA. The viral-protein coat remains outside the bacterial cell.

22. **(3)** The ameba reproduces by binary fission, an asexual method of reproduction. No sex cells are necessary, so reduction division (meiosis) does not take place. Each daughter cell is an exact duplicate of the original parent cell, as there is only one set of genes.

23. **(3)** Chloroplasts are membranous cell organelles with stacked membranes called grana. The grana contain the chlorophyll responsible for the initiation of photosynthetic chemistry.

24. **(1)** Mitochondria are double-membrane cell

organelles whose inner membrane is thrown into folds for increased surface area activity related to oxidative phosphorylation. The folds are called cristae.

25. **(2)** Endoplasmic reticulum is a complex membrane structure in cell cytoplasm which, when associated with ribosomes, is called rough endoplasmic reticulum. The ribosomes are the sites of protein synthesis.

26. **(4)** Cilia are cell organelles responsible for locomotion in some cells. Cilia are found to contain groups of microtubules in a typical $9 + 2$ arrangement.

27. **(2)** The body temperature is controlled and regulated by the thalamus of the brain. A heat-loss center in the hypothalamus receives information from cutaneous thermal receptors regarding environmental temperature.

28. **(1)** In any cross, in order for *all* offspring to be hybrids it is necessary for one parent to be homozygous dominant and the other parent to be homozygous recessive for the same characteristic. Only (A) meets this requirement.

29. **(2)** The blastula is an embryonic stage of development. It contains a hollow space (coele-cavity).

30. **(1)** The morula is a solid ball of cells formed by a number of mitotic divisions of the zygote. These divisions are referred to as cleavages.

31. **(3)** Gastrulation is a complex process of germ-layer formation leading to a three-layered gastrula.

32. **(1)** See answer for question 30.

33. **(1)** Two neurons are involved—the sensory neuron and the motor neuron. This is a simple monosynaptic reflex arc.

34. **(4)** The primary use of bile is to reduce the surface tension of the fat, and produce a colloidal suspension (emulsification) of the fat in the digestive tract, so that digestive enzymes can get at more of it. Otherwise, the enzymes would have to work on large fat globules, and would be unable to reach most of the fat before it passes out of the system.

35. **(4)** Gill-like and tail-like structures appear during the development of the human embryo.

36. **(2)** The two antiparallel strands of the DNA molecule are held together by the hydrogen bonds that are formed between complimentary nitrogenous bases.

37. **(3)** Lysosomes contain enzymes that, upon fusion with a food vacuole, aid in the digestion of the vacuole's contents.

38. **(3)** Facultative anaerobes can live in the presence or absence of oxygen. In the former case, they make use of oxidative phosphorylation in the manufacture of ATP.

39. **(2)** The structures are homologous because they share a common ancestry. They are functionally dissimilar, however, and as such cannot be considered analogous.

40. **(4)** (1), (2), and (3) all arise from the mesoderm, which is the middle layer of cells in the gastrula.

41. **(1)** If 10 percent are guanine, 10 percent must be cytosine for these two bases to bond gether. This leaves 80 percent of the total content in nitrogenous bases, 40 percent of which must be thymine and 40 percent of which must be adenine.

42. **(4)** Invertebrates, fish, and amphibians inhabit pond waters. The eggs of the female are discharged into the water, where the male discharges sperm over them, accomplishing fertilization. Since this process occurs outside the body of the female, external fertilization is said to take place.

43. **(2)**

	A	a
B	AB	aB
b	Ab	ab

As can be seen from the Punnett square above, ¼ of the gametes will be ab.

44. **(1)** In the dark reactions of photosynthesis, CO_2 is metabolized to carbohydrate, and water is produced. In the light reactions, water is broken down into O_2 and H^+.

45. **(3)** The stepwise (lengthwise) configuration of the single and double-ring compounds arranged within the DNA molecule determines the genetic code, its meaning, and net effect.

Chemistry

1. **(3)** According to Le Châtelier's principle, when a system at equilibrium is perturbed, the equilibrium will shift so as to diminish the effect of the perturbation. Thus, the addition of NH_3 will drive the reaction to the right, as written. This will decrease the amont of NH_3 produced.

2. **(1)** Ketones are of the formula $\begin{smallmatrix} R \\ R' \end{smallmatrix} \!\!\diagdown\!\! \, C = O$

   They cannot result from the oxidation of an alcohol in which the oxydryl (–OH) group is attached to a carbon that is itself attached to only one radical (R) (i.e., a primary alcohol).

3. **(2)** 5/29 is equivalent to 10/58. Since the molecular weight of the compound is 58, it must contain 10 atoms of hydrogen.

   That leaves $\dfrac{(58 - 10)}{12} = 4$ atoms of carbon.

4. **(2)** The "L" shell of an atom contains one "s" and three "p" orbitals. According to the Pauli exclusion principle, each of these orbitals can contain a maximum of 2 electrons (2 from "s" $+ 2 \times 3$ "p" $= 8$).

5. **(2)** The action of a catalyst is *only to change the rate of a reaction*. Catalysts do not affect the products or the equilibrium of products at all.

6. **(3)** The water molecule donates one of its protons to the ammonia molecule and becomes a hydroxide ion; therefore, it functions as an acid.

7. **(4)** By observing the X-ray scattering pattern of gold foil, Rutherford was able to show in 1912 that the positive charge of an atom was associated with most of the mass at the central core or nucleus, with enough negative charge distributed around the nucleus to render the whole atom neutral. This formulation is known as the nuclear atom model.

8. **(2)** Regardless of the physical characteristics of the cell, the flow of charge proceeds only insofar as the anode and cathode reactions proceed. The amount of charge that has flowed is therefore a direct measure of the mass of material deposited on the cathode.

9. **(4)** As one goes from left to right in the second period of the Periodic Table, electrons are added to "s" and "p" orbitals, which have the same effective radii and cannot shield each other from the increasing nuclear charge. This progressive increase in the positive charge draws in the orbital electrons and causes a progressive decrease in the effective radius of the elements.

10. **(2)** Recalling that one mole of an ideal gas occupies 22.4 liters at standard temperature and pressure, the molecular weight of the gas is found from

    $$\text{M.W.} = (1.25 \text{ g/l})(22.4 \text{ l/mole})$$
    $$= 28 \text{ g/mole}$$

    A molecular weight of 28 is consistent with compound (2).

11. **(2)** There are three equivalents of H_3PO_4 per mole and two equivalents of $Ca(OH)_2$ per mole so that the normalities of the two solutions are

    $$N(H_3PO_4) = 3(0.25) = 0.75 = N_1$$
    $$N(Ca(OH)_2) = 2(0.30) = 0.60 = N_2.$$

    Using the equation $N_1V_1 = N_2V_2$, with $V_2 = 25$ ml, yields $V_1 = 20$ ml.

12. **(3)** Naphthalene is a nonpolar molecule of relatively low molecular weight. Using the general rule of thumb, "like dissolves like," it is seen that benzene is the best choice due to its lack of polarity, as well as its similar structure.

13. **(3)** A balanced chemical equation must have the same amount of each element on both sides. In choice (3) there are 3C, 8H, and 10O on both sides of the equation.

14. **(1)** Upon the capture of a particle of atomic number 6 and mass number 13, the $_{96}C^{240}$ nucleus is converted into $_{102}No^{253}$ (No = Nobelium). The nuclear reaction may be represented as

    $$_{96}Cm^{240} + {_6}X^{13} \rightarrow {_{102}}No^{253}$$

15. **(4)** Beta emission involves the loss of an electron from a neutron and results in the production of a proton. The net result of beta emission, therefore, is an increase by one of the number of protons in the nucleus, and, consequently, of the atomic number of the atom.

16. **(1)** At S.T.P. one mole of any gas occupies 22.4 liters. Therefore, 11.2 liters of any gas contain ½ mole of that gas. One mole of ammonia contains 7 grams of nitrogen.

17. **(3)** Gamma rays are electromagnetic rays which

have higher energy than X rays. The photon, the unit of electromagnetic radiation, has a rest mass of zero and a charge of zero.

18. **(4)** An electrolyte is a substance that when added to water will conduct an electric current (very pure water will not do this). In order to conduct the current it must: (1) dissolve and (2) carry an electrical charge (i.e., be ionic). Therefore, the prime characteristic for an electrolyte is that it be ionic in solution.

19. **(1)** Carbon monoxide, with a molecular weight of 28, is the lightest of the gases listed. The molecular weights of the other gases are: sulfur dioxide, 64; hydrogen sulfide, 34; and fluorine, 38.

20. **(2)** This question can be answered when one pictures the actions of molecules on a molecular level. They are continually vibrating and colliding. The addition of very fine particles will cause collisions between these particles and the molecules of the liquid, resulting in the movement of the particles. This behavior is called *Brownian motion*.

21. **(2)** By definition, the half-life of a first order reaction is the time required for half of a given amount of starting material to react. Therefore, after 20 days ½ of the radioisotope would be left. After another 20 days, ½ of ½, or ¼, of pure radioisotope would be left.

22. **(2)** Since the reaction is endothermic, Le Châtelier's principle would predict that an increase in temperature would drive it from left to right. Also, since these volumes of reactant yield two volumes of product, an increase in pressure would aid the forward reaction.

23. **(1)** Zinc oxide is an example of an amphoteric compound. With acids, it forms zinc salts:

$$ZnO + 2HCl \rightarrow ZnCl_2 + H_2O$$

And with alkalis, it forms zincates:

$$ZnO + 2NaOH \rightarrow Na_2ZnO_2 + H_2O$$

24. **(4)** The efficiency of a reversible Carnot cycle is independent of the working substance, and is always 100% of the thermodynamic efficiency, which is determined only by the operating temperatures.

25. **(3)** Bronsted defines a base as a substance that can

accept a proton. Thus, since such electrically neutral substances as H_2O and NH_3 can accept protons to give H_3O^+ and NH_4^+, they are also defined as bases.

26. **(3)** Electrovalent bonding confers high melting points on substances since the ionic particles are held into rigid crystalline structures by strong electrostatic forces. Also, the ionic nature of the particles makes the transport of electricity possible in the liquid state.

27. **(2)** Compounds which have the same crystalline form are said to be isomorphic. The property of isomorphism, as expressed in Mitscherlich's Law—the same number of atoms combined in the same manner produce the same crystalline form—was widely used in the early days of the atomic theory to determine atomic weights.

28. **(1)** With solutions containing nonvolatile solutes, such properties as (a) the vapor pressure lowering of the solvent, (b) the boiling point elevation, (c) the freezing point depression, and (d) the osmotic pressure of the solution are found to depend only on the number of particles in solution, and not on their nature. These properties of the solution are referred to as colligative properties.

29. **(4)** Chemical equilibrium is dynamic rather than static. This means that the apparent stopping of a reaction at equilibrium is due to equal rates of reaction in the forward and reverse directions.

30. **(2)** Hot concentrated sulfuric acid is a moderately strong oxidizing agent that can be reduced by such metals as copper to sulfur dioxide. The reaction constitutes a laboratory method of preparing sulfur dioxide:

$$Cu + 2H_2SO_4 = CuSO_4 + 2H_2O + SO_2$$

31. **(4)** Fusion is a process in which two or more nuclei join together to form a heavier nucleus.

32. **(3)** If f is the surface pressure and A the surface area (per molecule), then the product fA for the two-dimensional case is analogous to PV in the three-dimensional case and the 2-D ideal gas law will be $fA = kT$. This can be derived from kinetic theory just as the 3-D ideal gas law.

33. **(4)** Tungsten and molybdenum both exist in oxides in the +6 oxidation state (WO_3 and MoO_3). These

oxides are reduced to the pure metals by hydrogen at high temperatures.

34. (2) In running across each of the long periods of the Periodic Table, it is seen that two "s" orbitals, ten "d" orbitals, and six "p" orbitals are filled consecutively.

35. (2) For every rubidium atom with mass 87, there are three with mass 85. Therefore, the average mass of a rubidium atom is:

$$\frac{3 \times 85 + 1 \times 87}{4} = 85.5$$

36. (4) The reactivity of the alkali metals is due to the ease with which they can be oxidized; that is, the ease with which they lose the lone electron in the outermost valence orbital. For cesium, this orbital is of higher energy than are the analogous orbitals on the other elements under consideration. In addition, the attractive force between this outermost electron and the nucleus is smaller for cesium because the inner filled shells act as a shield. These two factors render cesium more electropositive than the other elements listed.

37. (1) Potassium reacts violently with cold water to liberate hydrogen. Copper and mercury, being less electropositive than hydrogen, cannot liberate the latter from dilute acids. Iron reacts slowly with dilute hydrochloric acid to liberate hydrogen; and with steam, hot iron reacts according to the equation:

$$3Fe + 4H_2O \rightarrow Fe_3O_4 + 4H_2$$

38. (1) The reaction between $AgNO_3$ and KCl is:

$$AgNO_3 + KCl \rightarrow AgCl + K^+ + NO_3$$

Thus the total quantity of NO_3^- remains constant. Since the starting concentration is 0.1N in 500 ml and the final volume is 1000 ml, the final concentration of NO_3^- is:

$$\frac{0.1 \times 500}{1000} = 0.05N$$

39. (4) The addition of H_2S to an acidic solution of metallic ions leads t the precipitation of ions in Group II of the analytical tables. In the list, cadmium, copper and mercury ions belong in this group. Strontium belongs in Group IV, for which the group reagent is basic ammonium carbonate. The reagent for Group III, the iron group, is H_2S in the presence of NH_3 and NH_4Cl.

40. (3) The valence of the ion is the same as the charge on the complex, since the ligands are neutral. The coordination number is defined as the number of ligands around the central ion. In $Cu(NH_3)_4^{++}$, this number is obviously 4.

41. (1) The conjugate base of any substance is obtained by the removal of a proton from the substance. Removal of a proton from NH_4^+ leaves NH_3, which is the conjugate base of NH_4^+.

42. (1) Industrial alcohol can be prepared by the fermentation of sucrose from molasses or other suitable sources. The fermentation can be viewed as occurring in two steps:

1. $C_{12}H_{22}O_{11} + H_2O \xrightarrow{\text{sucrase}} \underset{\text{glucose}}{C_6H_{12}O_6} + \underset{\text{fructose}}{C_6H_{12}O_6}$

2. $\underset{\substack{\text{glucose} \\ \text{or} \\ \text{fructose}}}{C_6H_{12}O_6} \xrightarrow{\text{zymase}} 2CO_2 + \underset{\text{ethanol}}{2C_2H_5OH}$

43. (3) Salts such as NaCl and KCl are ionic even in the crystalline state. CCl_4 and CH_4, though covalent, are not polar due to the tetrahedral symmetry around the carbon atom. Because of unequal sharing of the electron pair, HCl gas is both polar and covalent.

44. (4) The compound, as written, is electrically neutral. Since there are a total of six negative charges (five on the chlorines and one on the hydroxyl group) and two positive charges on potassium, there will have to be four positive charges on ruthenium to create electrical neutrality.

45. (4) Addition of HCl to a solution of metallic ions causes the precipitation of the Group I ions, which are Ag^+, Pb^{++} and Hg^+.

Quantitative Ability

1. **(2)** Since the perimeter of a square is four times the length of a side, it is

$$4 \times \left(\frac{2x+1}{3}\right), \text{ or } \frac{8x+12}{3}$$

2. **(2)** If the circumference is 60 inches, since $C = 2\pi r$, substitute $C = 60$; therefore, $r = \frac{60}{2\pi}$.

3. **(1)** The radii of the pipe are 1.42 inches and 0.97 inches. The thickness is their difference, or .45 inches.

4. **(4)**

$$(4x)^3 - (3x)^3 = 296;$$
$$64x^3 - 27x^3 = 296;$$
$$x^3 = 8;$$
$$x = 2.$$

Therefore, the side of the smaller cube is $3 \times 2 = 6$.

5. **(1)** The area of the circle is π times the square of the radius, or 9π. The area of the square is 36. Thus, the ratio is $\frac{9\pi}{36}$, or $\frac{\pi}{4}$. Approximating π as 3.14, we divide and obtain .785, which is closest to $\frac{4}{5}$.

6. **(2)** In the first hour the motorist travels 120 miles at 60 MPH, which takes 2 hours. On the way back, he travels the same distance at 40 MPH, which takes 3 hours. His average rate is the total distance (240 miles) divided by the total time (5 hours), which yields 48 MPH.

7. **(1)**

$$\text{Angle DOC} = 6 + x$$
$$\text{Angle AOC} = (6 + x) + x = 180 - 20$$
$$6 + 2x = 160$$
$$2x = 154$$
$$x = 77$$

8. **(3)** Let C = the capacity in gallons. Then $\frac{1}{3}C + 3 = \frac{1}{2}C$. Multiplying through by 6, we obtain:

$$2C + 18 = 3C$$
$$\text{or } C = 18$$

9. **(4)**

$$\frac{91 + 88 + 86 + 78 + x}{5} = 85$$
$$343 + x = 425$$
$$x = 82$$

10. **(3)**

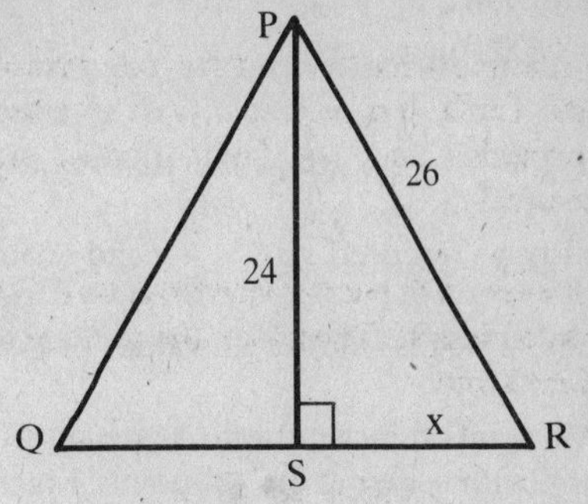

In the figure above, PS⊥QR. Then, in right triangle PSR,

$$x^2 + 24^2 = 26^2$$
$$x^2 = 26^2 - 24^2$$
$$= (26 + 24)(26 - 24)$$
$$x^2 = 50 \times 2 = 100$$
$$x = 10$$

Thus, QR = 20.

11. **(2)** Use a proportion comparing pencils to cents. Change $2D$ dollars to $200D$ cents

$$\frac{p}{200D} = \frac{x}{c}$$
$$\frac{pc}{200D} = x$$

12. **(3)** $\text{Rate} = \frac{\text{distance}}{\text{time}} = \frac{\frac{2}{5}\text{ mile}}{\frac{5}{60}\text{ hour}} = \frac{\frac{2}{5}}{\frac{1}{12}}$

$\text{Rate} = \frac{2}{5} \cdot \frac{12}{1} = \frac{24}{5} = 4\frac{4}{5}$ MPH.

13. **(4)** Draw the altitudes indicated. A rectangle and two right triangles are produced. From the figure, the base of each triangle is 20 feet. By the Pythagorean theorem, the altitude is 15 feet. Hence, the area

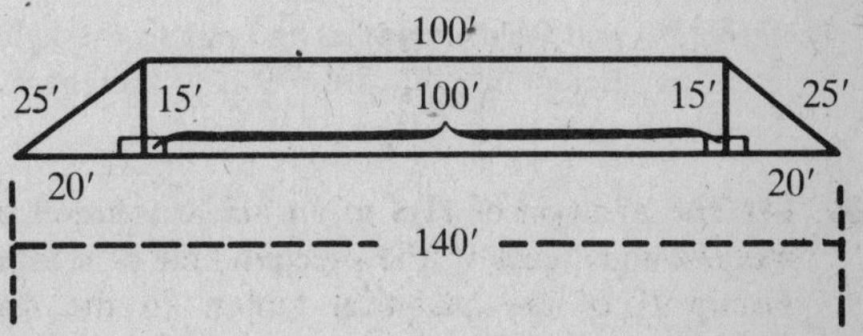

$K = \frac{1}{2} \cdot 15 \ (100 + 140)$
$= \frac{1}{2} \cdot 15 \cdot 240$
$= 15 \cdot 120$
$= 1800$ square feet

14. **(4)** If $1 + \dfrac{1}{t} = \dfrac{t + 1}{1}$, then the right-hand fraction can also be reduced to $1 + \dfrac{1}{t}$, and we have an identity, which is true for all values of t except 0.

15. **(4)** All points 6 inches from A are on a circle of radius 6 with center at A. All points 1 inch from b are on 2 straight lines parallel to b and 1 inch from it on each side. These two parallel lines intersect the circle in 4 points.

16. **(4)** Let $R = 5P$ and $S = 5Q$ where P and Q are integers.
Then $R - S = 5P - 5Q = 5(P - Q)$ is divisible by 5.
$RS = 5P \cdot 5Q = 25PG$ is divisible by 25.
$R + S = 5P + 5Q = 5(P + Q)$ is divisible by 5.
$R + S = 5P + 5Q = 5(P + Q)$, which is not necessarily divisible by 10.

17. **(1)** $\frac{1}{2} \cdot 7 \cdot h = \pi \cdot 7^2$
Dividing both sides by 7, we get $\frac{1}{2}h = 7\pi$, or $h = 14\pi$.

18. **(3)**

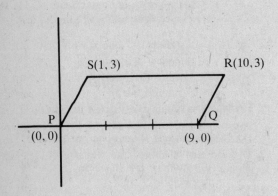

Since PQ and RS are parallel and equal, the figure is a parallelogram of base = 9 and height = 3. Hence, area = $9 \cdot 3 = 27$.

19. **(1)**

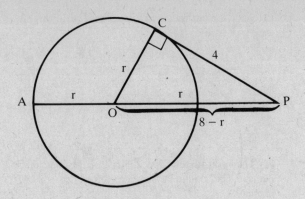

From the figure, in right $\triangle$ PCO,
$$PO^2 = r^2 + 4^2$$
$$(8 - r)^2 = r^2 + 16$$
$$64 - 16r + r^2 = r^2 + 16$$
$$48 = 16r$$
$$r = 3$$
$$\text{Diameter} = 6$$

20. **(2)** Area of wall = $4 \cdot 6\frac{0}{3} = 4 \cdot 20 = 80$ sq. yd.
Cost = $80 \times \$10.50 = \$840.00$.

21. **(3)** Distance of (4,4) from origin $= \sqrt{16 + 16}$
$= \sqrt{32} < 7$.
Distance of (5,5) from origin $= \sqrt{25 + 25}$
$= \sqrt{50} < 7$.
Distance of (4,5) from origin $= \sqrt{16 + 25}$
$= \sqrt{41} < 7$.
Distance of (4,6) from origin $= \sqrt{16 + 36}$
$= \sqrt{52} < 7$.
Hence, only II and IV are outside circle.

22. **(1)** Let x = the cost. Then,

$$x + \tfrac{1}{4}x = 80$$
$$4x + x = 320$$
$$5x = 320$$
$$= \$64 \text{ (cost)}$$

$$\frac{\text{Cost}}{\text{S.P.}} = {}^{64}\!/_{80}$$
$$= {}^{4}\!/_{5}$$

23. (2)

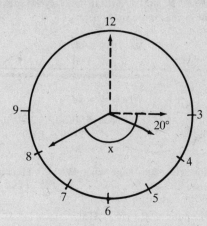

At 3:00, the large hand is at 12 and the small hand is at 3. During the next 40 minutes, the large hand moves to 8 and the small hand moves $^{40}/_{60} = ^{2}/_{3}$ of distance between 3 and 4; $^{2}/_{3} \times 30° = 20°$. Since there are 30° between two numbers of clock $<x = 5$ $(30°) - 20° = 150° - 20° = 130°$.

24. (1) Area of sector $= ^{120}/_{360} \cdot \pi \cdot 15^2$
$= ^{1}/_{3} \cdot \pi \cdot 15 \cdot 15$
$= 75\pi$

25. (4) Since $x + 2x + y = 180°$, it follows that

$$3x + y = 180$$
$$y = 180 - 3x$$

26. (1) $^{18}/_{33} = ^{6}/_{11} = \dfrac{\sqrt{6^2}}{\sqrt{11^2}} = \dfrac{\sqrt{6^2}}{\sqrt{11^2}}$

$$\dfrac{\sqrt{36}}{\sqrt{121}}$$

Missing denominator is $\sqrt{121}$

27. (3) There are 20 numbers that contain 7 in the unit's place. There are 20 more that contain 7 in the ten's place. Thus, there are 40 numbers with 7 in either unit's or ten's place. But the numbers 277 and 377 must be rejected, and they have each been counted twice. Hence, $40 - 4 = 36$

28. (1) $(r + s)^2 - r^2 - s^2 = r^2 + 2rs + s^2$
$\qquad\qquad - r^2 - s^2 = 2rs$

29. (1) As Q moves from R to S, PQ get smaller. Its largest possible value would be 9. Hence, $9 \geq PQ \geq 6$.

30. (4) Selling price per article $= \dfrac{K}{8}$. Cost per article $= \dfrac{K}{12}$.

Profit per article $= \dfrac{K}{8} - \dfrac{K}{12} = \dfrac{3K - 2K}{24} = \dfrac{K}{24}$.

31. (3) Analyze this by means of the diagram below.

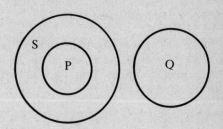

From the figure, we readily see that no P are Q.

32. (2) The sum of the four numbers is $45 \times 4 = 180$. For the average to remain the same, the sum must remain unchanged. If one number is increased by 6, then each of the other three must be reduced by 2.

33. (3) The papers drawn will be numbered 4, 11, 18, 25, 32, 39. Hence, number 39 will be the last.

34. (3) Let the angles be 2x, 3x, and 5x.
$$2x + 3x + 5x = 180°$$
$$10x = 180°$$
$$x = 18$$
Hence, $5x = 90°$ and the triangle is right.

35. (1) The dimensions of the open box become:
length $= 24 - 10 = 14$ in
width $= 18 - 10 = 8$ in
height $= 5$ in

Hence, $V = 14 \cdot 8 \cdot 5 = 560$ cu in

36. (2) VT $= 32$ feet so that ST $= ^{1}/_{2}$ TV $= 16$ feet. Thus, in right triangle QST, the legs are $12 = 4(3)$ and $16 = 4(4)$, so that hypotenuse QT $= 4(5) = 20$ feet. Add 1 foot for the extension and we get QR $= 21$ feet.

37. (2) Form the proportion $\dfrac{^{3}/_{4}}{9} = \dfrac{^{7}/_{8}}{x}$, where x is the side

in miles. Then ¾ x = ⅞·9 Multiply both sides by 8.

$$6x = 7·9 = 63$$
$$x = 10½ \text{ miles}$$

$$\text{Area} = x^2 = \frac{21}{2} \cdot \frac{21}{2} = \frac{441}{4} = 110¼ \text{ square miles.}$$

38. (1) Given V = fL, divide both sides by f, giving

$$L = \frac{V}{f}.$$

39. (4) The ten's digit of a number has a place value which is ten times the value of the digit. Hence, the number may be represented as 10t + u.

40. (4) There are nine numbers containing 5 in the unit's digit. From 50 to 59, there are 10 more numbers where 5 appears. Thus, the number 5 will be written 20 times.

41. (2) The fast clock gains 24 minutes. The slow clock loses 12 minutes. The minute hand of the fast clock reads 12:24. The minute hand of the slow clock reads 11:48. The minute hands are thus 24 minutes apart.

42. (1) Let side of square = 5. Then diagonal = $5\sqrt{2}$.
    Sum of 2 adjacent edges = 10
    Distance saved = $10 - 5\sqrt{2}$
    Fraction saved =

$$\frac{10 \ 5\sqrt{2}}{10} = \frac{10 \ 7.07}{10} = \frac{2.93}{10}$$

Percent saved = $\frac{29.3}{100}$ = 29% (approx.)

43. (1) Most of the blocks will have one, two, or three painted faces. Only *one* small block in the geometric center of the large block has no faces exposed to the outside and will show no paint at all.

44. (2) The divisors of 28 are 14, 7, 4, 2, 1. The sum of these is 28, making it a perfect number. This does not apply to the other numbers listed.

45. (3) Let x = number of minutes per period.
    There are 4 class periods and 3 passing periods from 9 AM to 11:51, or in 2 hr. 51 minutes. Hence,

$$4x + 3(5) = 120 + 51$$
$$4x + 15 = 171$$
$$4x = 156$$
$$x = 39$$

46. (4) Since the perimeter involves 3 fenced-in sides, it is true that L + 2W = 90. Also, the area is LW. If we solve the first equation for L, we obtain L = 90 − 2W. Now substitute in area = LW, giving area = W(90 − 2W) = 90W − 2W². Let W = 20 in this equation, giving area = 1000. Hence A, B, and C are all true. Now substitute L = W in the first equation;

$$W + 2W = 90$$
$$3W = 90$$
$$W = 30$$

When W = 30

$$\text{area} = 90(30) - 2(30^2)$$
$$= 2700 - 1800$$
$$= 900$$

But this area is less than when W = 20. Hence, 3 is not true.

47. (2) Discount = 90 − 75 = $15
    Rate of Discount = ¹⁵/₉₀ = ⅙ = 16⅔%

48. (3) The two semicircles make up the circumference of one circle of diameter 60 yd. Hence the circumference = π 60. The sum of the two lengths of the rectangle is 200. Thus the perimeter is equal to 200 + 60 π.

49. (2) 45 miles per hour = 45 × 5280 ft. per hour

$$= \frac{45 \times 5280 \text{ feet per hour}}{3600 \text{ seconds in one hour}}$$

$$= 66 \text{ ft per second}$$

50. (4) If angle P were 90°, x would equal $5\sqrt{2}$. If angle P were 180°, x would equal 10. It assumes all values between these 2 extremes. Hence, $5\sqrt{2} < x < 10$.

Study–Reading

1. (4) At the end of the first paragraph, it is stated that the 80 bones of the axial skeleton include those of the skull, vertebral column, and thorax.

2. (3) According to the first paragraph, the study of joints is called arthrology. Thus, an arthrologist is one who works specifically with skeletal joints and joint-related diseases.

3. (3) This is stated explicitly in the first paragraph.

4. (1) In paragraph two, it is stated that one of the major functions of human bones is to serve as centers of blood cell formation. Thus, the circula-

tory system would be directly influenced by a change in the skeletal system.

5. **(2)** This is listed as one of the four major functions of human bones.

6. **(2)** The axial skeleton is made up of 29, 26, and 25 bones of the skull, vertebral column, and thorax, respectively.

7. **(4)** This is stated explicitly in paragraph two.

8. **(4)** This is stated explicitly in the first sentence of paragraph three.

9. **(3)** In paragraph three, it is stated that the calcification process of bone formation is dependent on adequate supplies of calcium, phosphorus, vitamin D, and parathyroid hormone.

10. **(4)** It is not surprising that calcium is the most important element of those listed.

11. **(1)** In paragraph four, it is stated that the teeth of the oral cavity are set in three of the facial bones.

12. **(3)** Since these bones help make up the skull, they belong to the axial skeleton.

13. **(2)** In paragraph five, it is stated that the gingivae are composed of dense, fibrous connective tissue.

14. **(2)** Since the peridontal membrane binds each tooth to the alveolar wall, its destruction would be responsible for the loosening of teeth in the alveolus.

15. **(2)** This continuity is displayed graphically in the illustration.

16. **(3)** In paragraph four, it is stated that 16 alveoli are equally distributed in the two maxillae.

17. **(2)** This is implied in paragraph five.

18. **(2)** The teeth aid in chewing, an essential part of the digestive process.

19. **(1)** The apical foramen serves as the passageway for the nerves that enter and leave the pulp cavity, wherein lies the dental pulp.

20. **(4)** This is implied in paragraphs seven and eight.

21. **(2)** It is expected that the reader assumes that the

inferior dental arch holds one-half of the 20 deciduous teeth in a child.

22. **(4)** This is stated explicitly in the first sentence of paragraph seven.

23. **(3)** This is stated at the end of paragraph six.

24. **(2)** In paragraph seven, it is stated that the pulp is richly innervated (and the dentin is not).

25. **(3)** This is stated explicitly in paragraph seven.

26. **(1)** This is stated explicitly in paragraph eight.

27. **(3)** This is stated in paragraph three (for bones), and in paragraph eight (for teeth).

28. **(2)** Paragraph seven states that 80 percent of a tooth's dry weight is due to dentin, which is made up mostly of calcium.

29. **(2)** This is stated in paragraph nine.

30. **(3)** This is stated in paragraph nine.

31. **(1)** This is stated in paragraph nine.

32. **(2)** According to the last sentence in paragraph eleven, 12 molars are included in a full set of permanent teeth. It is expected that the reader assume that one-half of these are housed by the inferior dental arch.

33. **(4)** This is stated in paragraph eleven.

34. **(3)** As stated in paragraph eleven, the second molars do not generally come in until a child reaches the age of 20 months.

35. **(3)** This is stated in paragraph eleven.

36. **(2)** The inferior dental arch would account for one-half of the permanent teeth listed in the last sentence of paragraph eleven.

37. **(4)** It is stated in paragraph twelve that permanent teeth initiate development around the fourth month after conception.

38. **(2)** This is listed in paragraph twelve as one of the mechanisms through which fetal tooth calcium is derived.

39. **(2)** This is stated in paragraph thirteen.

40. **(2)** The second paragraph states that short bones are tubular and have no one dimension that significantly exceeds any other.

41. **(3)** The point of the statement is that it is an amazing coincidence that the upper and lower limbs contain the same number of bones.

42. **(4)** We may assume that the parathyroid gland secretes parathyroid hormone, a constituent vital to the calcification process.

43. **(2)** The neck is stated to be that part of the tooth at the gum line. According to the illustration, the interface between enamel and cementum is also located at that level.

44. **(3)** This is stated in paragraph eight.

45. **(2)** Upon considering the information presented in paragraphs three, seven, and nine, it appears that enamel is harder than bone because it contains more calcium.

46. **(1)** There is an indication in paragraphs eleven and twelve that the pattern of tooth development is precise. The other choices are neither mentioned nor alluded to in the passage.

47. **(4)** All of the choices except (4) are mentioned or alluded to in the passage.

48. **(2)** The initial section of the passage is devoted entirely to a discussion of the development of the structure and function of the skeletal system.

49. **(1)** A large portion of the closing section is devoted to a discussion of the development of teeth. It should be included in the title.

50. **(3)** This is the most appropriate of the titles listed, because the passage discusses elements of both the skeletal and dental systems, not just one of these subjects.

Part Three

MEDICAL COLLEGE ADMISSION TEST (MCAT)

MEDICAL COLLEGE ADMISSION TEST (MCAT)

The Medical College Admission Test is designed to measure an applicant's preparation in the natural sciences and in data interpretation. The examination is composed of four separate subtests entitled Science Knowledge; Science Problems; Skills Analysis—Reading; and Skills Analysis—Quantitative. The Science Knowledge and Science Problems sections are made up of questions from the material taught in introductory college-level biology, chemistry, and physics courses.

MCAT ANALYSIS AND TIMETABLE		
Subtest	*Number of Questions*	*Testing Time*
SCIENCE KNOWLEDGE		
Biology	38	25 minutes (suggested)
Chemistry	49	60 minutes (suggested)
Physics	38	50 minutes (suggested)
Subtotals	125	135 minutes
SCIENCE PROBLEMS		
Biology	18	
Chemistry	27	
Physics	21	
Subtotals	66	85 minutes
SKILLS ANALYSIS: READING	68	85 minutes
SKILLS ANALYSIS: QUANTITATIVE	68	85 minutes
TOTALS	327 questions	390 minutes (6 hours 30 minutes)

You will be given 10-minute breaks between each section of the MCAT and a one-hour lunch break after the science sections.

In the Science Knowledge section, there are three separate subsections—biology, chemistry, and physics. The Science Problems section contains questions in the same subject areas; however, questions in these areas are intermingled throughout the entire section instead of being set off in separate subsections.

When your MCAT is scored, you will receive six separate scores in the following categories: biology, chemistry, physics, science problems, reading skills, and quantitative skills. The biology, chemistry, and physics scores are based on your responses to questions in both the Science Knowledge and Science Problems sections. The science problems score is based on your responses to all of the questions in the Science Problems section.

Because your MCAT scores are based only on the number of correct answers, it is to your advantage to answer every question. Guess even when you are not sure of the answer—no points are deducted from your scores for wrong answers.

ANSWER SHEET FOR THE MCAT PRACTICE EXAMINATION

Section 1: Science Knowledge

1 Ⓐ Ⓑ Ⓒ Ⓓ Ⓔ	26 Ⓐ Ⓑ Ⓒ Ⓓ Ⓔ	51 Ⓐ Ⓑ Ⓒ Ⓓ Ⓔ	76 Ⓐ Ⓑ Ⓒ Ⓓ Ⓔ	101 Ⓐ Ⓑ Ⓒ Ⓓ Ⓔ
2 Ⓐ Ⓑ Ⓒ Ⓓ Ⓔ	27 Ⓐ Ⓑ Ⓒ Ⓓ Ⓔ	52 Ⓐ Ⓑ Ⓒ Ⓓ Ⓔ	77 Ⓐ Ⓑ Ⓒ Ⓓ Ⓔ	102 Ⓐ Ⓑ Ⓒ Ⓓ Ⓔ
3 Ⓐ Ⓑ Ⓒ Ⓓ Ⓔ	28 Ⓐ Ⓑ Ⓒ Ⓓ Ⓔ	53 Ⓐ Ⓑ Ⓒ Ⓓ Ⓔ	78 Ⓐ Ⓑ Ⓒ Ⓓ Ⓔ	103 Ⓐ Ⓑ Ⓒ Ⓓ Ⓔ
4 Ⓐ Ⓑ Ⓒ Ⓓ Ⓔ	29 Ⓐ Ⓑ Ⓒ Ⓓ Ⓔ	54 Ⓐ Ⓑ Ⓒ Ⓓ Ⓔ	79 Ⓐ Ⓑ Ⓒ Ⓓ Ⓔ	104 Ⓐ Ⓑ Ⓒ Ⓓ Ⓔ
5 Ⓐ Ⓑ Ⓒ Ⓓ Ⓔ	30 Ⓐ Ⓑ Ⓒ Ⓓ Ⓔ	55 Ⓐ Ⓑ Ⓒ Ⓓ Ⓔ	80 Ⓐ Ⓑ Ⓒ Ⓓ Ⓔ	105 Ⓐ Ⓑ Ⓒ Ⓓ Ⓔ
6 Ⓐ Ⓑ Ⓒ Ⓓ Ⓔ	31 Ⓐ Ⓑ Ⓒ Ⓓ Ⓔ	56 Ⓐ Ⓑ Ⓒ Ⓓ Ⓔ	81 Ⓐ Ⓑ Ⓒ Ⓓ Ⓔ	106 Ⓐ Ⓑ Ⓒ Ⓓ Ⓔ
7 Ⓐ Ⓑ Ⓒ Ⓓ Ⓔ	32 Ⓐ Ⓑ Ⓒ Ⓓ Ⓔ	57 Ⓐ Ⓑ Ⓒ Ⓓ Ⓔ	82 Ⓐ Ⓑ Ⓒ Ⓓ Ⓔ	107 Ⓐ Ⓑ Ⓒ Ⓓ Ⓔ
8 Ⓐ Ⓑ Ⓒ Ⓓ Ⓔ	33 Ⓐ Ⓑ Ⓒ Ⓓ Ⓔ	58 Ⓐ Ⓑ Ⓒ Ⓓ Ⓔ	83 Ⓐ Ⓑ Ⓒ Ⓓ Ⓔ	108 Ⓐ Ⓑ Ⓒ Ⓓ Ⓔ
9 Ⓐ Ⓑ Ⓒ Ⓓ Ⓔ	34 Ⓐ Ⓑ Ⓒ Ⓓ Ⓔ	59 Ⓐ Ⓑ Ⓒ Ⓓ Ⓔ	84 Ⓐ Ⓑ Ⓒ Ⓓ Ⓔ	109 Ⓐ Ⓑ Ⓒ Ⓓ Ⓔ
10 Ⓐ Ⓑ Ⓒ Ⓓ Ⓔ	35 Ⓐ Ⓑ Ⓒ Ⓓ Ⓔ	60 Ⓐ Ⓑ Ⓒ Ⓓ Ⓔ	85 Ⓐ Ⓑ Ⓒ Ⓓ Ⓔ	110 Ⓐ Ⓑ Ⓒ Ⓓ Ⓔ
11 Ⓐ Ⓑ Ⓒ Ⓓ Ⓔ	36 Ⓐ Ⓑ Ⓒ Ⓓ Ⓔ	61 Ⓐ Ⓑ Ⓒ Ⓓ Ⓔ	86 Ⓐ Ⓑ Ⓒ Ⓓ Ⓔ	111 Ⓐ Ⓑ Ⓒ Ⓓ Ⓔ
12 Ⓐ Ⓑ Ⓒ Ⓓ Ⓔ	37 Ⓐ Ⓑ Ⓒ Ⓓ Ⓔ	62 Ⓐ Ⓑ Ⓒ Ⓓ Ⓔ	87 Ⓐ Ⓑ Ⓒ Ⓓ Ⓔ	112 Ⓐ Ⓑ Ⓒ Ⓓ Ⓔ
13 Ⓐ Ⓑ Ⓒ Ⓓ Ⓔ	38 Ⓐ Ⓑ Ⓒ Ⓓ Ⓔ	63 Ⓐ Ⓑ Ⓒ Ⓓ Ⓔ	88 Ⓐ Ⓑ Ⓒ Ⓓ Ⓔ	113 Ⓐ Ⓑ Ⓒ Ⓓ Ⓔ
14 Ⓐ Ⓑ Ⓒ Ⓓ Ⓔ	39 Ⓐ Ⓑ Ⓒ Ⓓ Ⓔ	64 Ⓐ Ⓑ Ⓒ Ⓓ Ⓔ	89 Ⓐ Ⓑ Ⓒ Ⓓ Ⓔ	114 Ⓐ Ⓑ Ⓒ Ⓓ Ⓔ
15 Ⓐ Ⓑ Ⓒ Ⓓ Ⓔ	40 Ⓐ Ⓑ Ⓒ Ⓓ Ⓔ	65 Ⓐ Ⓑ Ⓒ Ⓓ Ⓔ	90 Ⓐ Ⓑ Ⓒ Ⓓ Ⓔ	115 Ⓐ Ⓑ Ⓒ Ⓓ Ⓔ
16 Ⓐ Ⓑ Ⓒ Ⓓ Ⓔ	41 Ⓐ Ⓑ Ⓒ Ⓓ Ⓔ	66 Ⓐ Ⓑ Ⓒ Ⓓ Ⓔ	91 Ⓐ Ⓑ Ⓒ Ⓓ Ⓔ	116 Ⓐ Ⓑ Ⓒ Ⓓ Ⓔ
17 Ⓐ Ⓑ Ⓒ Ⓓ Ⓔ	42 Ⓐ Ⓑ Ⓒ Ⓓ Ⓔ	67 Ⓐ Ⓑ Ⓒ Ⓓ Ⓔ	92 Ⓐ Ⓑ Ⓒ Ⓓ Ⓔ	117 Ⓐ Ⓑ Ⓒ Ⓓ Ⓔ
18 Ⓐ Ⓑ Ⓒ Ⓓ Ⓔ	43 Ⓐ Ⓑ Ⓒ Ⓓ Ⓔ	68 Ⓐ Ⓑ Ⓒ Ⓓ Ⓔ	93 Ⓐ Ⓑ Ⓒ Ⓓ Ⓔ	118 Ⓐ Ⓑ Ⓒ Ⓓ Ⓔ
19 Ⓐ Ⓑ Ⓒ Ⓓ Ⓔ	44 Ⓐ Ⓑ Ⓒ Ⓓ Ⓔ	69 Ⓐ Ⓑ Ⓒ Ⓓ Ⓔ	94 Ⓐ Ⓑ Ⓒ Ⓓ Ⓔ	119 Ⓐ Ⓑ Ⓒ Ⓓ Ⓔ
20 Ⓐ Ⓑ Ⓒ Ⓓ Ⓔ	45 Ⓐ Ⓑ Ⓒ Ⓓ Ⓔ	70 Ⓐ Ⓑ Ⓒ Ⓓ Ⓔ	95 Ⓐ Ⓑ Ⓒ Ⓓ Ⓔ	120 Ⓐ Ⓑ Ⓒ Ⓓ Ⓔ
21 Ⓐ Ⓑ Ⓒ Ⓓ Ⓔ	46 Ⓐ Ⓑ Ⓒ Ⓓ Ⓔ	71 Ⓐ Ⓑ Ⓒ Ⓓ Ⓔ	96 Ⓐ Ⓑ Ⓒ Ⓓ Ⓔ	121 Ⓐ Ⓑ Ⓒ Ⓓ Ⓔ
22 Ⓐ Ⓑ Ⓒ Ⓓ Ⓔ	47 Ⓐ Ⓑ Ⓒ Ⓓ Ⓔ	72 Ⓐ Ⓑ Ⓒ Ⓓ Ⓔ	97 Ⓐ Ⓑ Ⓒ Ⓓ Ⓔ	122 Ⓐ Ⓑ Ⓒ Ⓓ Ⓔ
23 Ⓐ Ⓑ Ⓒ Ⓓ Ⓔ	48 Ⓐ Ⓑ Ⓒ Ⓓ Ⓔ	73 Ⓐ Ⓑ Ⓒ Ⓓ Ⓔ	98 Ⓐ Ⓑ Ⓒ Ⓓ Ⓔ	123 Ⓐ Ⓑ Ⓒ Ⓓ Ⓔ
24 Ⓐ Ⓑ Ⓒ Ⓓ Ⓔ	49 Ⓐ Ⓑ Ⓒ Ⓓ Ⓔ	74 Ⓐ Ⓑ Ⓒ Ⓓ Ⓔ	99 Ⓐ Ⓑ Ⓒ Ⓓ Ⓔ	124 Ⓐ Ⓑ Ⓒ Ⓓ Ⓔ
25 Ⓐ Ⓑ Ⓒ Ⓓ Ⓔ	50 Ⓐ Ⓑ Ⓒ Ⓓ Ⓔ	75 Ⓐ Ⓑ Ⓒ Ⓓ Ⓔ	100 Ⓐ Ⓑ Ⓒ Ⓓ Ⓔ	125 Ⓐ Ⓑ Ⓒ Ⓓ Ⓔ

Section 2: Science Problems

1 Ⓐ Ⓑ Ⓒ Ⓓ Ⓔ 15 Ⓐ Ⓑ Ⓒ Ⓓ Ⓔ 29 Ⓐ Ⓑ Ⓒ Ⓓ Ⓔ 43 Ⓐ Ⓑ Ⓒ Ⓓ Ⓔ 57 Ⓐ Ⓑ Ⓒ Ⓓ Ⓔ

2 Ⓐ Ⓑ Ⓒ Ⓓ Ⓔ 16 Ⓐ Ⓑ Ⓒ Ⓓ Ⓔ 30 Ⓐ Ⓑ Ⓒ Ⓓ Ⓔ 44 Ⓐ Ⓑ Ⓒ Ⓓ Ⓔ 58 Ⓐ Ⓑ Ⓒ Ⓓ Ⓔ

3 Ⓐ Ⓑ Ⓒ Ⓓ Ⓔ 17 Ⓐ Ⓑ Ⓒ Ⓓ Ⓔ 31 Ⓐ Ⓑ Ⓒ Ⓓ Ⓔ 45 Ⓐ Ⓑ Ⓒ Ⓓ Ⓔ 59 Ⓐ Ⓑ Ⓒ Ⓓ Ⓔ

4 Ⓐ Ⓑ Ⓒ Ⓓ Ⓔ 18 Ⓐ Ⓑ Ⓒ Ⓓ Ⓔ 32 Ⓐ Ⓑ Ⓒ Ⓓ Ⓔ 46 Ⓐ Ⓑ Ⓒ Ⓓ Ⓔ 60 Ⓐ Ⓑ Ⓒ Ⓓ Ⓔ

5 Ⓐ Ⓑ Ⓒ Ⓓ Ⓔ 19 Ⓐ Ⓑ Ⓒ Ⓓ Ⓔ 33 Ⓐ Ⓑ Ⓒ Ⓓ Ⓔ 47 Ⓐ Ⓑ Ⓒ Ⓓ Ⓔ 61 Ⓐ Ⓑ Ⓒ Ⓓ Ⓔ

6 Ⓐ Ⓑ Ⓒ Ⓓ Ⓔ 20 Ⓐ Ⓑ Ⓒ Ⓓ Ⓔ 34 Ⓐ Ⓑ Ⓒ Ⓓ Ⓔ 48 Ⓐ Ⓑ Ⓒ Ⓓ Ⓔ 62 Ⓐ Ⓑ Ⓒ Ⓓ Ⓔ

7 Ⓐ Ⓑ Ⓒ Ⓓ Ⓔ 21 Ⓐ Ⓑ Ⓒ Ⓓ Ⓔ 35 Ⓐ Ⓑ Ⓒ Ⓓ Ⓔ 49 Ⓐ Ⓑ Ⓒ Ⓓ Ⓔ 63 Ⓐ Ⓑ Ⓒ Ⓓ Ⓔ

8 Ⓐ Ⓑ Ⓒ Ⓓ Ⓔ 22 Ⓐ Ⓑ Ⓒ Ⓓ Ⓔ 36 Ⓐ Ⓑ Ⓒ Ⓓ Ⓔ 50 Ⓐ Ⓑ Ⓒ Ⓓ Ⓔ 64 Ⓐ Ⓑ Ⓒ Ⓓ Ⓔ

9 Ⓐ Ⓑ Ⓒ Ⓓ Ⓔ 23 Ⓐ Ⓑ Ⓒ Ⓓ Ⓔ 37 Ⓐ Ⓑ Ⓒ Ⓓ Ⓔ 51 Ⓐ Ⓑ Ⓒ Ⓓ Ⓔ 65 Ⓐ Ⓑ Ⓒ Ⓓ Ⓔ

10 Ⓐ Ⓑ Ⓒ Ⓓ Ⓔ 24 Ⓐ Ⓑ Ⓒ Ⓓ Ⓔ 38 Ⓐ Ⓑ Ⓒ Ⓓ Ⓔ 52 Ⓐ Ⓑ Ⓒ Ⓓ Ⓔ 66 Ⓐ Ⓑ Ⓒ Ⓓ Ⓔ

11 Ⓐ Ⓑ Ⓒ Ⓓ Ⓔ 25 Ⓐ Ⓑ Ⓒ Ⓓ Ⓔ 39 Ⓐ Ⓑ Ⓒ Ⓓ Ⓔ 53 Ⓐ Ⓑ Ⓒ Ⓓ Ⓔ

12 Ⓐ Ⓑ Ⓒ Ⓓ Ⓔ 26 Ⓐ Ⓑ Ⓒ Ⓓ Ⓔ 40 Ⓐ Ⓑ Ⓒ Ⓓ Ⓔ 54 Ⓐ Ⓑ Ⓒ Ⓓ Ⓔ

13 Ⓐ Ⓑ Ⓒ Ⓓ Ⓔ 27 Ⓐ Ⓑ Ⓒ Ⓓ Ⓔ 41 Ⓐ Ⓑ Ⓒ Ⓓ Ⓔ 55 Ⓐ Ⓑ Ⓒ Ⓓ Ⓔ

14 Ⓐ Ⓑ Ⓒ Ⓓ Ⓔ 28 Ⓐ Ⓑ Ⓒ Ⓓ Ⓔ 42 Ⓐ Ⓑ Ⓒ Ⓓ Ⓔ 56 Ⓐ Ⓑ Ⓒ Ⓓ Ⓔ

Section 3: Skills Analysis—Reading

1 Ⓐ Ⓑ Ⓒ Ⓓ Ⓔ 15 Ⓐ Ⓑ Ⓒ Ⓓ Ⓔ 29 Ⓐ Ⓑ Ⓒ Ⓓ Ⓔ 43 Ⓐ Ⓑ Ⓒ Ⓓ Ⓔ 57 Ⓐ Ⓑ Ⓒ Ⓓ Ⓔ

2 Ⓐ Ⓑ Ⓒ Ⓓ Ⓔ 16 Ⓐ Ⓑ Ⓒ Ⓓ Ⓔ 30 Ⓐ Ⓑ Ⓒ Ⓓ Ⓔ 44 Ⓐ Ⓑ Ⓒ Ⓓ Ⓔ 58 Ⓐ Ⓑ Ⓒ Ⓓ Ⓔ

3 Ⓐ Ⓑ Ⓒ Ⓓ Ⓔ 17 Ⓐ Ⓑ Ⓒ Ⓓ Ⓔ 31 Ⓐ Ⓑ Ⓒ Ⓓ Ⓔ 45 Ⓐ Ⓑ Ⓒ Ⓓ Ⓔ 59 Ⓐ Ⓑ Ⓒ Ⓓ Ⓔ

4 Ⓐ Ⓑ Ⓒ Ⓓ Ⓔ 18 Ⓐ Ⓑ Ⓒ Ⓓ Ⓔ 32 Ⓐ Ⓑ Ⓒ Ⓓ Ⓔ 46 Ⓐ Ⓑ Ⓒ Ⓓ Ⓔ 60 Ⓐ Ⓑ Ⓒ Ⓓ Ⓔ

5 Ⓐ Ⓑ Ⓒ Ⓓ Ⓔ 19 Ⓐ Ⓑ Ⓒ Ⓓ Ⓔ 33 Ⓐ Ⓑ Ⓒ Ⓓ Ⓔ 47 Ⓐ Ⓑ Ⓒ Ⓓ Ⓔ 61 Ⓐ Ⓑ Ⓒ Ⓓ Ⓔ

6 Ⓐ Ⓑ Ⓒ Ⓓ Ⓔ 20 Ⓐ Ⓑ Ⓒ Ⓓ Ⓔ 34 Ⓐ Ⓑ Ⓒ Ⓓ Ⓔ 48 Ⓐ Ⓑ Ⓒ Ⓓ Ⓔ 62 Ⓐ Ⓑ Ⓒ Ⓓ Ⓔ

7 Ⓐ Ⓑ Ⓒ Ⓓ Ⓔ 21 Ⓐ Ⓑ Ⓒ Ⓓ Ⓔ 35 Ⓐ Ⓑ Ⓒ Ⓓ Ⓔ 49 Ⓐ Ⓑ Ⓒ Ⓓ Ⓔ 63 Ⓐ Ⓑ Ⓒ Ⓓ Ⓔ

8 Ⓐ Ⓑ Ⓒ Ⓓ Ⓔ 22 Ⓐ Ⓑ Ⓒ Ⓓ Ⓔ 36 Ⓐ Ⓑ Ⓒ Ⓓ Ⓔ 50 Ⓐ Ⓑ Ⓒ Ⓓ Ⓔ 64 Ⓐ Ⓑ Ⓒ Ⓓ Ⓔ

9 Ⓐ Ⓑ Ⓒ Ⓓ Ⓔ 23 Ⓐ Ⓑ Ⓒ Ⓓ Ⓔ 37 Ⓐ Ⓑ Ⓒ Ⓓ Ⓔ 51 Ⓐ Ⓑ Ⓒ Ⓓ Ⓔ 65 Ⓐ Ⓑ Ⓒ Ⓓ Ⓔ

10 Ⓐ Ⓑ Ⓒ Ⓓ Ⓔ 24 Ⓐ Ⓑ Ⓒ Ⓓ Ⓔ 38 Ⓐ Ⓑ Ⓒ Ⓓ Ⓔ 52 Ⓐ Ⓑ Ⓒ Ⓓ Ⓔ 66 Ⓐ Ⓑ Ⓒ Ⓓ Ⓔ

11 Ⓐ Ⓑ Ⓒ Ⓓ Ⓔ 25 Ⓐ Ⓑ Ⓒ Ⓓ Ⓔ 39 Ⓐ Ⓑ Ⓒ Ⓓ Ⓔ 53 Ⓐ Ⓑ Ⓒ Ⓓ Ⓔ 67 Ⓐ Ⓑ Ⓒ Ⓓ Ⓔ

12 Ⓐ Ⓑ Ⓒ Ⓓ Ⓔ 26 Ⓐ Ⓑ Ⓒ Ⓓ Ⓔ 40 Ⓐ Ⓑ Ⓒ Ⓓ Ⓔ 54 Ⓐ Ⓑ Ⓒ Ⓓ Ⓔ 68 Ⓐ Ⓑ Ⓒ Ⓓ Ⓔ

13 Ⓐ Ⓑ Ⓒ Ⓓ Ⓔ 27 Ⓐ Ⓑ Ⓒ Ⓓ Ⓔ 41 Ⓐ Ⓑ Ⓒ Ⓓ Ⓔ 55 Ⓐ Ⓑ Ⓒ Ⓓ Ⓔ

14 Ⓐ Ⓑ Ⓒ Ⓓ Ⓔ 28 Ⓐ Ⓑ Ⓒ Ⓓ Ⓔ 42 Ⓐ Ⓑ Ⓒ Ⓓ Ⓔ 56 Ⓐ Ⓑ Ⓒ Ⓓ Ⓔ

Section 4: Skills Analysis—Quantitative

1 Ⓐ Ⓑ Ⓒ Ⓓ Ⓔ   15 Ⓐ Ⓑ Ⓒ Ⓓ Ⓔ   29 Ⓐ Ⓑ Ⓒ Ⓓ Ⓔ   43 Ⓐ Ⓑ Ⓒ Ⓓ Ⓔ   57 Ⓐ Ⓑ Ⓒ Ⓓ Ⓔ

2 Ⓐ Ⓑ Ⓒ Ⓓ Ⓔ   16 Ⓐ Ⓑ Ⓒ Ⓓ Ⓔ   30 Ⓐ Ⓑ Ⓒ Ⓓ Ⓔ   44 Ⓐ Ⓑ Ⓒ Ⓓ Ⓔ   58 Ⓐ Ⓑ Ⓒ Ⓓ Ⓔ

3 Ⓐ Ⓑ Ⓒ Ⓓ Ⓔ   17 Ⓐ Ⓑ Ⓒ Ⓓ Ⓔ   31 Ⓐ Ⓑ Ⓒ Ⓓ Ⓔ   45 Ⓐ Ⓑ Ⓒ Ⓓ Ⓔ   59 Ⓐ Ⓑ Ⓒ Ⓓ Ⓔ

4 Ⓐ Ⓑ Ⓒ Ⓓ Ⓔ   18 Ⓐ Ⓑ Ⓒ Ⓓ Ⓔ   32 Ⓐ Ⓑ Ⓒ Ⓓ Ⓔ   46 Ⓐ Ⓑ Ⓒ Ⓓ Ⓔ   60 Ⓐ Ⓑ Ⓒ Ⓓ Ⓔ

5 Ⓐ Ⓑ Ⓒ Ⓓ Ⓔ   19 Ⓐ Ⓑ Ⓒ Ⓓ Ⓔ   33 Ⓐ Ⓑ Ⓒ Ⓓ Ⓔ   47 Ⓐ Ⓑ Ⓒ Ⓓ Ⓔ   61 Ⓐ Ⓑ Ⓒ Ⓓ Ⓔ

6 Ⓐ Ⓑ Ⓒ Ⓓ Ⓔ   20 Ⓐ Ⓑ Ⓒ Ⓓ Ⓔ   34 Ⓐ Ⓑ Ⓒ Ⓓ Ⓔ   48 Ⓐ Ⓑ Ⓒ Ⓓ Ⓔ   62 Ⓐ Ⓑ Ⓒ Ⓓ Ⓔ

7 Ⓐ Ⓑ Ⓒ Ⓓ Ⓔ   21 Ⓐ Ⓑ Ⓒ Ⓓ Ⓔ   35 Ⓐ Ⓑ Ⓒ Ⓓ Ⓔ   49 Ⓐ Ⓑ Ⓒ Ⓓ Ⓔ   63 Ⓐ Ⓑ Ⓒ Ⓓ Ⓔ

8 Ⓐ Ⓑ Ⓒ Ⓓ Ⓔ   22 Ⓐ Ⓑ Ⓒ Ⓓ Ⓔ   36 Ⓐ Ⓑ Ⓒ Ⓓ Ⓔ   50 Ⓐ Ⓑ Ⓒ Ⓓ Ⓔ   64 Ⓐ Ⓑ Ⓒ Ⓓ Ⓔ

9 Ⓐ Ⓑ Ⓒ Ⓓ Ⓔ   23 Ⓐ Ⓑ Ⓒ Ⓓ Ⓔ   37 Ⓐ Ⓑ Ⓒ Ⓓ Ⓔ   51 Ⓐ Ⓑ Ⓒ Ⓓ Ⓔ   65 Ⓐ Ⓑ Ⓒ Ⓓ Ⓔ

10 Ⓐ Ⓑ Ⓒ Ⓓ Ⓔ   24 Ⓐ Ⓑ Ⓒ Ⓓ Ⓔ   38 Ⓐ Ⓑ Ⓒ Ⓓ Ⓔ   52 Ⓐ Ⓑ Ⓒ Ⓓ Ⓔ   66 Ⓐ Ⓑ Ⓒ Ⓓ Ⓔ

11 Ⓐ Ⓑ Ⓒ Ⓓ Ⓔ   25 Ⓐ Ⓑ Ⓒ Ⓓ Ⓔ   39 Ⓐ Ⓑ Ⓒ Ⓓ Ⓔ   53 Ⓐ Ⓑ Ⓒ Ⓓ Ⓔ   67 Ⓐ Ⓑ Ⓒ Ⓓ Ⓔ

12 Ⓐ Ⓑ Ⓒ Ⓓ Ⓔ   26 Ⓐ Ⓑ Ⓒ Ⓓ Ⓔ   40 Ⓐ Ⓑ Ⓒ Ⓓ Ⓔ   54 Ⓐ Ⓑ Ⓒ Ⓓ Ⓔ   68 Ⓐ Ⓑ Ⓒ Ⓓ Ⓔ

13 Ⓐ Ⓑ Ⓒ Ⓓ Ⓔ   27 Ⓐ Ⓑ Ⓒ Ⓓ Ⓔ   41 Ⓐ Ⓑ Ⓒ Ⓓ Ⓔ   55 Ⓐ Ⓑ Ⓒ Ⓓ Ⓔ

14 Ⓐ Ⓑ Ⓒ Ⓓ Ⓔ   28 Ⓐ Ⓑ Ⓒ Ⓓ Ⓔ   42 Ⓐ Ⓑ Ⓒ Ⓓ Ⓔ   56 Ⓐ Ⓑ Ⓒ Ⓓ Ⓔ

PERIODIC TABLE OF THE ELEMENTS

1a	2a	3b	4b	5b	6b	7b	8	8	8	1b	2b	3a	4a	5a	6a	7a	0
1 H 1.0097																	2 He 4.0026
3 Li 6.939	4 Be 9.0122											5 B 10.811	6 C 12.01115	7 N 14.0067	8 O 15.9994	9 F 18.9984	10 Ne 20.183
11 Na 22.9898	12 Mg 24.312											13 Al 26.9815	14 Si 28.086	15 P 30.9738	16 S 32.064	17 Cl 33.453	18 Ar 39.948
19 K 39.102	20 Ca 40.08	21 Sc 44.956	22 Ti 47.90	23 V 50.942	24 Cr 51.996	25 Mn 54.9380	26 Fe 55.847	27 Co 58.9332	28 Ni 58.71	29 Cu 63.546	30 Zn 63.37	31 Ga 69.72	32 Ge 72.59	33 As 74.9216	34 Se 78.96	35 Br 79.904	36 Kr 83.80
37 Rb 85.47	38 Sr 87.62	39 Y 88.905	40 Zr 91.22	41 Nb 92.906	42 Mo 95.94	43 Tc (97)	44 Ru 101.07	45 Rh 102.905	46 Pd 106.4	47 Ag 107.868	48 Cd 112.40	49 In 114.82	50 Sn 118.69	51 Sb 121.75	52 Te 127.60	53 I 126.9044	54 Xe 131.30
55 Cs 132.905	56 Ba 137.34	57* La 138.91	72 Hf 178.49	73 Ta 180.948	74 W 183.85	75 Re 186.2	76 Os 190.2	77 Ir 192.2	78 Pt 195.09	79 Au 196.967	80 Hg 200.59	81 Tl 204.37	82 Pb 207.19	83 Bi 208.980	84 Po (209)	85 At (210)	86 Rn (222)
87 Fr (223)	88 Ra (236)	89** Ac (227)															

Transition Elements — Group 8

104 –

*Lanthanides	58 Ce 140.12	59 Pr 140.907	60 Nd 144.24	61 Pm (145)	62 Sm 150.35	63 Eu 151.96	64 Gd 157.25	65 Tb 158.924	66 Dy 162.50	67 Ho 164.930	68 Er 167.26	69 Tm 168.934	70 Yb 173.04	71 Lu 174.97
**Actinides	90 Th (232)	91 Pa (231)	92 U (238)	93 Np (237)	94 Pu (244)	95 Am (243)	96 Cm (247)	97 Bk (247)	98 Cf (251)	99 Es (254)	100 Fm (257)	101 Md (256)	102 No (254)	103 Lw (254)

Numbers in parentheses are mass numbers of most stable isotope of that element.

MCAT PRACTICE EXAMINATION

Section 1: SCIENCE KNOWLEDGE

Time: **135 minutes**
125 questions

Directions: Each question is followed by three to five lettered choices. Choose the one best answer to each question. A Periodic Table of the Elements appears on page 86. Consult it whenever you wish. You will be given 135 minutes to answer all 125 questions; suggested times for the biology, chemistry, and physics sections are provided as a guideline.

Biology

(*Suggested time: 25 minutes*)

1. Which of the following would be a meaningful distinction between the ribosomes that are associated with the rough endoplasmic reticulum and the so-called free ribosomes, which are not?
   (A) Rough E.R. ribosomes are involved in the synthesis of proteins that will leave the cell, while free ribosomes are not.
   (B) Free ribosomes are involved in the synthesis of proteins that will leave the cell while rough E.R. ribosomes are not.
   (C) Free ribosomes are inactive until they become associated with the rough E.R.
   (D) Only the rough E.R. ribosomes are involved in producing steriods.
   (E) none of the above

2. Which of the following types of cells would be the LEAST appropriate choice for studying nuclear phenomena?
   (A) smooth muscle cells
   (B) mature red blood cells
   (C) nerve cells
   (D) sperm cells
   (E) liver cells

3. Damage to the Golgi apparatus might

   (A) interfere with the addition of sulfate groups to newly synthesized proteins
   (B) inhibit assembly of the nuclear membrane
   (C) disturb the packaging of protein products
   (D) block protein synthesis
   (E) more than one of the above

4. The actual incidence of hemophilia is less than the theoretically predictable level because
   (A) hemophilia is sex-linked
   (B) of adverse marriage selection pressure against hemophiliacs
   (C) the gene for hemophilia is recessive
   (D) homozygosity is seldom found in the female
   (E) the gene for hemophilia is dominant

5. A bacteriophage and a yeast cell are alike in that both
   (A) carry on intracellular digestion
   (B) can carry on aerobic respiration
   (C) contain nucleic acids
   (D) have a cell wall
   (E) must have living cells to grow on

6. Darwin discovered and formulated the theory of evolution, popularized as "the survival of the fittest." Which of the following traits would Darwin regard as the most important for survival in the long run?
   (A) strength
   (B) intelligence
   (C) agility
   (D) economy
   (E) adaptability

7. Cellophane membranes permeable to water molecules and impermeable to sugar mole-

cules are filled according to the table that follows. They are then suspended in beakers filled with water or sugar and water according to the table. Assume that temperatures are constant and all sugar/water solutions were obtained from the same source.

BEAKER	MEMBRANE CONTENTS	BEAKER CONTENTS
1	water	water
2	sugar water	water
3	water	sugar water

Which of the following will occur in beaker two?
(A) The bag will shrink.
(B) Water molecules will diffuse out of the bag.
(C) Sugar molecules will diffuse out of the bag.
(D) Water molecules will diffuse into the bag.
(E) There is no movement of molecules.

8. The equation below represents

(A) dehydration synthesis
(B) hydrolysis
(C) protein digestion
(D) cellular respiration
(E) assimilation

9. If motor neurons are cut, the individual
(A) cannot hear or see
(B) cannot feel or sense anything
(C) loses all sense of balance
(D) is incapable of making voluntary motions
(E) both A and C

10. Final cellular differentiation within a developing embryo is
(A) determined by the physical and chemical environment surrounding the cell
(B) entirely dependent upon the germ layer from which the cell is derived
(C) dependent upon the specific chromosomes the cell receives
(D) controlled by the cytoplasm of the unfertilized egg
(E) determined before gastrulation of the embryo

11. If one parent belongs to blood group B and the other belongs to blood group AB, the children could belong to
(A) A, B, AB only
(B) A or B only
(C) A, B, O, or AB
(D) B or O only
(E) A or O only

12. Although the amount of any given base found in DNA varies considerably from one species to another, the amount of thymine is always equal to the amount of
(A) cytosine
(B) guanine
(C) uracil
(D) adenine
(E) none of the above

13. "Leaky" lysosomal membranes that permit inappropriate release of the organelle contents into the surrounding cytoplasm might be responsible for
(A) inhibiting storage of lipids
(B) destruction of cellular components
(C) release of glucose
(D) decreased synthesis of nucleic acids
(E) increased synthesis of acid hydrolases

14. A cell concerned with synthesizing and secreting large quantities of protein would be expected to have
(A) many lysosomes and mitochondria, with cristae possessing an abnormally large number of folds
(B) many more chromosomes than the average human cell

(C) large numbers of mitochondria and ribosomes and a well-developed Golgi apparatus

(D) a nuclear membrane with an abnormally large number of pores

(E) none of the above

15. Mammalian embryos float in an isotonic fluid which serves the important function of
(A) food supplier
(B) mutagen enhancer
(C) shock absorber
(D) cardiac arrester
(E) all of the above

16. The fluid mosiac model of the cell membrane suggests that
(A) cell membranes are three-layered sandwiches of lipid/protein/lipid
(B) cell membranes are a sea of double layers of lipid molecules in which protein molecules are floating
(C) cell membranes are rigid structures composed of cellulose and pectin
(D) cell membranes are trilaminar and contain only primary and secondary proteins
(E) all cell membrane components are completely soluble in polar solvents

17. Neurons that conduct impulses from the central nervous system to a muscle or a gland are known as
(A) apolar neurons
(B) sensory neurons
(C) motor neurons
(D) afferent neurons
(E) association neurons

18. During mitosis, daughter nuclei are formed in the
(A) interphase
(B) prophase
(C) metaphase
(D) anaphase
(E) telophase

19. Which of the following structures does not include nucleic acid?
(A) gene
(B) chromosome

(C) centriole
(D) ribosome
(E) chromatin

20. Complete obstruction of the bile duct in a patient might be expected to
(A) inhibit protein digestion
(B) increase stool fat content
(C) increase pH of duodenal contents
(D) decrease the synthesis of pancreatic lipase
(E) cause the liver to take over as the site of bile synthesis

21. A form of binary fission, in which one of the two offspring is smaller than the other, is called
(A) spermatogenesis
(B) budding
(C) mitosis
(D) parthenogenesis
(E) cogenesis

22. Which layer of tissue is adjacent to the gastrocoele?
(A) zygoderm
(B) ectoderm
(C) mesoderm
(D) endoderm
(E) cortoderm

23. The organism interaction in which one species benefits from the association while the other is essentially unaffected is known as
(A) commensalism
(B) mutualism
(C) parasitism
(D) competition
(E) autotrophism

24. The common factor in mutation, gene flow, and genetic drift is that
(A) they all affect the individual
(B) they can all contribute to gene pool change
(C) they can all contribute to evolution
(D) all of the above
(E) both B and C are correct

25. Which of the following statements about vasopressin is true?

(A) It tends to increase urine osmolarity.

(B) It generally acts to lower blood pressure.

(C) It is produced by the posterior pituitary gland.

(D) It is known to stimulate contraction of uterine smooth muscle as its predominant physiologic action.

(E) None of the above statements is true.

26. Adding ribonuclease to cells would effectively inhibit which one of the following processes?
(A) protein synthesis
(B) diffusion
(C) catalysis
(D) lipogenesis
(E) none of these

27. The second meiotic division is essentially a mitosis except for the product which is
(A) haploid
(B) diploid
(C) triploid
(D) heterozygous
(E) achromatic

28. The theory of endosymbiosis states that
(A) animal cells were plant cells that lost their mitochondria
(B) organelles were originally independent cells
(C) all cells are parasitic
(D) organelles arose through a partitioning off of cell membrane
(E) all of these

29. The type of muscle tissue found within the walls of blood vessels and internal organs is
(A) smooth muscle
(B) skeletal muscle
(C) cardiac muscle
(D) voluntary muscle
(E) striated muscle

30. Homologous structures commonly exhibit
(A) structural diversity
(B) functional similarity
(C) genetic relationship
(D) genetic diversity
(E) functional diversity

31. Which of the following is *not* promptly reabsorbed in the villi?
(A) carbohydrates
(B) lipids
(C) water
(D) vitamins
(E) amino acids

32. Which of the following does *not* contain both DNA and RNA?
(A) blue-green algae
(B) bacteria
(C) bacteriophages
(D) protozoa
(E) none of the above

33. Motile sperm cells are found in all of the following plants *except*
(A) pine
(B) ginkgo
(C) mosses
(D) ferns
(E) liverworts

34. A section of the circulatory system which plays an important role in fishes but which disappears in higher land animals is the
(A) hepatic portal system
(B) renal portal system
(C) renal arteries
(D) hepatic arteries
(E) hepatic veins

35. When bronchioles are obstructed, fresh oxygen is most directly kept from reaching the
(A) bronchial tubes
(B) ciliated epithelium
(C) larynx
(D) trachea
(E) alveolar capillaries

36. To determine whether a black guinea pig is pure black or hybrid black, it should be crossed with which of the following kinds of guinea pigs?
(A) white
(B) pure black
(C) hybrid white
(D) an unknown
(E) hybrid black

37. The evidence that untrained planaria worms, when fed chopped planaria worms that had learned a maze, were able to learn a maze faster than the controls is consistent with the notion that learning is
    (A) associated with reflexes
    (B) not at present fully understood
    (C) an instinct
    (D) a conditioned activity
    (E) associated with RNA

38. Most of the oxidative enzymes of the cell and of the tricarboxylic acid cycle are concentrated within which one of the following?
    (A) grana of chloroplasts
    (B) cristae of mitochondria
    (C) ergastoplasm
    (D) Golgi apparatus
    (E) microsomes

Chemistry

(Suggested time: 60 minutes)

39. According to the Bohr model of the hydrogen atom, which of the following transitions by an electron will result in a photon of the highest frequency?
    (A) n = 4 to n = 3
    (B) n = 3 to n = 2
    (C) n = 2 to n = 1
    (D) n = 5 to n = 4
    (E) None of these transitions can take place because the Bohr model refers to the lowest (ground state) orbit only.

40. Given the following thermochemical equations,

    $Zn + \frac{1}{2}O_2 = ZnO + 84{,}000$ cals
    $Hg + \frac{1}{2}O_2 = HgO + 21{,}700$ cals

    what is the heat of reaction for the following reaction? $Zn + HgO = ZnO + Hg + heat$
    (A) 105,700 cals
    (B) 61,000 cals
    (C) 105,000 cals
    (D) 62,300 cals
    (E) 106,000 cals

41. The molecular property of a gas that is the same for all gases at a particular temperature is the
    (A) momentum
    (B) velocity
    (C) kinetic energy
    (D) potential energy
    (E) angular momentum

42. A substance that increases in volume upon freezing has a melting point that
    (A) is lowered with an increase in external pressure
    (B) is raised with an increase in external pressure
    (C) is unaltered by an increase in external pressure
    (D) may be either lowered or raised depending upon its chemical composition
    (E) is called a eutectic substance

43. Of the following diagrams, the one representing the work done by a gas during adiabatic expansion is (P = pressure, V = volume)

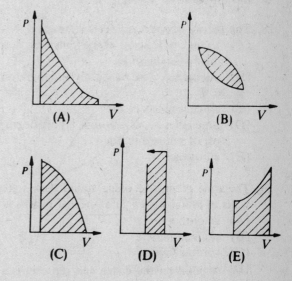

44. Which of the following properties makes water indispensable to life as we know it?
    (A) Water expands at temperatures below 4°C.
    (B) Water has an extremely high surface tension.

(C) Water has a very high heat capacity, heat of vaporization, and heat of fusion.

(D) Water has a high dielectric constant.

(E) All of the above are essential.

45. In an attempt to determine the identity of an unknown compound, elemental analysis was performed. This revealed the following information:

K: 77% by weight of the entire sample
O: 23% by weight of the entire sample

The molecular weight of the compound was determined to be 408 grams/mole (Atomic weights: K = 39; O = 16).
What is the empirical formula of the compound?

(A) K_2O_3
(B) K_4O_3
(C) K_4O_5
(D) K_3O_4
(E) K_2O_5

46. Consider the *PV* diagram that follows and select a correct statement derived from it (*P* = pressure, *V* = volume).

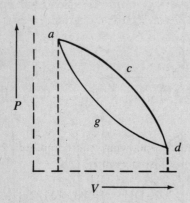

(A) A point on the curve *agd* represents a higher temperature than a point on the curve *acd*.

(B) Heat is lost to the environment during the process represented by pathway *agd*.

(C) The magnitude of the work done by the system undergoing the process represented by the path *agd* is greater than that done by the system undergoing the process represented by *acd*.

(D) Pathway *acd* and *agd* represent isothermal conditions.

(E) The area *acdga* represents the work done by the system for the process shown.

47. The minimum energy required to ionize a hydrogen atom from its ground state is about

(A) 1.36 *eV*
(B) 0.136 *eV*
(C) 13.6 *eV*
(D) 136 *eV*
(E) 1.36 *eV*

48. An aqueous solution of which of the following compounds has the highest pH? Assume all concentrations to be equal.

(A) $NaCl$
(B) Na_2CO_3
(C) NH_4Cl
(D) $NaHCO_3$
(E) CH_3COOH

49. Given that a radioactive species decays according to the exponential law $N = N_0exp(-\lambda t)$, what is the half-life of the species?

(A) λ
(B) $N_0\lambda$
(C) $\lambda/\ln(2)$
(D) $N_0/2\lambda$
(E) $\ln(2/\lambda)$

50. Sp^3d hybridization results in which of the following geometrical configurations?

(A) trigonal plane
(B) trigonal pyramid
(C) tetrahedral
(D) tetragonal plane
(E) bipyramid

51. The greatest amount of CO_2 can be dissolved in water under conditions of

(A) high pressure and low temperature
(B) high pressure and high temperature
(C) low pressure and low temperature
(D) low pressure and high temperature
(E) either high temperature or low pressure

52. U-235 may be separated from natural uranium by a process called
    (A) ionization
    (B) electrolysis
    (C) precipitation
    (D) gaseous diffusion
    (E) crystallization

53. A 0.1 N solution of sodium bicarbonate has a pH value of
    (A) 5.6
    (B) 7.0
    (C) 8.4
    (D) 13.0
    (E) 4.0

54. A brass cylinder (specific gravity = 6.8) is floating in a pool of mercury (specific gravity = 13.6). The fraction of the volume of the cylinder submerged is
    (A) ¼
    (B) ⅓
    (C) ½
    (D) ¾
    (E) ⅕

55. The height to which a liquid will rise in a capillary tube which it wets is inversely proportional to the
    (A) temperature
    (B) air pressure
    (C) surface tension
    (D) viscosity of the liquid
    (E) radius of the tube

56. The element whose atoms have the greatest number of electrons in their outer shell is the element whose atomic number is
    (A) 2
    (B) 7
    (C) 11
    (D) 12
    (E) 4

57. The statement "If 0.003 moles of gas are dissolved in 900 grams of water under 1 atmosphere pressure, 0.006 moles will be dissolved if the pressure is 2 atmospheres" illustrates
    (A) Dalton's Law of Partition
    (B) Graham's Law

(C) Raoult's Law
(D) Boyle's Law
(E) Henry's Law

58. Acetic acid may be made by the
    (A) oxidation of ethyl alcohol
    (B) destructive distillation of soft coal
    (C) polymerization of ethylene
    (D) esterification of propionic acid
    (E) reduction of acetone

59. $_{20}Ca^{40}$ and $_{18}Ar^{40}$ are examples of
    (A) isotopes
    (B) isomers
    (C) isobars
    (D) lanthanides
    (E) isotones

60. The number of molecules of water needed to convert one molecule of P_2O_5 into orthophosphoric acid, H_3PO_4, is
    (A) 1
    (B) 2
    (C) 3
    (D) 4
    (E) 5

61. The most probable valence of an element with an electronic distribution of $1s^2 2s^2 2p^6 3s^2 3p^1$ is
    (A) + 1
    (B) + 2
    (C) + 3
    (D) − 1
    (E) − 2

62. Of the following, the compound possessing optical isomerism is
    (A) $CH_3 \cdot CH_2OH$
    (B) $CH_2OH \cdot CHOH \cdot CH_2OH$
    (C) CCl_2F_2
    (D) CCl_2BrF_2
    (E) $CH_3 \cdot CHOH \cdot C_2H_5$

63. An element X is found to combine with oxygen to form a compound with the molecular formula X_4O_6. If 8.40 g of the element X combine with 6.50 g of oxygen, the atomic weight of the element is
    (A) 24.0 a.m.u.
    (B) 31.0 a.m.u.

(C) 50.4 a.m.u.
(D) 118.7 a.m.u.
(E) 70.3 a.m.u.

64. Which one of the following is an illustration of a reversible reaction?
(A) $Pb(NO_3)_2 + 2NaI \rightarrow PbI_2 + 2NaNO_3$
(B) $AgNO_3 + NaCl \rightarrow AgCl + NaNO_3$
(C) $2Na + 2HOH \rightarrow 2NaOH + H_2$
(D) $AgNO_3 + HBr \rightarrow AgBr + HNO_3$
(E) $KNO_3 + NaCl \rightarrow KCl + NaNO_3$

65. Approximately how many grams of copper will be deposited from a solution of $CuSO_4$ by 0.5 faraday of electricity? (Atomic weights: $Cu = 64$; $S = 32$; $O = 16$)
(A) 16
(B) 32
(C) 48
(D) 64
(E) 128

66. If the dissociation constant of NH_4OH is 1.8×10^{-5}, the concentration of OH^- ions, in moles per liter, of a 0.1 molar NH_4OH solution is
(A) 1.80×10^{-6}
(B) 1.34×10^{-3}
(C) 4.20×10^{-3}
(D) 5.00×10^{-2}
(E) 1.80×10^{-4}

67. The volume of 0.25 molar H_3PO_4 necessary to neutralize 25 ml of 0.30 molar $Ca(OH)_2$ is
(A) 8.3 ml
(B) 20 ml
(C) 50 ml
(D) 75 ml
(E) 40 ml

68. The mole fraction of methanol in a water solution containing 80% methanol (Atomic weights: $C = 12$; $H = 1$; $O = 16$) is closest to
(A) 0.3
(B) 0.5
(C) 0.2
(D) 0.9
(E) 0.8

69. Which one of the following statements about $AgNO_3$ is true?

(A) $AgNO_3$ has a negative heat of solution.
(B) The precipitation of $AgNO_3$ is endothermic.
(C) The hydration energy of $AgNO_3$ is negative.
(D) The hydration energy of $AgNO_3$ exceeds its lattice energy.
(E) $AgNO_3$ is paramagnetic.

70. When $CaCN_2$ reacts with steam or hot water, the nitrogen compound formed is
(A) N_2O
(B) NO
(C) NO_2
(D) NH_3
(E) $(CN)_2$

71. Of the following, the compound that obeys the *octet* rule is
(A) CO_2
(B) BCl_3
(C) PCl_5
(D) OsF_8
(E) SiF_6

72. The heaviest of the following particles is
(A) S^{-2}
(B) S^0
(C) S^{+4}
(D) S^{+6}
(E) S^{-4}

73. The substance among the following with the highest vapor pressure is
(A) solid $Na_2SO_4 \cdot 10H_2O$
(B) liquid CS_2
(C) liquid H_2SO_4
(D) solid I_2
(E) CH_4

74. Real gases will approach the behavior of an ideal gas at
(A) low temperatures and high pressures
(B) high temperatures and low pressures
(C) low temperatures and low pressures
(D) high temperatures and high pressures
(E) none of the above

75. Of the following, a particle which *cannot* be accelerated in a particle accelerator is
(A) an alpha particle

(B) an electron
(C) an ion of carbon
(D) a neutron
(E) a proton

76. The mole fraction of nitrogen in a mixture containing 70 grams of nitrogen, 128 grams of oxygen, and 44 grams of carbon dioxide is
(A) 0.29
(B) 0.33
(C) 0.36
(D) 0.50
(E) 0.12

77. When the temperature of 23 ml of dry CO_2 gas is increased from 10°C to 30°C, at a constant pressure of 760 mm, the volume of gas becomes closest to which one of the following?
(A) 7.7 ml
(B) 21.5 ml
(C) 24.6 ml
(D) 69 ml
(E) 35 ml

78. An element that has a specific heat of .166 cal/gm$^-$°C has an atomic weight of approximately
(A) 28 grams/mole
(B) 14 grams/mole
(C) 56 grams/mole
(D) 36 grams/mole
(E) 96 grams/mole

79. How many are the possible results for the measurement of the z component of the orbital angular momentum for a hydrogen atom in a 3d state (n = 3, 1 = 2)?
(A) 1
(B) 2
(C) 3
(D) 4
(E) 5

80. H_2O has its boiling point at 100 and H_2Se has its boiling point at −42°C. This could be explained by
(A) Van der Waal's force considerations
(B) covalent bonding considerations
(C) ionic bonding considerations

(D) molecular weight differences
(E) hydrogen bonding considerations

81. The smallest ionic radius belongs to which one of the following ions? (Periodic Table appears on page 88.)
(A) K^+
(B) Ca^{++}
(C) Sc^{+++}
(D) Ti^{+++}
(E) Ti^{++++}

82. The most acidic among the following is
(A) $C_6H_5SO_3H$
(B) C_2H_5OH
(C) CH_3CHO
(D) CH_3COCH_3
(E) $(CH_3)_3CH$

83. Assuming that the NH^+_3 radical is planar and has three equivalent hydrogen atoms, the hybridization of the bonding should be
(A) sp^3
(B) sp
(C) sp^2
(D) sd^2
(E) sd^3

84. When KNO_3 dissolves in a beaker of water, it dissociates according to the equation $KNO_3 + 8500$ Cal. $\rightarrow K^+ + NO_3^-$. It follows that
(A) the ions contain less energy than molecular KNO_3
(B) the water will become warmer
(C) 8500 calories will be given off during the ionization of 1 gram molecular weight of KNO_3
(D) the beaker will become cooler
(E) the temperature of the beaker will be kept constant

85. The slow partial oxidation of ethyl alcohol results in the formation of
(A) acetone
(B) acetic acid
(C) butyric acid
(D) propionic acid
(E) acetaldehyde

86. An example of a buffer solution is

(A) $HC_2H_3O_2 + NaC_2H_3O_2$
(B) $HCl + HC_2H_3O_2$
(C) $NaOH + NH_4OH$
(D) $HCl + NaCl$
(E) $NaOH + NaCl$

87. If a system is caused to change reversibly from an initial state to a final state by adiabatic means only,
(A) the work done is different for different adiabatic paths connecting the two states
(B) the work done is the same for all adiabatic paths connecting the two states
(C) there is no work done since there is no transfer of heat energy
(D) the total internal energy of the system will not change
(E) the total internal energy of the system will change according to different paths

Physics

(*Suggested time: 50 minutes*)

88. An object of mass m_1 dropped from height h_1 strikes the ground at velocity v_1. Another object of mass m_2 is then dropped from a height h_2 equal to $4h_1$. It will strike the ground at a velocity v_2 equal to (neglect air resistance)
(A) v_1
(B) $2v_1$
(C) $4v_1$
(D) $\frac{1}{2}v_1$
(E) cannot be determined from the information given

89. The velocity of light in a dense medium is found to be equal to 1×10^{10} cm/sec. What is the index of refraction of the medium (the velocity of light in a vacuum is 3×10^{10} cm/sec)?
(A) $\frac{1}{3}$
(B) $\frac{2}{3}$
(C) $\frac{3}{2}$
(D) $\frac{3}{1}$
(E) $\frac{9}{1}$

90. The force of gravitational attraction between two bodies is F. If the distance between them is doubled and their masses are doubled,
(A) F will double
(B) F will halve
(C) F will remain the same
(D) F will quadruple
(E) F will be quartered

91. A block of wood floats in liquid A with 20% of its volume above the surface. If the specific gravities of liquids A and B are in the ratio 2:3, what percent of the block's volume will float above the surface in liquid B?
(A) 20%
(B) 30%
(C) 40%
(D) $13\frac{1}{3}\%$
(E) 50%

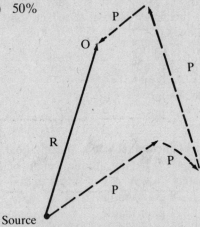

92. In the preceding diagram are represented two sound waves, both of which are produced by the same source. Wave R's path is represented by a solid line, whereas that of wave P is represented by a dotted line. Assuming that this diagram is drawn to scale, which of the following statements is not likely to be accurate regarding the sound intensity at point 0?
(A) It is greater for wave P than for wave R.
(B) It is greater for wave R than for wave P.
(C) It is equal for both waves.
(D) It cannot be determined without knowing the frequency of the sound.
(E) It cannot be determined without knowing the medium's characteristics.

93. Given a charge, q, and an electric field, E, at

a given point in space, what else is necessary to determine the force on q?

(A) the distance, r, to the charge distribution that has created the electric field
(B) the value of the potential, v, at the given point in space
(C) both the distance to the charge distribution and the potential are necessary
(D) information as to whether the charge is positive or negative
(E) none of the above

94. After two days, 6.25% of a sample of radioactive nuclei remains. What is the half-life of the element?
(A) 24 hours
(B) 18 hours
(C) 16 hours
(D) 12 hours
(E) 6 hours

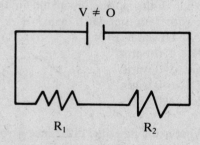

95. What is the ratio of the current through R_1 to the current through R_2 in the preceding diagram?
(A) R_1/R_2
(B) R_2/R_1
(C) $R_1 + R_2/R_1R_2$
(D) $R_1R_2/R_1 + R_2$
(E) none of the above

96. Above is a representation of two equipotential surfaces due to an electric species. What

is the general direction of the electric field in this area of space?

(A)
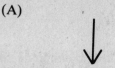

(B)
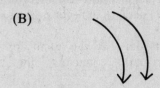

(C)
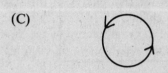

(D)
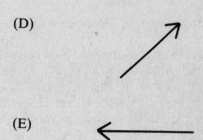

(E)

97. A string that can sustain a tension of 25 newtons is fastened to a mass of 2 kg lying on a smooth table. The largest acceleration in m/sec^2 that can be imparted to the mass without breaking the string is equal to
(A) 6.25
(B) 12.5
(C) 27
(D) 36
(E) 50

98. A 180-pound man stands in an elevator. The force, in pounds, that the floor exerts on the man when the elevator is moving upward, but decelerating at 8 ft/sec^2, is closest to which one of the following?

(A) 23
(B) 90
(C) 180
(D) 225
(E) 135

(C) $_{86}Rn^{223}$

(D) $_{86}Rn^{222}$

(E) $_{80}Rn^{222}$

Use the illustration that follows to answer questions 99 and 100:

The frictionless incline below has been placed at the surface of the earth. (Do not neglect air friction.)

Use the illustration that follows to answer questions 102 and 103:

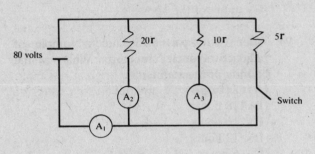

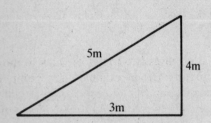

(Acceleration due to gravity = 9.8 m/sec).

99. How much work is necessary to move a 5-kilogram block to the top of the incline?
    (A) 160 Kg−m^2/sec^2
    (B) 184 Kg−m^2/sec^2
    (C) 196 Kg−m^2/sec^2
    (D) 210 Kg−m^2/sec^2
    (E) It cannot be determined from the information given.

100. Suppose that the block is dropped from the top of the plane and reaches the ground at a velocity of 8 m/sec. Approximately what percent of its energy was lost while falling through the air?
    (A) 0
    (B) 5
    (C) 10
    (D) 20
    (E) It cannot be determined from the information given.

101. The emission of an alpha particle from the nucleus of $_{88}Ra^{226}$ will produce
    (A) $_{88}Ra^{222}$
    (B) $_{87}Fr^{222}$

102. What is the power dissipated in the 10 r resistor with the switch open?
    (A) 60 watts
    (B) 120 watts
    (C) 360 watts
    (D) 640 watts
    (E) 800 watts

103. What is the potential difference across the 5 r resistor with the switch closed?
    (A) 16 volts
    (B) 32 volts
    (C) 68 volts
    (D) 80 volts
    (E) none of the above

104. A current of 5 amp exists in a 10-ohm resistance for 4 min. How many coulombs pass through any cross section of the resistor in this time?
    (A) 1.2 coul
    (B) 12 coul
    (C) 120 coul
    (D) 1200 coul
    (E) 12,000 coul

105. A parallel-plate capacitor is charged and then disconnected from the charging battery. If the plates of the capacitor are then

moved farther apart by the use of insulated handles, which one of the following results?
(A) The charge on the capacitor increases.
(B) The charge on the capacitor decreases.
(C) The capacitance of the capacitor increases.
(D) The voltage across the capacitor remains the same.
(E) The voltage across the capacitor increases.

106. A piece of copper wire is cut into ten equal parts. These parts are connected in parallel. The joint resistance of the parallel combination will be equal to the original resistance of the single wire, multiplied by a factor of
(A) .01
(B) .10
(C) 10
(D) 100
(E) .20

Use the diagram that follows to answer questions 107 and 108:

An object is placed inside the focal length of a convex lens, as shown below.

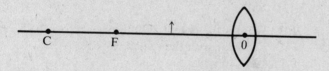

C = the center of the curvature of the lens
F = the focal point

107. The image formed will be
(A) virtual and erect
(B) virtual and inverted
(C) real and erect
(D) real and inverted
(E) none of the above

108. Suppose now that the object, as shown in the diagram, is 10 cm from the lens, and that the image formed is 40 cm on the other side of the lens. What else is necessary to determine the size of the object?
(A) the focal length, f
(B) the magnification, M
(C) the size of the image, Si
(D) both the focal length, f, and the magnification, M
(E) the focal length, f, the magnification, M, and the size of the image, Si

109. The capacitance between two parallel plates is 2x and the potential difference across the plates is 4x. What is the energy stored in the capacitor?
(A) $2x^2$
(B) $4x^2$
(C) $8x^2$
(D) $16x^3$
(E) $2x^3$

110. If it requires two joules of work to move 20 coulombs from point A to point B, a distance of 0.2 meter, the potential difference between points A and B, in volts, is
(A) 2×10^{-2}
(B) 4×10^{-2}
(C) 4×10^{-1}
(D) 8
(E) 1×10^{-1}

111. A parallel-plate capacitor with 0.3 cm thickness of air between its two plates has a capacitance of 15 $\mu\mu f$. When the air is replaced by mica (dielectric constant = 6), the capacitance, in $\mu\mu f$, becomes
(A) 5
(B) 15
(C) 90
(D) 300
(E) 2.5

112. The potential at a point 0.5×10^{-8} cm from a proton whose positive charge is 4.8×10^{-10} esu, is (1 statvolt = 300 volts)
(A) 28.8 volts
(B) 288 volts
(C) 2.88 volts
(D) 0.288 volts
(E) 0.0288 volts

113. Classically, an electron of a hydrogen atom moves in a circular orbit of radius 0.53×10^{-8} cm with a frequency of 6.6×10^{15} sec^{-1}. The current in this orbit is

(A) 1.05×10^{-4} amp
(B) 1.05×10^{-3} amp
(C) 1.05×10^{-1} amp
(D) 1.05×10^{-5} amp
(E) 1.05×10^{-2} amp

114. Two series-connected capacitors of capacitance 0.5 μf and 1.0 μf are connected to a 220 V d.c. source. The net charge on each capacitor plate is
(A) 6.30×10^{-9} coulomb
(B) 7.3×10^{-5} coulomb
(C) 3.15×10^{-7} coulomb
(D) 3.15×10^{-3} coulomb
(E) 3.15×10^{-1} coulomb

115. How long does it take a radioactive isotope to lose at least 99% of its radioactivity?
(A) two half-lives
(B) four half-lives
(C) seven half-lives
(D) fifteen half-lives
(E) twenty half-lives

116. In order for a 30-volt lamp to work properly when inserted in a 120-volt dc line, it should have in series with it a resistor whose resistance, in ohms, is
(A) 10
(B) 20
(C) 30
(D) 40
(E) 50

117. A ray of light in a dense liquid, index of refraction = 1.4, approaches the boundary surface between the liquid and air at an angle of incidence whose sine = 0.8. Which of the following statements best apply?
(A) It is impossible to predict the behavior of the light ray on the basis of the information supplied.
(B) The sine of the angle of refraction of the emergent ray will be less than 0.8.
(C) The ray will be internally reflected.
(D) The sine of the angle of refraction of the emergent ray will be greater than 0.8.
(E) The ray will be totally absorbed.

118. What is particle Z in the nuclear reaction below?

$$iH + 96 \text{ cm} \rightarrow 97Bk \quad Z$$

$$97 \text{ Bk} \rightarrow 98 \text{ Cf} + iH + y$$

(A) an electron
(B) a positron
(C) a proton
(D) an alpha particle
(E) a neutron

119. If a parallel beam of light of energy density U falls normally on an object and is totally reflected, the pressure it exerts on the object is given by

(A) $p = U/c$
(B) $p = \frac{1}{3}U$
(C) $p = Uc$
(D) $p = 2U$
(E) $p = U/2c$

120. Two men together hold a uniform rod (or plank). At the instant one of the men lets go of his end of the rod, the other feels the force on his hand changed to (W = weight of rod)

(A) $\frac{1}{3} W$
(B) $\frac{1}{4} W$
(C) $\frac{1}{6} W$
(D) $\frac{1}{2} W$
(E) $\frac{3}{4} W$

121. The resistance of a metallic element whose temperature is lowered
(A) is always increased
(B) is always decreased
(C) may be either increased or decreased
(D) is at first increased and then decreased
(E) always remains constant

122. A ball is thrown vertically into the air. When it reaches its zenith, which of the following statements is most correct?

(A) The potential energy is at a minimum and the kinetic energy is at a maximum.

(B) The potential energy is at a maximum and the kinetic energy is at a minimum

(C) The potential energy and the kinetic energy are both at a maximum.

(D) The potential energy and the kinetic energy are both at a minimum

(E) The potential energy and the kinetic energy are equal.

123. If a sphere and a cylinder start from rest at the same position and roll down the same incline (moments of inertia: cylinder = $\frac{1}{2}MR^2$; sphere = $\frac{2}{5}MR^2$),

(A) the cylinder will reach the bottom first.

(B) the sphere will reach the bottom first

(C) they will reach the bottom at the same time

124. A gravitational field is a conservative field. The work done in this field by transporting an object from one point to another

(A) depends on the end points only

(B) depends on the path along which the object is transported

(C) depends on both the end points and the path between these points.

125. Assume that two capacitors, one of 3 microfarads and the other of 6 microfarads, are connected in series and charged to a difference of potential of 120 volts. The potential difference, in volts, across the 3 microfarad capacitor is

(A) 40

(B) 50

(C) 80

(D) 180

(E) 360

STOP

END OF SCIENCE KNOWLEDGE QUESTIONS

Section 2: SCIENCE PROBLEMS

Time: 85 minutes
66 questions

Directions: There are 22 sets of problems, each containing three related questions. Choose the one best answer from the lettered choices that follow each question.

Consider the following reaction and the results of four independent measurements made in an experiment to determine the relationship between reactant concentration and reaction rate.

$$A(g) \rightarrow B(g) + C(g)$$

	Measurement # 1	Measurement # 2	Measurement # 3	Measurement # 4
Concentration of A (moles/liter)	.10	.20	.30	.40
Rate of reaction (moles/liter = seconds)	.030	.120	.270	.480

1. What is the order of the reaction with respect to $A(g)$?
   - (A) 0
   - (B) 1
   - (C) 2
   - (D) 3
   - (E) 4

2. What is the rate constant for the reaction?
   - (A) 1 liter/mole = sec
   - (B) 2 liters/mole = sec
   - (C) 3 liters/mole = sec
   - (D) 4 liters/mole = sec
   - (E) 5 liters/mole = sec

3. Suppose the reaction were zero order with respect to A(g). A plot of reaction rate versus [A(g)] would be
   - (A) linear in nature
   - (B) quadratic in nature
   - (C) exponential in nature

An optical fiber, index of refraction n_2, is submerged in human tissue, index of refraction $n_1 < n_2$. Angle β is sufficiently great such that there is total internal reflection of the monochromatic red light (represented by the connecting arrows).

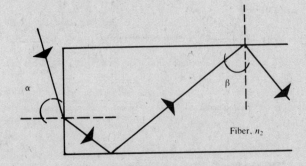

4. What is the index of refraction of the tissue, n_1, in terms of α, β, and n_2?
   (A) $n_1 = n_2 \sin \beta / \sin \alpha$
   (B) $n_1 = n_2 \sin \alpha / \sin \beta$
   (C) $n_1 = n_2 \sin \beta / n_2 \sin \alpha$
   (D) $n_1 = n_2 \cos \beta / \sin \alpha$
   (E) $n_1 = n_2 \sin \beta / \cos \alpha$

5. Which of the following did *not* occur when the light entered the optical fiber?
   (A) its wavelength decreased
   (B) its velocity decreased
   (C) its frequency remained the same
   (D) its period decreased
   (E) none of the above

6. What effect, if any, would using blue light instead of red have on the angle β?
   (A) Angle β would increase.
   (B) Angle β would decrease.
   (C) Angle β would remain the same.

When the straight chain molecule D–glucose undergoes self-conversion to its ring form, C1 becomes chiral and the need arises to distinguish between the resulting anomers.

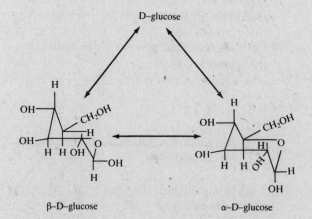

D–glucose

β–D–glucose   α–D–glucose

The molecule is constantly flipping back and forth from its ring to its straight chain form.

7. Upon conversion from the straight chain to the ring, the molecule must react "with itself." Which two carbons are most directly involved in this reaction?
   (A) C1 and C5
   (B) C1 and C6
   (C) C2 and C5
   (D) C2 and C6
   (E) C3 and C4

8. Unequal amounts of α and β–D–glucose are placed in the same beaker. Comparing the absolute amounts of the anomers *after* equilibrium has been established, one finds that
   (A) there will be more α than β
   (B) there will be more β than α
   (C) there will be equal amounts of α and β

9. Six-membered rings like α and β–D–glucose are called pyranoses. Five-membered rings are called furanoses. One would expect to find, generally, that
   (A) pyranoses are more reactive than furanoses
   (B) furanoses are more reactive than pyranoses
   (C) they are of equal reactivity

A culture of eukaryotic cells was grown in a medium containing the following radioactively labeled species.

    I.   uracil
   II.   cytosine
  III.   glucose
  IV.   glycine (an amino acid)

10. It was later discovered that several mitochondria were labeled. Which of the above could have been responsible?
    (A) species I only
    (B) species II only
    (C) species III only
    (D) species II and III only

11. Which of the following organelles would you

expect to have been labeled by species IV?
(A) Golgi bodies
(B) smooth endoplasmic reticulum
(C) rough endoplasmic reticulum
(D) Golgi bodies and rough endoplasmic reticulum
(E) Golgi bodies, smooth endoplasmic reticulum, and rough endoplasmic reticulum

12. Suppose now that bacteria had been grown in the same medium. Which of the species could have been responsible for labeling the bacteria?
(A) I, II, and III only
(B) II, III, and IV only
(C) I, III, and IV only
(D) I, II, and IV only
(E) I, II, III, and IV

In an attempt to lower the body temperature of a patient with an excessively high fever, a cooling bath of distilled water was prepared.

13. If the nurse in charge of the task begins with 100 kilograms of water at 40°C, how many grams of water at 10°C must he or she add to lower the temperature of the bath to 30°C?
(A) 25,000
(B) 50,000
(C) 100,000
(D) 150,000
(E) none of these

14. When it was determined that the patient's body temperature was not decreasing at a rapid enough rate, a decision was made to place 10,000 grams of ice into the bath. By how many degrees centigrade will a 100-kilogram bath at 30°C be lowered upon melting 10,000 grams of ice? (The heat of fusion of ice is 80 cal/gram.)
(A) 2
(B) 4
(C) 6
(D) 8
(E) 10

15. After the ice was added, there was no futher human intervention. The system (patient plus

bath plus added water and ice) then underwent
(A) an increase in entropy
(B) a decrease in entropy
(C) no change in entropy

The graph that follows depicts the decay of a radioactive tracer.

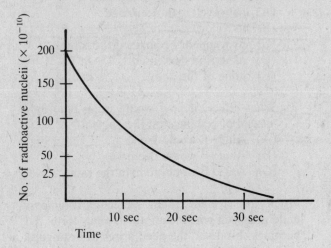

16. What is the half-life of the tracer?
(A) 10 sec
(B) 15 sec
(C) 20 sec
(D) 30 sec
(E) none of these

17. After 40 sec, what percent of the radioactive nuclei will remain?
(A) 25%
(B) 12½%
(C) 6¼%
(D) 3⅛%
(E) It cannot be determined from the information given.

18. Approximately how long will it take for all of the nuclei to decay?
(A) 50 sec
(B) 60 sec
(C) 70 sec
(D) 80 sec
(E) none of these

A blood vessel segment was taken from a woman suffering from blockage of the arteries. In the cross section that follows, the shaded portion represents the material that has accumulated on the vessel wall.

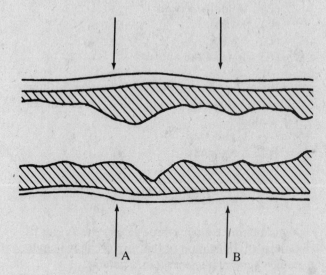

A   B

19. In an experiment to determine the effects of the blockage, blood was passed through the vessel. At point A (radius = 10 μm) the blood traveled at 30 ft/sec. At what speed did the blood travel at point B (radius = 5 μm)?
    (A) 15 ft/sec
    (B) 30 ft/sec
    (C) 60 ft/sec
    (D) 120 ft/sec
    (E) 240 ft/sec

20. A blood platelet (weight in vacuum = 3×10^{-3} dynes) was removed from the patient. It weighed 2×10^{-3} dynes when allowed to submerge in water and 1×10^{-3} dynes when allowed to submerge in blood plasma. What is the specific gravity of the blood plasma?

    (A) $\frac{2}{3}$
    (B) $1\frac{1}{3}$
    (C) $1\frac{2}{3}$
    (D) 2
    (E) $2\frac{2}{3}$

21. Suppose that the blood velocity is equal to

zero at all points in a circulatory system. The pressure at any point depends on
    (A) the density of the blood only
    (B) the depth as measured from the top of the containing system only
    (C) both the density of the blood and the depth as measured from the top of the containing system

22. A large number of homozygous polled (hornless) red bulls were mated to horned white cows. Their offspring were polled roan. Roan is a color that is intermediate between red and white. Which of the following is most likely correct?
    (A) Polled is dominant and roan shows incomplete dominance.
    (B) Polled and roan are linked traits.
    (C) Polled is hybrid and roan is a pure trait.

23. Producing an F_2 from the preceding progeny would result in which one of the following ratios?
    (A) 3:2:2:1
    (B) 1:2:2:1
    (C) 9:6:6:1
    (D) 6:3:3:1
    (E) 9:3:3:1

24. The F_2 offspring of the cross of polled roan cattle referred to above give evidence of which one of the following?
    (A) epistasis
    (B) linkage
    (C) dominance
    (D) independent assortment
    (E) segregation

Consider the generalized equilibrium that follows:

$$A + B \rightleftharpoons C$$

25. What effect does increasing the pressure have on the reaction?
    (A) The reaction is driven to the left.
    (B) The reaction is driven to the right.
    (C) The reaction is not affected.
    (D) It cannot be determined from the information given.

26. Suppose that the reaction were exothermic.

What effect would raising the temperature have?
(A) The reaction would be driven to the left.
(B) The reaction would be driven to the right.
(C) The reaction would not be affected.
(D) It cannot be determined from the information given.

27. Which of the following will drive the reaction to the right?
(A) addition of A
(B) removal of B
(C) addition of C
(D) none of these

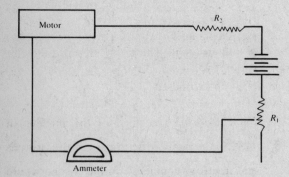

The type of circuit diagrammed above is useful in the design of the latest generation of electronic cardiac pacemakers. In this particular circuit, a 16-volt battery supplies a motor whose resistance is 4 ohms. The motor is in series with the "indicator resistor" R_2 and a variable resistor R_1, which controls the frequency of the impulses.

28. R_1 is set so that the ammeter reads 1 ampere. What would be the combined resistance of R_1 and R_2 under these conditions?
(A) 4 ohms
(B) 8 ohms
(C) 12 ohms

(D) 16 ohms
(E) none of the above

29. The power dissipated by the motor when the ammeter reads 1 ampere is
(A) 4 joules
(B) 16 joules/second
(C) 8 watts
(D) 4 watts
(E) none of the above

30. When the ammeter reads 0.5 amperes, how much will pass through the motor in 10 seconds?
(A) 1 coulomb
(B) 5 coulombs
(C) 10 coulombs
(D) 25 coulombs
(E) 50 coulombs

A gas mixture contains three gases—gas A, gas B, and gas C. Inhalation of this mixture may help to induce general anesthesia in a patient.

Gas	Partial Pressure (mm Hg)
gas A	500
gas B	300
gas C	720

31. If ideal gas behavior is assumed, what is the approximate mole fraction of gas B in the mixture?
(A) 1/10
(B) 1/5
(C) 1/4
(D) 1/3
(E) 1/2

32. What is the pressure of the gas mixture if it is administered as above?
(A) 0.25 atm
(B) 0.50 atm
(C) 1.00 atm
(D) 2.00 atm
(E) 3.00 atm

33. The mixture is administered at a rate of 11 liters/minute. If gas C makes up 12% of the mixture, approximately how many moles/minute of gas C are being administered?

(Assume ideal gas properties and STP conditions.)
(A) .06
(B) .12
(C) 1.0
(D) 1.1
(E) 1.2

Colchicine is a drug that has been demonstrated to be an inhibitor of mitosis when applied to human cells in vitro. It has, therefore, been proposed that colchicine may be used in the treatment of cancer, a disease for which a disorderly and frequently unrestricted multiplication of cells is perhaps the cardinal feature.

34. A newly-fertilized human egg is immediately transferred to an in vitro culture system. Approximately how many hours after fertilization occurs could attainment of the two-cell stage be expected, assuming that the culture system allows for precise replication of normal in vivo results?
(A) 10 hours
(B) 20 hours
(C) 30 hours
(D) 40 hours
(E) 48 hours

35. It has been demonstrated repeatedly that the mitotic disturbance associated with colchicine always occurs during the metaphase stage. On this basis, which of the following is the most likely action of colchicine?
(A) destruction of DNA polymerase
(B) disruption of the cleavage furrow
(C) disruption of synapsis
(D) impairment of the formation of the spindle apparatus
(E) destruction of the nucleolus

36. Concern has been expressed that in vivo administration of colchicine may produce considerable damage in normal as well as in cancer cells. Which of the following human cell types could be expected to show the *least* effect from in vivo colchicine administration?
(A) red blood cell precursors in the bone marrow
(B) mature liver cells

(C) mature nerve cells
(D) mature intestinal lining cells possessing villi
(E) None of the above are likely to be affected by colchicine administration.

$$^{131}_{53}X \longrightarrow {}^{131}_{54}Y + Z$$

The half life of $^{131}_{53}X$ is 9 seconds.

37. How long does it take for 75% of a small sample of $^{131}_{53}X$ to decay by this process?
(A) 4.5 seconds
(B) 9 seconds
(C) 18 seconds
(D) 27 seconds
(E) 36 seconds

38. On comparing the mass of the nucleus of $^{131}_{53}X$ to the sum of the masses of the protons and neutrons contained within it, one would find that
(A) the mass of the nucleus is greater than the sum of its parts (protons and neutrons)
(B) the mass of the nucleus is less than the sum of its parts (protons and neutrons)
(C) the mass of the nucleus is equal to the sum of its parts (protons and neutrons)

39. Combination of $^{131}_{54}Y$ with a positron yields only a new element, the atomic and mass numbers of which are, respectively,
(A) 53, 132
(B) 55, 132
(C) 56, 135
(D) 55, 131
(E) 54, 132

B is color-blind and heterozygous for brown eyes. A does not carry any genes for color blindness. She has green eyes.

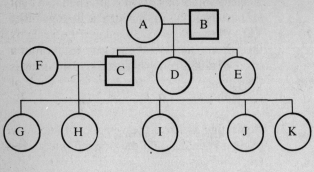

$\square$ = Male
$\bigcirc$ = Female

40. Which best represents the genetic makeup for eye color of H?
    (A) homozygous brown
    (B) homozygous green
    (C) heterozygous brown
    (D) heterozygous green
    (E) It cannot be determined from the information given.

41. If E marries a male who is color-blind, which statement is true?
    (A) All of her sons will be color-blind.
    (B) All of her daughters will carry at least one gene for color blindness.
    (C) All of her daughters will be color-blind.
    (D) 50% of her sons may be color-blind, but none of her daughters may be color-blind.

42. The probability that the next child born to F and C will be male is closest to which of the following?
    (A) 0%
    (B) 16%
    (C) 83%
    (D) 50%
    (E) 100%

Blood is one of the many buffered body fluids. Significant deviations from its normal pH value of 7.4 are sometimes life-threatening.

Consider a generalized buffer solution containing the very weak acid HA and its conjugate base, A^-.

$$HA \rightarrow H^+ + A^- \qquad K_a = 1 \times 10^{-5}$$

43. If a 1-liter solution contains .22 moles of HA and .22 moles of A^-, what is its pH?
    (A) 4.4
    (B) 4.6
    (C) 4.8
    (D) 5.0
    (E) 5.2

44. Suppose that .18 mole of HCl is added to the solution above. What is the resulting pH? (Assume that all of the HCl that dissociates, reacts.)
    (A) 4.8
    (B) 5.4
    (C) 5.8
    (D) 6.0
    (E) 6.4

45. Approximately how may equivalents are present in 12 g of HCl (atomic weights: H = 1, Cl = 35.5)?
    (A) .17
    (B) .33
    (C) .50
    (D) .66
    (E) .75

A new device has been devised to allow physicians to visualize directly the minute blood vessels found on the retina of the eye. The device consists of a light source and a concave mirror. An examination using this device may reveal vascular changes associated with hypertension and diabetes mellitus.

46. Many of the incoming light rays regularly processed by the human eye are parallel. Where are incoming parallel light rays normally brought to a focus by a concave mirror?
    (A) between F and 2F on the opposite side of the mirror
    (B) at F on the same side of the mirror
    (C) at 2F on the opposite side of the mirror
    (D) at F on the opposite side of the mirror
    (E) beyond 2F on the opposite side of the mirror

47. A concave mirror
    (A) usually produces virtual images
    (B) acts to diverge incoming rays of light

(C) has optical effects similar to those of a convex lens

(D) more than one of the above

(E) none of the above

48. Which of the following statements about the normal human eye is *incorrect*?
(A) The parasympathetic nervous system promotes constriction of the pupils.
(B) More of the refraction of incoming light rays is performed by the cornea than by the lens.
(C) The optic nerve has both motor and sensory functions.
(D) more than one of the above
(E) none of the above

The diagram that follows depicts the phase changes of water.

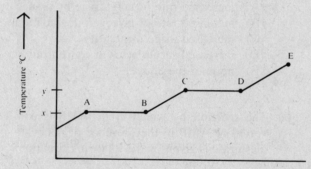

49. "$x = 0°C.$" This statement is
(A) supported by the given information
(B) contradicted by the given information
(C) neither supported nor contradicted by the given information

50. What is the point of greatest entropy?
(A) A
(B) B
(C) C
(D) D
(E) E

51. As the temperature is being increased from $x°C$ to $y°C$,
(A) ice is melting
(B) ice is increasing in temperature
(C) water is boiling
(D) none of these

A small object of mass m is attached to a light string which passes through a hollow tube. The tube is held by one hand and the string by the other. The object is set into rotation in a circle of radius r_1 with a speed s_1. The string is then pulled down, shortening the radius of the path to r_2.

52. Neglecting gravity, the relation of the new angular speed ω_2 and the original one ω_1 is
(A) $\omega_2 = (r_1/r_2)\omega_1$
(B) $\omega_2 = (r_1/r_2)^2\omega_1$
(C) $\omega_2 = (r_2/r_1)\omega_1$
(D) $\omega_2 = (r_2/r_1)^2\omega_1$
(E) $\omega_2 = \omega_1$

53. The ratio of the new kinetic energy to the original kinetic energy is
(A) $(r_1/r_2)^2$
(B) r_1/r_2
(C) 1
(D) r_2/r_1
(E) $(r_2/r_1)^2$

54. Again neglecting gravity and assuming that the radius, r_1, and the speed, s_1, remain constant, what can be concluded about the linear acceleration, $\vec{a}_1$?
(A) $\vec{a}_1$ varies in magnitude but not in direction.
(B) $\vec{a}_1$ varies in direction but not in magnitude.
(C) $\vec{a}_1$ varies in both magnitude and direction.
(D) $\vec{a}_1$ remains constant in magnitude and direction.

Diagram X represents the nucleus of a mature plant spermatocyte. The following questions relate to the six *numbered* diagrams immediately below diagram X.

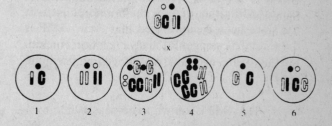

55. A functional sperm nucleus from a pollen grain produced by this plant could resemble
    (A) 1
    (B) 2
    (C) 5
    (D) 4
    (E) 6

56. If meiotic division had *not* accompanied the formation of both gametes, a nucleus of the zygote formed would most likely have resembled
    (A) 1
    (B) 2
    (C) 3
    (D) 4
    (E) 5

57. If, during meiosis, crossing over occurred between a single pair of homologous chromosomes, the nucleus of the resulting gamete would most likely resemble
    (A) 2
    (B) 3
    (C) 4
    (D) 6
    (E) 1

A major breakthrough in the elucidation of the mechanism of hormone action came about as an outgrowth of studies started in the 1950s. At that time, a molecule known as cyclic AMP was identified. It was shown that cyclic AMP is formed from ATP by the action of a membrane-bound enzyme known as adenyl cyclase. It was proposed that cyclic AMP acts as a "second messenger" in the action of some hormones, the first messenger being the hormone itself. An important feature of this "second messenger" model is that the hormone need not enter the cell. Its impact is made at the cell membrane, where adenyl cyclase is stimulated by the hormone to generate cyclic AMP. The biologic effects of the hormone are then mediated inside the cell by cyclic AMP rather than by the hormone itself. It has since been demonstrated that cyclic AMP is the second messenger for many hormones, including thyroxine and thyroid-stimulating hormone (TSH).

58. Cyclic AMP is known to be deactivated by a specific phosphodiesterase enzyme, which hydrolyzes cyclic AMP to AMP. It has been shown that the drug theophylline is an inhibitor of this phosphodiesterase enzyme. Which of the following is a likely effect of an overdose of theophylline in a patient with normal thyroxine and TSH levels?
    (A) decreased basal metabolic rate
    (B) diminished knee-jerk reflexes
    (C) decreased heart rate
    (D) decreased breathing rate
    (E) none of the above

59. It is known that cyclic AMP also acts as a second messenger for epinephrine, glucagon, norepinephrine, vasopressin, and parathyroid hormone. On this basis, which of the following is *not* among the likely effects of cyclic AMP?
    (A) increased rate of fat storage by tissues
    (B) increased rate of glycogen degradation
    (C) increased urine osmolarity
    (D) increased serum calcium concentration
    (E) none of the above

60. The reaction by which cyclic AMP is converted to AMP in the presence of phosphodiesterase is given by the following equation:

$$\text{cyclic AMP} + H_2O \xrightarrow[\text{phosphodiesterase}]{Mg} AMP + H^+$$

The $\triangle G^0$ for this reaction is -12 kcal/mol. What does this value suggest?
    (A) This reaction, as written, is endothermic.
    (B) AMP is an inherently unstable molecule.
    (C) This reaction, as written, will proceed spontaneously.
    (D) The entropy of the products is greater than that of the reactants.
    (E) None of the above apply.

Base your answers on the pedigree chart that follows, where individual B is a hemophiliac male who is heterozygous for brown eyes and individual A is his blue-eyed wife who does *not* carry any genes for hemophilia.

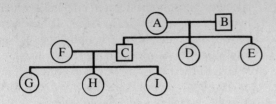

○ = female
□ = male

61. What is the probability that individual D is a hemophiliac?
(A) 0
(B) ¹⁄₁
(C) ½
(D) ⅓
(E) ¼

62. What is the probability that individual D is a carrier for hemophilia and has blue eyes?
(A) 0
(B) ¹⁄₁
(C) ½
(D) ⅓
(E) ¼

63. What is the probability that individual E is blue-eyed?
(A) ½
(B) ¼
(C) ⅛
(D) ⅓
(E) It cannot be determined from the information given.

A 20-kilogram box slides from the top of an inclined plane that is 20 meters long and 10 meters high and has an angle of inclination of 30°. The box starts from rest and strikes the ground with a velocity of 10 meters per second. (Assume that the acceleration due to gravity is 9.8 meters/sec².)

64. What is the work done by friction as the box descends the plane?
(A) 480 joules
(B) 680 joules
(C) 720 joules
(D) 960 joules
(E) none of the above

65. Which of the following is a correct expression for the coefficient of sliding friction here (m = mass of the box; g = acceleration due to gravity; F_f = force of friction; h = height of box)?

(A) $\dfrac{F_f}{mg \sin 30°}$

(B) $\dfrac{F_f}{mg \cos 30°}$

(C) $(F_f)(mg \sin 30°)$
(D) $(F_f)(mg \cos 30°)$
(E) none of the above

66. Assuming that friction does not act upon the box, what velocity would the box attain at the bottom of the incline?
(A) 10 meters/second
(B) 14 meters/second
(C) 15 meters/second
(D) 17 meters/second
(E) 20 meters/second

STOP

END OF SCIENCE PROBLEMS QUESTIONS

Section 3: SKILLS ANALYSIS—READING

Time: 85 minutes
68 questions

Directions: Select the one best answer from the lettered choices that follow each question. Each group of questions is preceded by and concerns some descriptive material presented in verbal format.

Questions 1–7

When an animal is presented with food, he will salivate. If a bell is repeatedly rung shortly before the food is administered, the animal will begin to salivate soon after the sound of the bell, even if the food is not offered. With repeated trials of the bell followed by the food (conditioning trials), the latency of the response (that is, the time interval between the advent of the bell and the beginning of salivation) decreases. This process is called conditioning, and salivation to the sound of the bell is termed the conditioned response. The conditioned response may be unlearned or extinguished if the bell is presented a number of times without being followed by food (extinction trials). Under such conditions, the latency of the conditioned response gradually increases until the response does not take place at all.

Trials that are separated by an interval of time are called distributed trials, while those which follow immediately one upon the other are called massed trials. One theory holds that after each conditioning trial a finite amount of excitation is left which facilitates the occurrence of the conditioned response, and also that a finite amount of inhibition is left which inhibits the occurrence of the conditioned response. During the conditioning trials, the excitation is built up faster than the inhibition, whereas during the extinction trials the reverse is held to be true. The strength of the conditioned response, as measured, for example, in terms of how quickly it begins after the bell is sounded, is said to be a function of the magnitude of the difference between the quantity of excitation and the quantity of inhibition. The inhibitory component disappears more quickly with the passage of time than does the excitatory component. It has been assumed that 50 percent of the inhibition is spontaneously dissipated after a few hours, while the excitation remains practically intact. The inhibitory component is also more readily destroyed upon the occurrence of some novel stimulus than is the excitatory component.

1. In experiment A the conditioning trials are massed, and in experiment B they are distributed. On the basis of the theory, after the same number of trials, the latency of the conditioned response in experiment A as compared with experiment B should be
   (A) longer
   (B) shorter
   (C) the same
   (D) unpredictable

2. If the conditioned response, salivation, is extinguished,
   (A) its latency decreases
   (B) the food was presented without the bell
   (C) the amount of inhibition is greater than the amount of excitation
   (D) the animal is no longer hungry

3. In experiment C the extinction trials are massed, and in experment D they are distributed. On the basis of the theory, the number of trials necessary to extinguish the conditioned response in experiment C as compared with experiment D should be
   (A) greater
   (B) predictable under certain conditions
   (C) the same
   (D) fewer

115

4. In experiment E an unusual tone was sounded immediately after the bell. On that trial the conditioned response failed to occur. This means that the tone was sufficiently loud to
   (A) dissipate all the excitation but none of the inhibition
   (B) dissipate all the excitation and leave some of the inhibition
   (C) dissipate all the excitation and all the inhibition
   (D) increase the excitation, but increase the inhibition more

5. On the basis of the theory, the rapidity with which a hungry animal should adopt a conditioned response as compared with a satiated animal should be
   (A) less
   (B) greater
   (C) the same
   (D) unpredictable

6. If after a series of extinction trials the animal is permitted to rest for an hour, the latency of the conditioned response on the trial following the rest as compared with the trial preceding the rest should be
   (A) less
   (B) greater
   (C) the same
   (D) unpredictable

7. After the bell sounds, the conditioned response of trial 7 of the conditioning series as compared with trial 30 should take place
   (A) more quickly
   (B) more slowly
   (C) after the same interval
   (D) sometimes more quickly and sometimes more slowly

Questions 8–14

Barring substantial climatic change, the world water supply estimate should remain constant throughout the near future, while water withdrawals climb steadily with population and rising agricultural and industrial output. Even if water withdrawals were to increase by a factor of 7 by the year 2000, only about 50 percent of aggregate supply would be withdrawn, and about 15 percent actually consumed.

Comforting as such figures may be, they are misleading. In fact, any significant increase in the rate of water withdrawal, even a doubling by the year 2000, is virtually certain to cause major water supply problems. The use of energy and other resources by the water supply sector will increase dramatically. Water shortages will become more frequent, and their effects will be more widespread and more severe. The availability of water will become an even more binding constraint on the location of economic development. The notion of water as a free good available in essentially limitless quantities will have disappeared throughout much of the world.

These less encouraging predictions stem from recognition of the intensely local nature of a water resource. There exists no world water economy, and it is rarely meaningful to speak of a national water economy. Most water economies exist within smaller hydrologic provinces, in single river basins, adjoining basins connected by water transmission facilities and the like. When the supply in such a limited area falls short of the attempted withdrawals, water shortages occur, regardless of the quantities of water available in neighboring basins. It may also be true that attempted water withdrawals cannot be maintained during a period of low streamflow, even though adequate water is available in the same stream at other times.

This nonuniform distribution of water, both in space and in time, is the fundamental cause of the uniquely local nature of water supply problems. When data are summed or averaged over a number of water supply areas, the nonuniformity is concealed, and water resources may appear to be adequate when, in fact, serious shortages are likely to occur.

When shortages do occur or are considered likely to occur, a number of steps can be taken. First, the supply may be augmented.

One approach to augmentation consists of transferring water in space and/or time so as to meet the requirements of attempted withdrawals. Water is transferred in space by constructing or employing transportation facilities (such as water transmission mains) to move water from an area where it is not required to the area of potential shortage. Water is transferred in time by constructing storage facilities, usually major impoundments on existing streams. Due to the very large quantities of water involved, transmission over large distances is very expensive, requiring large commitments of energy. Major storage projects are also expensive, and have the added disadvantage of increasing total evaporation, thus reducing the total supply available. Both actions have the potential of permanently altering natural landscapes, and of creating ecological disruptions. However, water shortages that result from a lack of adequate storage capacity may entail high economic and social costs.

Another means of supply augmentation requires increased reuse of return flows from other water users. This may require rearranging the sequence of uses so that those requiring the highest quality come first, followed by users who are increasingly tolerant of lower-quality water. More often, reuse may be increased by the installation of improved treatment facilities, either at the first user's effluent or the second user's intake. Such measures are costly, and they consume significant quantities of energy and, perhaps, various chemicals. Changes in the quality of the environment may occur directly, or as the result of decreased streamflows below the region of more intensive water use.

The second step taken in the case of water shortage involves reducing rates of water use. This may occur through economic incentive, as increasing scarcity drives the price of water higher, encouraging water users to substitute other goods or other inputs for the use of water. It may occur administratively, as users either voluntarily invoke water conservation practices or do so because of regulation or because of reductions in water allocations. Water use may also be reduced by stimulating the introduction of new, less water-intensive technology (cooling towers for power plants, or drip irrigation).

Finally, when possibilities for supply augmentation and for water-use reduction have been exhausted, and withdrawals still threaten to exceed available supply, water must be allocated among several uses, so that the damages incurred as a result of shortage will be minimized. In the absence of such allocation, the available water is used on a first come, first served basis, until the water supply fails entirely. Supply failure creates a potential for public health problems, industrial shutdowns, and massive crop failures (which also have human health implications).

Some of the measures outlined here can only be implemented after relatively long-term planning and construction (water transmission and storage facilities, for example); others are available on an immediate short-term basis (water-use reduction techniques not involving new technology). The measures requiring construction have the potential of creating adverse environmental effects, and some may imply large increases in the use of energy. It may be advantageous to engage in still longer-term planning, so as to facilitate the location of future water-using activities in areas better able to provide the necessary water. Again, these considerations and findings depend upon specific, area-by-area analyses of water supply and demand; they cannot be obtained from national aggregate data.

The statements that follow are related to the information presented above. Select

(A) if the statement is supported by the given information
(B) if the statement is contradicted by the given information
(C) if the statement is neither supported nor contradicted by the given information

8. Local water shortages can be predicted by examining the national water supply as a whole.

9. Salt- to freshwater processing plants may be introduced to alleviate water shortages.

10. Reduction of water use is superior to water reuse as a strategy in case of water shortage.

11. Water withdrawals are expected to remain constant throughout the near future.

12. The amount of water in a stream supplying a given area remains fairly constant over time.

13. Water shortages are likely to increase in frequency.

14. As far as total water supply is concerned,

transmission is superior to storage as a solution to water shortages.

Questions 15–21

Originally, fermentation used some of the most primitive forms of plant life as cell factories. Bacteria were used to make yogurt and antibiotics, yeasts to ferment wine, and the filamentous fungi or molds to produce organic acids. More recently, fermentation technology has begun to use cells derived from higher plants and animals under growth conditions known as cell or tissue culture. In all cases, large quantities of cells with uniform characteristics are grown under defined, controlled conditions.

In its simplest form, fermentation consists of mixing a micro-organism with a liquid broth and allowing the components to react. More sophisticated large-scale processes require control of the entire environment so that fermentation proceeds efficiently and, more importantly, so that it can be repeated exactly, with the same amounts of raw materials, broth, and micro-organisms producing the same amount of product. Strict control is maintained of such variables as pH, temperature, and oxygen supply. The newest fermenter models are regulated by sensors that are monitored by computers. The capacity of industrial-sized fermenters can reach 50,000 gallons or more. The one-shot system of fermentation is called batch fermentation—i.e., fermentation in which a single batch of material is processed from start to finish.

In continuous fermentation, an improvement on the batch process, fermentation goes on without interruption, with a constant input of raw materials and other nutrients and an attendant output of fermented material. The most recent approaches use micro-organisms that have been immobilized in a supporting structure. As the solution containing the raw material passes over the cells, the micro-organisms process the material and release the products into the solution flowing out of the fermenter.

In general, products obtained by fermentation also can be produced by chemical synthesis; to a lesser extent, they can be isolated by extraction from whole organs or organisms. A fermentation process is usually most competitive when the chemical process requires several individual steps to complete the conversion. In a chemical synthesis, the raw material, *a*, might have to be transformed to an intermediate, *b*, which, in turn, might have to be converted to intermediates *c* and *d* before final conversion to the product *e*—each step necessitating recovery of its products before the next conversion. In fermentation technology, all steps take place within those miniature chemical factories, the micro-organisms; the microbial chemist merely adds the raw material *a* and recovers the product *e*.

A wide variety of carbohydrate raw materials can be used in fermentation. These can be pure substances (sucrose [or table sugar], glucose, or fructose) or complex mixtures still in their original form (cornstalks, potato mash, sugar cane, sugar beets, or cellulose). They can be of recent biological origin (biomass) or derived from fossil fuels (methane or oil). The availability of raw materials varies from country to country and even from region to region within a country; the economics of the production process varies accordingly.

The cost of the raw material can contribute significantly to the cost of production. Usually, the most useful micro-organisms are those that consume readily available, inexpensive raw materials. For large-volume, low-priced products (such as commodity chemicals), the relationship between the cost of the raw material and the cost of the end product is significant. For low-volume, higher-priced products (such as certain pharmaceuticals), the relationship is negligible.

The statements that follow are related to the information presented above. Select

(A) if the statement is supported by the given information
(B) if the statement is contradicted by the given information
(C) if the statement is neither supported nor contradicted by the given information

15. Continuous fermentation is superior to batch fermentation.

16. Fermentation products can only be produced by living organisms.

17. Sucrose is superior to potato mash as a fermentation starting material.

18. The kind of raw material available dictates to some extent the choice of micro-organisms employed.

19. There is currently a search for new fermentation processes.

20. A single enzyme situated within a living cell is needed to convert a raw material into a product.

21. The fermentation process always produces intermediate products that must be recovered by the chemist and purified before conversion can continue.

Questions 22–28

Hong Kong's size and association with Britain, and its position in relation to its neighbors in the Pacific, particularly China, determine the course of conduct it has to pursue. Hong Kong is no more than a molecule in the great substance of China. It was part of the large province of Kwangtung, which came under Chinese sovereignty about 200 B.C., in the period of the Han Dynasty. In size, China exceeds 3¾ million square miles, and it has a population estimated to be greater than 850 million. Its very immensity has contributed to its survival over a great period of time. Without probing into the origins of its remarkable civilization, we can mark that it has a continuous history of more than 4,000 years. And, through the centuries, it has always been able to defend itself in depth, trading space for time.

In this setting Hong Kong is minute. Its area is a mere 398 square miles, about one two-hundredth of the province of which it was previously part, Kwangtung. Fortunately, however, we cannot dispose of Hong Kong as simply as this. There are components in its complex and unique existence which affect its character and, out of all physical proportion, increase its significance.

Amongst these, the most potent are its people, their impressive achievements in partnership with British administration and enterprise, and the rule of law which protects personal freedom in the British tradition.

What is Hong Kong, and what is it trying to do?

In 1841 Britain acquired outright, by treaty, the Island of Hong Kong, to use as a base for trade with China, and, in 1860, the Kowloon Peninsula, lying immediately to the north, to complete the perimeter of the superb harbor, which has determined Hong Kong's history and character. In 1898 Britain leased for 99 years a hinterland on the mainland of China to a depth of less than 25 miles, much of it very hilly. Hong Kong prospered as a center of trade with China, expanding steadily until it fell to the Japanese in 1941. Although the rigors of a severe occupation set everything back, the Liberation in 1945 was the herald of an immediate and spectacular recovery in trade. People poured into the Colony, and this flow became a flood during 1949–50, when the Chinese National Government met defeat at the hands of the Communists. Three-quarters of a million people entered the colony at that stage, bringing the total population to 2⅓ million. Today the population is more than 4⅓ million.

Very soon two things affected commercial expansion. First, the Chinese Government restricted Hong Kong's exports to China, because she feared unsettled internal conditions, mounting inflation and a weakening of her exchange position. Secondly, during the Korean War, the United Nations imposed an embargo on imports into China, the main source of Hong Kong's livelihood. This was a crisis for Hong Kong; its China trade went overnight, and, by this time, it had over one million refugees on its hands. But something dramatic happened. Simply stated, it was this: Hong Kong switched from trading to manufacture. It did it so quickly that few people, even in Hong Kong, were aware at the time of what exactly was happening, and the rest of the world was not quickly convinced of Hong Kong's transformation into a center of manufactures. Its limited industry began to expand rapidly and, although more slowly, to diversify, and it owed not a little to the immigrants from Shanghai, who brought their capital, their experience and expertise with them. Today Hong Kong must be unique amongst so-called developing countries in the dependence of its economy on industrialization. No less than 40 percent of the labor force is engaged in the manufacturing industries; and of the products from these, Hong Kong exports 90 percent, and it does this despite the fact that its industry is exposed to the full competition of the industrially mature nations. The variety of its goods now ranges widely from the products of shipbuilding and ship-breaking, through textiles and plastics, to air-conditioners, transistor radios and cameras.

More than 70 percent of its exports are either manufactured or partly manufactured in Hong Kong and the value of its domestic exports in 1964 was about 750 million dollars. In recent years these figures have been increasing at about 15 percent a year. America is the largest market, taking 25 percent of the value of Hong Kong's exports; then follows the United Kingdom, Malaysia, West Germany, Japan, Canada and Australia; but all countries come within the scope of its marketing.

22. The article gives the impression that
    (A) English rule constituted an important factor in Hong Kong economy
    (B) refugees from China were a liability to the financial status of Hong Kong
    (C) Hong Kong has taken a developmental course comparable to that of the new African nations
    (D) British forces used their military might imperialistically to acquire Hong Kong
    (E) there is a serious dearth of skilled workers in Hong Kong

23. The economic stability of Hong Kong is mostly attributable to
    (A) its shipbuilding activity
    (B) businessmen and workers from Shanghai who settled in Hong Kong
    (C) its political separation from China
    (D) its exports to China
    (E) a change in the area of business concentration

24. Hong Kong's commerce was adversely affected by
    (A) the Han Dynasty
    (B) Japanese occupation
    (C) British administration
    (D) the defeat of the Chinese National Government
    (E) the conversion from manufacturing to trading

25. Hong Kong's population is about _____ that of China.

(A) $1/50$
(B) $1/100$
(C) $1/200$
(D) $1/500$
(E) $1/1000$

26. The author states or implies that
    (A) the United States imports more goods from Hong Kong than all the other nations combined
    (B) about three-quarters of Hong Kong's exports are made exclusively in Hong Kong
    (C) Malaysia, Canada, and West Germany provide excellent markets for Hong Kong goods
    (D) approximately one-half of the Hong Kong workers are involved with manufacturing
    (E) the United Nations has consistently co-operated to improve the economy of Hong Kong

27. Hong Kong first came under Chinese rule approximately
    (A) a century ago
    (B) eight centuries ago
    (C) fourteen centuries ago
    (D) twenty-one centuries ago
    (E) forty centuries ago

28. According to the passage, which of the following did *not* contribute to Hong Kong's transformation from a trading to a manufacturing economy?
    (A) the Korean War
    (B) the immigration of many Chinese to Hong Kong after the defeat of the Chinese National Government
    (C) the restriction of Hong Kong's exports to China
    (D) the Japanese invasion of Hong Kong in 1941
    (E) unstable internal conditions in China

Questions 29–34

It is a measure of how far the Keynesian revolution has proceeded that the central thesis of "The General Theory" now sounds rather commonplace. Until it appeared, economists in the classical (or non-socialist) tradition had assumed that the economy, if left to itself, would find its equilibrium at full employment. Increases or decreases in wages and interest rates would occur as necessary to bring about this pleasant result. If people were unemployed, their wages would fall in relation to prices. With lower wages and wider margins, it would be profitable to employ those from whose toil an adequate return could not previously have been made. It followed that steps to keep wages at artificially high levels, such as might result from the ill-considered efforts by unions, would cause unemployment. Such efforts were deemed to be the principal cause of unemployment.

Movements in interest rates played a complementary role by insuring that all income would ultimately be spent. Thus, were people to decide for some reason to increase their savings, the interest rates on the now more abundant supply of loanable funds would fall. This, in turn, would lead to increased investment. The added outlays for investment goods would offset the diminished outlays by the more frugal consumers. In this fashion, changes in consumer spending or in investment decisions were kept from causing any change in total spending that would lead to unemployment.

Keynes argued that neither wage movements nor changes in the rate of interest had, necessarily, any such agreeable effect. He focused attention on the total of purchasing power in the economy—what is now called "aggregate demand." Wage reductions might not increase employment; in conjunction with other changes, they might merely reduce this aggregate demand. And he held that interest was not the price that was paid to people to save but the price they got for exchanging holdings of cash, or its equivalent, their normal preference in assets, for less liquid forms of investment. And it was difficult to reduce interest beyond a certain level. Accordingly, if people sought to save more, this wouldn't necessarily mean lower interest rates and a resulting increase in investment. Instead, the total demand for goods might fall, along with employment and also investment, until savings were brought back into line with investment by the pressure of hardship which had reduced saving in favor of consumption. The economy would find its equilibrium not at full employment but with an unspecified amount of unemployment.

Out of this diagnosis came the remedy. It was to bring aggregate demand back up to the level where all willing workers were employed, and this could be accomplished by supplementing private expenditure with public expenditure. This should be the policy wherever intentions to save exceeded intentions to invest. Since public spending would not perform this offsetting role if there were compensating taxation (which is a form of saving), the public spending should be financed by borrowing—by incurring a deficit. So far as Keynes' theory can be condensed into a few paragraphs, this is the substance of his ideas.

29. Keynes emphasized that
    (A) unemployment was largely caused by high wages
    (B) interest rate fluctuations were desirable
    (C) lowering salaries would eventually create more jobs
    (D) the government should go into debt, if necessary, to provide jobs
    (E) an internal laissez-faire policy is advantageous

30. The writer's attitude toward the Keynesian economic philosophy seems to be
    (A) antagonistic
    (B) questioning
    (C) favorable
    (D) mocking
    (E) bombastic

31. It is undeniable that Keynes would
    (A) favor the full employment of only those who wished to be employed
    (B) favor full employment at the cost of forcing unwilling workers to work
    (C) oppose government spending in conjunction with private spending
    (D) oppose a government deficit
    (E) force people to work

32. The main purpose of the passage is to
    (A) describe a theory that provides for government spending as a means of economic control
    (B) show how traditional economists fail to provide for full employment

    (C) criticize an economic theory that provides workers with a less than adequate return on their investment

    (D) show ways economists have failed to account for variations in consumer spending

    (E) analyze the role interest rates play in reducing aggregate demand

33. The following statements are not in correct chronological order. Place them in the correct order.

    I.   A rise in investment would follow.

    II.   The rate of interest would fluctuate so that people would eventually spend what they had earned.

    III. There was assurance, therefore, that fluctuations in investment and/or purchasing would not throw workers out of jobs.

    IV. Accordingly, as a person decided to save more, the rate of interest on loans would decrease.

    (A) IV, III, I, II
    (B) II, IV, I, III
    (C) III, I, IV, II
    (D) I, IV, III, II
    (E) IV, III, II, I

34. According to the passage, classical economists reasoned that

    (A) a lack of union efforts to keep wages high would increase unemployment

    (B) as people save more, interest rates increase

    (C) full employment is impossible to achieve

    (D) lower interest rates would cause an increase in investments

    (E) private expenditures should be supplemented with public expenditures to insure that all willing workers are employed

Questions 35–40

Antimicrobial agents for the treatment of infectious diseases have been the largest selling prescription pharmaceuticals in the world for the past three decades. Most of these agents are antibiotics—antimicrobials naturally produced by micro-organisms rather than by chemical synthesis or by isolation from higher organisms. However, one major antibiotic, chloramphenicol—originally produced by a micro-organism—is now synthesized by chemical methods. The field of antibiotics, in fact, provides most of the precedent for employing microbial fermentation to produce useful medical substances. The United States has been prominent in their development, production, and marketing, with the result that American companies account for about half of the roughly $5 billion worth of antimicrobial agents sold world-wide each year. The American market share has been growing as new antibiotics are developed and introduced every year.

For 30 years, high-yielding, antibiotic-producing micro-organisms have been identified by selection from among mutant strains. Initially, organisms producing new antibiotics are so isolated by soil sampling and other broad screening efforts. They are then cultured in the laboratory, and efforts are made to improve their productivity.

Antibiotics are complex, usually nonprotein, substances that are generally the end products of a series of biological steps. While knowledge of molecular details in metabolism has made some difference, not a single antibiotic has had its complete biosynthetic pathway elucidated. This is partly because there is no *single* gene that can be isolated to produce an antibiotic. However, mutations can be induced within the original micro-organism so that the *level* of production can be increased.

Other methods can also increase production, and possibly create new antiobiotics. Microbial mating, for example, which leads to natural recombination, has been widely investigated as a way of developing vigorous, high-yielding antibiotic producers. However, its use has been limited by the mating incompatibility of many industrially important higher fungi, the presence of chromosomal aberrations in micro-organisms improved by mutation, and a number of other problems. Furthermore, natural recombination is most advantageous when strains of extremely diverse origins are mated; the proprietary secrets protecting commercial strains usually prevent the sort of divergent "competitor" strains most likely to produce vigorous hybrids from being brought together.

The technique of protoplast, or cell, fusion provides a convenient method for establishing a recombinant system in strains, species, and genera that lack an efficient natural means for mating. For example, as many as four strains of the antibiotic-producing bacterium *Streptomyces* have been fused together in a single step to yield recombinants that inherit genes from four parents. The technique is applicable to nearly all antibiotic producers. It will help combine the benefits developed in divergent lines by mutation and selection.

In addition, researchers have compared the quality of an antibiotic-producing fungus, *Cephalosporium acremonium*, produced by mating to one produced by protoplast fusion. They concluded that protoplast fusion was far superior for that purpose. What is more, protoplast fusion can give rise to hundreds of recombinants—including one isolate that consistently produced the antibiotic cephalosporin C in 40 percent greater yield than the best producer among its parents—without losing that parent strain's rare capacity to use inorganic sulfate, rather than expensive methionine, as a source of sulfur. It also acquired the rapid growth and sporulation characteristics of its less-productive parent. Thus, desirable attributes from different parents were combined in an important industrial organism that had proved resistant to conventional crossing.

Even more significant are the possibilities for preparation by protoplast fusion between different species or genera of hybrid strains, which could have unique biosynthetic capacities. One group is reported to have isolated a novel antibiotic, clearly not produced by either parent, in an organism created through fusion of actinomycete protoplasts. The value of protoplast fusion, therefore, lies in potentially broadening the gene pool.

Protoplast fusion is genetic recombination on a large scale. Instead of one or a few genes being transferred across genus and species barriers, entire sets of genes can be moved. Success is not assured, however; a weakness today is the inherited instability of the "fused" clones. The preservation of traits and long-range stability has yet to be resolved. Furthermore, it seems that one of the most daunting problems is screening—

determining what to look for and how to recognize it.

Recombinant DNA techniques are also being examined for their ability to improve strains. Many potentially useful antibiotics do not reach their commercial potential because the microorganisms cannot be induced to produce sufficient quantities by traditional methods. The synthesis of certain antibiotics is controlled by plasmids, and it is believed that some plasmids may nonspecifically enhance antibiotic production and excretion.

It may also be possible to transfer as a group, all the genes needed to produce an antibiotic into a new host. However, increasing the number of copies of critical genes by phage or plasmid transfer has yet to be achieved in antibiotic producing organisms because little is known of the potential vectors. The genetic systems of commercial strains will have to be understood before the newer genetic engineering approaches can be used.

The following statements are related to the information presented above. Select

(A)   if the statement is supported by the given information
(B)   if the statement is contradicted by the given information
(C)   if the statement is neither supported nor contradicted by the given information

35. The output rate of antibiotics by micro-organisms is fixed.

36. Occasionally, the biosynthetic pathway leading to an antibiotic is determined, so that the antibiotic may be synthesized by chemical methods.

37. Irradiation is employed to induce mutations within existing micro-organisms, thereby increasing the level of antibiotic production.

38. Mutation induction sometimes produces deleterious effects on microbial mating.

39. Assuming parent compatibility, microbial

mating is always superior to protoplast fusion as a production method for antibiotics.

40. Once the problem of screening is solved, the method of protoplast fusion will be virtually faultless.

Questions 41–45

The interest in augmenting the world's supply of protein has focused attention on microbial sources of protein as food for both animals and humans. Since a large portion of each bacterial or yeast cell consists of proteins (up to 72 percent for some protein-rich cells), large numbers have been grown to supply single-cell protein (SCP) for consumption. The protein can be consumed directly as part of the cell itself or can be extracted and processed into fibers or meatlike items. By now, advanced food processing technologies can combine this protein with meat flavoring and other substances to produce nutritious food that looks, feels, and tastes like meat.

The idea of using SCP as animal feed or human food is not new; yeast has been used as food protein since the beginning of the century. However, in the past several years, there has been a dramatic increase in research on SCP and in the construction of large-scale plants for its production, especially for the production of yeast. Interest in this material is reflected in the numerous national and international conferences on SCP, the increasing number of proceedings and reviews published, and the number of patents issued in recent years.

The issues addressed have covered topics such as the economic and technological factors influencing SCP processes, nutrition and safety, and SCP applications to human or animal foods. Thus far, commercial use has been limited by several factors. For each bacterial, yeast, or algal strain used, technological problems (from the choice of micro-organisms to the use of corresponding raw material) and logistical problems of construction and location of plants have arisen. But the primary limitation so far has been the cost of production compared with the costs of competing sources of protein.

The costs of manufacturing SCP for animal feed in the United States are high, particularly relative to its major competing protein source, soybeans, which can be produced with little fertilizer and minimal processing. The easy availability of this legume severely limits microbial SCP production for animal feed or human food.

In fact, it is estimated that total foreign and domestic consumption of U.S. soybeans will grow seventy-three percent in the next two years.

Soybeans are primarily consumed as animal feed. But while only four percent of their annual production is directly consumed by humans, the market is growing significantly. The introduction of improved-textured soy protein found in cereals in meat substitutes and extenders and in dairy substitutes has increased the use of soy products. Nevertheless, the market does not demand soy products in particular but protein supplements, vegetable oils, feed grain supplements, and meat extenders in general. Other protein and oil sources could replace soybeans if the economics were attractive enough. Fish meal, dry beans, SCP, and cereals are all potential competitors. As long as a substitute can meet the nutritional, flavor, toxicity, and regulatory standards, competition will be based primarily on price.

The competition between soybeans and SCP illustrates one of the paradoxes of genetic engineering. While significant research is attempting the genetic improvement of soybeans, genetic techniques are also being explored to increase the production of SCP. Consequently, the same tool—genetic engineering—encourages competition between the two commodities.

The following statements are related to the information presented above. Select

(A) if the statement is supported by the given information
(B) if the statement is contradicted by the given information
(C) if the statement is neither supported nor contradicted by the given information

41. The taste of soy protein is superior to the taste of single-cell protein.

42. Soybeans are a cheaper source of protein than single-cell proteins.

43. Soy protein production is beginning to decline.

44. The maturation of the field of genetic engineering will likely increase the position of SCP relative to soy protein.

45. There are no particular problems associated with the manufacture of SCP.

Questions 46–53

Recent scientific discoveries are throwing new light on the basic nature of viruses and on the possible nature of cancer, genes and even life itself. These discoveries are providing evidence for relationships among these four subjects which indicates that one may be dependent upon another to an extent not fully appreciated heretofore. Too often one works and thinks within too narrow a range and hence fails to recognize the significance of certain facts for other areas. Sometimes the important new ideas and subsequent fundamental discoveries come from the borderline areas between two well-established fields of investigation. This will result in the synthesis of new ideas regarding viruses, cancer, genes and life. These ideas in turn will result in new experiments which may provide the basis for fundamental discoveries in these fields.

There is no doubt that of the four topics, life is the one most people would consider to be of the greatest importance. However, life means different things to different people and it is in reality difficult to define just what we mean by life. There is no difficulty in recognizing an agent as living so long as we contemplate structures like a man, a dog or even a bacterium, and at the nonliving extreme, a piece of iron or glass or an atom of hydrogen or a molecule of water. The ability to grow or reproduce and to change or mutate has long been regarded as a special property characteristic of living agents along with the ability to respond to external stimuli. These are properties not shared by bits of iron or glass or even by a molecule of hemoglobin. Now if viruses had not been discovered, all would have been well. The organisms of the biologist would have ranged from the largest of animals all the way down to the smallest of the bacteria, which are about 200 millimicra. There would have been a definite break with respect to size; the largest molecules known to the chemist were less than 20 millimicra in size. Thus life and living agents

would have been represented by those structures which possessed the ability to reproduce themselves and to mutate and were about ten times larger than the largest known molecule. This would have provided a comfortable area of separation between living and nonliving things.

Then came the discovery of the viruses. These infectious, disease-producing agents are characterized by their small size, by their ability to grow or reproduce within specific living cells, and by their ability to change or mutate during reproduction. This was enough to convince most people that viruses were merely still smaller living organisms. When the sizes of different viruses were determined, it was found that some were actually smaller than certain protein molecules. When the first virus was isolated in the form of a crystallizable material, it was found to be a nucleoprotein. It was found to possess all the usual properties associated with protein molecules yet was larger than any molecule previously described. Here was a molecule that possessed the ability to reproduce itself and to mutate. The distinction between living and nonliving things seemed to be tottering. The gap in size between 20 and 200 millimicra has been filled in completely by the viruses, with some actual overlapping at both ends, as some large viruses are larger than some living organisms.

Let us consider the relationship between genes and viruses, since both are related to life. Both genes and viruses seem to be nucleoproteins and both reproduce only within specific living cells. Both possess the ability to mutate. Although viruses generally reproduce many times within a given cell, some situations are known in which they appear to reproduce only once with each cell division. Genes usually reproduce once with each cell division, but here also the rate can be changed. Actually the similarities between genes and viruses are so remarkable that viruses were referred to as "naked genes" or "genes on the loose."

Despite the fact that today viruses are known to cause cancer in animals and in certain plants, there exists a great reluctance to accept viruses as being of importance in human cancer. Basic biological phenomena generally do not differ strikingly as one goes from one species to another. It should be recognized that cancer is a biological problem and not a problem that is unique for man. Cancer originates when a normal cell suddenly becomes a cancer cell which multiplies quickly and without apparent restraint. Cancer may originate in many different kinds of cells, but the cancer cell usually continues to carry certain traits of the cell of origin. Because the transformation of a normal cell into a cancer cell may have more than one kind of cause, there is good reason to consider the relationships that exist between viruses and cancer.

Since there is no evidence that human cancer, as generally experienced, is infectious, many persons believe that because viruses are infectious agents they cannot possibly be of importance in human cancer. However, viruses can mutate and examples are known in which a virus that never kills its host can mutate to form a new strain of virus that always kills its host. It does not seem unreasonable to assume than an innocuous latent virus might mutate to form a strain that causes cancer. Certainly the experimental evidence now available is consistent with the idea that viruses as we know them today could be the causative agents of most, if not all, cancer, including cancer in man.

46. People were convinced that viruses were small living organisms, because viruses
    (A) are disease-producing
    (B) reproduce within living cells
    (C) could be grown on artificial media
    (D) consist of nucleoproteins

47. Scientists very often do not apply the facts learned in one subject area to a related field of investigation because
    (A) the borderline areas are too close to both to give separate facts
    (B) scientists work in a very narrow range of experimentation
    (C) new ideas are synthesized only as a result of new experimentation
    (D) fundamental discoveries are based upon finding close relationships in related sciences

48. Before the discovery of viruses, it might have been possible to distinguish living things from nonliving things by the fact that
    (A) animate objects can mutate
    (B) nonliving substances cannot reproduce themselves

(C) responses to external stimuli are characteristic of living things
(D) living things were greater than 20 millimicra in size

49. The size of viruses is presently known to be
    (A) between 20 and 200 millimicra
    (B) smaller than any bacterium
    (C) larger than any protein molecule
    (D) larger than most nucleoproteins

50. That genes and viruses seem to be related might be shown by the fact that
    (A) both are ultra-microscopic
    (B) each can mutate but once in a cell
    (C) each reproduces but once in a cell
    (D) both appear to have the same chemical structure

51. Cancer should be considered to be a biological problem rather than a medical one because
    (A) viruses are known to cause cancers in animals
    (B) at present, human cancer is not believed to be contagious
    (C) there are many known causes for the transformation of a normal cell to a cancer cell
    (D) results of experiments on plants and animals do not vary greatly from species to species

52. The possibility that a virus causes human cancer is indicated by
    (A) the fact that viruses have been known to mutate
    (B) the fact that a cancer-immune individual may lose his immunity
    (C) the fact that reproduction of human cancer cells might be due to a genetic factor
    (D) the fact that man is host to many viruses

53. The best title for this passage is
    (A) New Light on the Cause of Cancer
    (B) The Newest Theory on the Nature of Viruses
    (C) Viruses, Genes, Cancer and Life
    (D) On the Nature of Life

Questions 54–61

Regarding physical changes that have been and are now taking place on the surface of the earth, the sea and its shores have been the scene of the greatest stability. The dry land has seen the rise, the decline, and even the disappearance of vast hordes of various types and forms within times comparatively recent, geologically speaking; but life in the sea is today virtually what it was when many of the forms now extinct on land had not been evolved. Also, it may be parenthetically stated here, the marine habitat has been biologically the most important in the evolution and development of life on this planet. Its rhythmic influence can still be traced in those animals whose ancestors have long since left that realm to abide far from their primary haunts. For it is now generally held as an accepted fact that the shore area of an ancient sea was the birthplace of life.

Still, despite the primitive conditions still maintained in the sea, its shore inhabitants show an amazing diversity, while their adaptive characters are perhaps not exceeded in refinement by those that distinguish the dwellers of dry land. Why is this diversity manifest? We must look for an answer into the physical factors obtained in that extremely slender zone surrounding the continents, marked by the rise and fall of the tides.

It will be noticed by the most casual observer that on any given seashore the area exposed between the tide marks may be roughly divided into a number of levels, each characterized by a certain assemblage of animals. Thus in proceeding from high- to low-water mark, new forms constantly become predominant while other forms gradually drop out. Now, provided that the character of the substratum does not change, these differences in the types of animals are determined almost exclusively by the duration of time that the individual forms may remain exposed to the air without harm. Indeed, so regularly does the tidal rhythm act on certain animals (the barnacles, for instance), that certain species have come to require a definite period of exposure in order to maintain themselves, and will die out if kept continuously submerged. Although there are some forms that actually require periodic exposure, the number of species

inhabiting the shore that are able to endure exposure every twelve hours, when the tide falls, is comparatively few.

With the alternate rise and fall of the tides, the successive areas of the tidal zone are subjected to the force of wave-impact. In certain regions waves often break with considerable force. Consequently, wave-shock has had a profound influence on the structure and habits of shore animals. It is characteristic of most shore animals that they shun definitely exposed places, and seek shelter in nooks and crannies and such refuges as are offered under stones and seaweed; particularly is this true of those forms living on rock and other firm foundations. Many of these have a marked capacity to cling closely to the substratum; some, such as anemones and certain snails, although without the grasping organs of higher animals, have special powers of adhesion; others, such as sponges and sea squirts, remain permanently fixed, and if torn loose from their base are incapable of forming a new attachment. But perhaps the most significant method of solving the problem presented by the surf has been in the adaptation of body-form to minimize friction. This is strikingly displayed in the fact that seashore animals are essentially flattened forms. Thus, in the typical shore forms, the sponges are of the encrusting type, the nonburrowing worms are leaflike, the snails and other mollusks are squat forms and are without the spines and other ornate extensions such as are often produced on the shells of many mollusks in deeper and quieter waters.

In sandy regions, because of the unstable nature of the substratum, no such means of attachment as indicated in the foregoing paragraph will suffice to maintain the animals in their almost ceaseless battle with the billows. Most of them must perforce depend on their ability to penetrate into the sand for safety. Some forms endowed with less celerity, such as the sand dollars, are so constructed that their bodies offer no more resistance to wave impact than does a flat pebble.

Temperature, also, is a not inconsiderable factor among those physical forces constantly operating to produce a diversity of forms among seashore animals. At a comparatively shallow depth in the sea, there is a small fluctuation of temperatures and life there exists in surround-

.ings of serene stability; however, as the shore is approached, the influence of the sun becomes more and more manifest and the variation is greater. This variation becomes greatest between the tide marks where, because of the very shallow depths and the fresh water from the land, this area is subjected to wide changes in both temperature and salinity.

Nor is a highly competitive mode of life without its bearing on structure as well as habits. In this phase of their struggle for existence, the animals of both the sea and the shore have become possessed of weapons for offense and defense that are correspondingly varied.

Although the life in the sea has been generally considered and treated as separate and distinct from the more familiar life on land, that supposition has no real basis in fact. Life on this planet is one vast unit, depending for its existence chiefly on the same sources of supply. That portion of animal life living in the sea, notwithstanding its strangeness and unfamiliarity, may be considered as but the aquatic fringe of the life on land. It is supported largely by materials washed into the sea, which are no longer available for the support of land animals. Perhaps we have been misled in these considerations of sea life because of the fact that approximately three times as many major types of animals inhabit salt water as live on the land: of the major types of animals no fewer than ten are exclusively marine, that is to say, nearly half again as many as land-dwelling types together. A further interesting fact is that, despite the greater variety in the form and structure of sea animals, about three-fourths of all known kinds of animals live on the land, while only one-fourth live in the sea. In this connection it is noteworthy that sea life becomes scarcer with increasing distance from land; toward the middle of the oceans it disappears almost completely. For example, the central south Pacific is a region more barren than is any desert area on land. Indeed, no life of any kind has been found in the surface water, and there seems to be none on the bottom.

Sea animals are largest and most abundant on those shores receiving the most copious rainfall. Particularly is this true on the most rugged and colder coasts where it may be assumed that the material from the land finds its way to the sea unaltered and in greater quantities.

54. The best title for this passage is
(A) Between the Tides
(B) Seashore Life
(C) The Tides
(D) The Seashore

55. Of the following adaptations, the one that would best enable an organism to live on a sandy beach is
(A) the ability to move rapidly
(B) the ability to burrow
(C) a flattened shape
(D) spiny extensions of the shell
(E) both (B) and (C)

56. The absence of living things in mid-ocean might be due to
(A) lack of rainfall in mid-ocean
(B) the distance from material washed into the sea
(C) larger animals feeding on smaller ones which must live near the land
(D) insufficient dissolved oxygen

57. A greater variety of living things exist on a rocky shore than on a sandy beach because
(A) rocks offer a better foothold than sand
(B) sandy areas are continually being washed by the surf
(C) temperature changes are less drastic in rocky areas
(D) the water in rock pools is less salty
(E) both A and B

58. Organisms found living at the high-tide mark are adapted to
(A) maintain themselves in the air for a long time
(B) offer no resistance to wave impact
(C) remain permanently fixed to the substratum
(D) burrow in the ground

59. The author holds that living things in the sea represent the aquatic fringe of life on land. This is so because
(A) there are relatively fewer marine forms of animals than there are land-living forms
(B) there is greater variety among land-living forms

(C) marine animals ultimately depend upon material from the land

(D) there are three times as many kinds of animals on land than there are in the sea

60. A scientist wishing to study a great variety of living things would do well to hunt for them
    (A) in shallow waters
    (B) on a rocky seashore
    (C) on a sandy seashore
    (D) on any shore between the tide lines

61. The most primitive forms of living things in the evolutionary scale are to be found in the sea because
    (A) the influence of the sea is found in land animals
    (B) the sea is relatively stable
    (C) many forms have become extinct on land
    (D) land animals are supposed to have evolved from sea organisms

Questions 62–68

In the initial period following a nuclear attack, severe medical care problems will occur on a nationwide scale because of (1) the massive increase in the number of people who will require medical care for burns, radiation sickness, blast effects, shock, and other injuries and (2) the unavailability of necessary medical services and supplies due to the wholesale destruction of hospital facilities, widespread deaths and injuries among medical personnel, and the almost total destruction of the drug industry.

Other serious health problems are likely to appear later. For example, while epidemics are unlikely to occur during the *early* post-attack period because the large reservoirs of disease carriers will be absent, crowded living situations could foster epidemics. Prolonged contact in crowded conditions necessitated by extended shelter life or fuel and housing conservation measures would therefore increase the long-term probability of epidemics. In addition, the appearance of diseases not normally seen in the United States, such as plague, typhus, cholera, etc., may generate fear (magnified by the post-attack atmosphere) which will cause spontaneous or planned isolation of specific areas, and diminish the effectiveness of post-attack recovery programs.

The most serious immediate post-attack medical problem will be treatment for injuries from burns, blast injuries, and radiation exposure. This will be complicated by the likelihood of multiple injuries, that is, combinations of burn, blast, and radiation injuries. Analysis of the data from the atomic bombings of Hiroshima reveals that some 40 percent of the survivors sustained multiple injuries. Radiation exposure complicates the treatment of other injuries because it decreases resistance to infection. Tests of animals with both burn and radiation injuries showed a significant increase in mortality over death caused from burn injuries alone, because of increased vulnerability to infection.

Yet, there are only 12 burn-care centers in the United States and, of the nation's 6,000 general hospitals, fewer than 100 provide specialized burn care. Though burn center care is important to survival rates for serious burn victims of all ages, flame injuries affect children more severely than adults. For eight-year-olds burned over 60 percent of their bodies, the survival rate in hospitals is only 20 percent, but it increases to 50 percent for those treated in burn-care centers. Few, if any, of these facilities will survive nuclear attacks on metropolitan areas.

The prognosis for the seriously exposed radiation cases or multiple injury patients will depend on nutrition, rest, and medical care. In radiation cases, the hematological system is seriously disturbed, including blood cell production by the bone marrow and storage by the spleen. Resistance to infection is severely limited. For patients with substantial radiation exposure, antibiotics, transfusions, and, in cases of exposure to over 300 R, the depression of the white blood count (leukopenia) can be successfully treated with sophisticated medical treatment, including bone marrow transplants. But the likelihood of the availability of this treatment on a large scale is inconceivable in a post-attack environment.

In summary, under post-attack conditions even basic care could be limited or completely unavailable in the urban-industrial areas. Given the magnitude of the casualties nationwide (20 to 30 million) and the loss of specialized medical facilities and personnel, even simple protection against infection will be difficult. Infection control would require antibiotics and other prophylactics, stocks of which would be exhausted immediately with little possibility of rapid supply due to the destruction of the drug industry in the attack.

The following statements are related to the preceding information. Select

(A) if the statement is supported by the given information
(B) if the statement is contradicted by the given information
(C) if the statement is neither supported nor contradicted by the given information

62. The chief cause of medical care problems following a nuclear attack will be the almost total destruction of the drug industry.

63. Widespread fear among the public will diminish the effectiveness of post-attack recovery programs.

64. The most serious immediate post-attack problem will be the increased likelihood of epidemics.

65. Virtually all of the survivors of a nuclear attack are likely to sustain multiple injuries.

66. Multiple injuries increase the likelihood of death among attack victims.

67. Limited resistance to disease infection is a direct result of serious radiation exposure.

68. Following a nuclear attack, the incidence of diseases not normally seen in the United States will increase.

STOP

END OF SKILLS ANALYSIS—READING QUESTIONS

Section 4: SKILLS ANALYSIS—QUANTITATIVE

Time: 85 minutes
67 questions

Directions: Select the one best answer from the lettered choices that follow each question. Each group of questions is preceded by and concerns some descriptive material presented in quantitative format.

NUMBER OF TELEPHONES PER PERSON; SELECTED CITIES, 1930–2000

Year	Chicago	Boston	Los Angeles
1930	.4	.2	.1
1940	1.0	.8	.2
1950	2.0	1.0	.6
1960	2.5	1.5	1.5
1970	3.0	2.0	3.0
1980	3.5	2.0	4.0
1990*	3.0	2.0	3.5
2000*	3.0	2.0	3.5

*projected

The following statements are related to the information in the preceding table. Select

(A) if the statement is supported by the given information
(B) if the statement is contradicted by the given information
(C) if the statement is neither supported nor contradicted by the given information

1. The number of people per telephone was greatest in Los Angeles in 1930.

2. The increase in the number of telephones per person from 1930 to 1980 was greater in Boston than in Chicago.

3. If, in 1970, there were two-thirds as many people living in Boston as in Los Angeles, the number of telephones in those cities was equal.

4. There were four times as many people per telephone in Chicago in 1930 as there were in Los Angeles in the same year.

5. If the population of Chicago doubles from the year 1990 to the year 2000, the projected number of telephones per person will halve during that time.

6. There was a 500 percent increase in the number of telephones per person in Boston from 1930 to 1950.

7. In Chicago from 1950 to 1980, the number of telephones per person increased by the same amount for each successive ten-year period.

8. If the data from 1930 to 1980 were displayed on a Cartesian coordinate system with "Year" on the horizontal axis and "Number

of Telephones per Person" on the vertical axis, and a line were drawn connecting the 1930 to the 1980 data for each city, the line for Los Angeles would have the greatest slope.

9. From 1930 to 1940, the number of telephones in Los Angeles doubled.

10. There was no increase in the number of telephones per person in Chicago from 1970 to 1990.

AVERAGE EXPECTED LIFE SPAN AT VARIOUS AGES

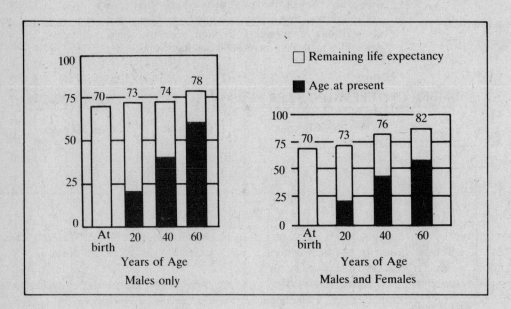

The following statements are related to the information in the preceding graphs. Select

(A) if the statement is supported by the given information
(B) if the statement is contradicted by the given information
(C) if the statement is neither supported nor contradicted by the given information

11. The average expected life span of 60-year-old females is 86.

12. The average 20-year-old male will live about 53 more years.

13. The average 20-year-old female will live about 53 more years.

14. The older a female gets, the more likely it is that she will live longer than the average male.

15. The average 40-year-old male has longer remaining to live than the average male who has just been born.

16. Females have a greater life expectancy at birth than do males.

17. The older an individual gets, the more likely it is that he or she will have a longer life.

18. The percentage of 60-year-old males who live past 80 years is greater than the percentage of 40-year-old males who live past 80 years.

School	Department	Under-graduates	Graduates	Alumni	Totals
SCIENCE		68 (7)	36 (13)	6 (5)	110 (25)
	Biology	10 (2)	4 (4)	1 (0)	15 (6)
	Chemistry	15 (1)	12 (0)	0 (2)	27 (3)
	Mathematics	22 (0)	14 (0)	1 (1)	37 (1)
	Nutrition	2 (4)	6 (9)	0 (2)	8 (15)
	Physics	19 (0)	0 (0)	4 (0)	23 (0)
HUMANITIES		34 (19)	10 (4)	14 (8)	58 (31)
	Business	5 (1)	4 (1)	0 (0)	9 (2)
	History	2 (1)	0 (1)	4 (1)	6 (3)
	Linguistics	1 (4)	0 (0)	1 (1)	2 (5)
	Management	6 (2)	0 (0)	1 (1)	7 (3)
	Political Science	7 (1)	4 (1)	2 (1)	13 (3)
	Literature	7 (7)	0 (0)	6 (2)	13 (9)
	Economics	4 (0)	2 (0)	0 (1)	6 (1)
	Philosophy	2 (3)	0 (1)	0 (1)	2 (5)

The preceding table contains data regarding the plight of a recent group of medical school applicants at a large northeastern university. In each position there are two numerical entries. The first indicates the number of applicants accepted to at least one medical school. The second, which is in parentheses, indicates the number of applicants who were not accepted at any medical school. Based on this information, select

(A) if the statement is supported by the given information
(B) if the statement is contradicted by the given informtion
(C) if the statement is neither supported nor contradicted by the given information

19. 250% more applicants affiliated with the Department of Philosophy were not accepted anywhere than were accepted by at least one school.

20. Biology undergraduates had a lower percentage of applicants not accepted anywhere than did all students affiliated with the Department of Economics.

21. Mathematics undergraduates tend to be smarter than literature alumni.

22. 50% of the history undergraduates were not accepted at any school.

23. Physics undergraduates were accepted by more schools than were literature graduates.

24. There were more undergraduate chemistry acceptances than political science applicants.

25. 40% of the School of Humanities graduate students were not accepted at any school.

26. More than one-half of the applicants affiliated with the School of Humanities were not accepted by any school.

Questions 27–30 refer to the description and results of an experiment followed by statements about the experiment. Analyze each statement solely on the basis of the experiment. From the information given about the experiment, mark your answer sheet

(A) if the experiment proves the statement is true

(B) if the experiment shows that the statement is probably true

(C) if the experiment does not show whether the statement is true or false

(D) if the experiment shows that the statement is probably false

(E) if the experiment shows that the statement is false

As shown in the following table, five sugar cubes coated with different chemicals (labeled A–E) are placed in widely separated locations in an enclosed room. One hundred flies are introduced into the room and the length of time necessary for the flies to reach one of the cubes, and which cube each reaches, is carefully recorded.

Chemical	*A*	*B*	*C*	*D*	*E*
No flies landed	8	8	6	76	2
Length of time (min.) to get to sugar	12.2	12.5	16.6	1.36	19.7
Boiling point of chemical °C	100	87	97	52	68

27. Some of the chemicals used affect both the length of time necessary for the flies to land on the sugar cubes as well as which ones they select.

28. The boiling point of a chemical determines which cube the flies will choose.

29. The length of time required for a fly to reach the differently coated sugar cubes is proportional to the melting point of the chemical.

30. Some flies landed on one chemically treated sugar cube and then flew to another.

In a previous publication it was reported that intravenous injections of crystalline L. casei factor led to complete regressions of spontaneous breast cancers in mice, in about one-third of the animals. Drs. Hutchings and Stokstad indicate that the correct tentative designation of this substance is fermentation L. casei factor. The isolation of this compound was announced, and its microbiological activity and other properties were described by Hutchings. More recently, Angier reported the synthesis of a compound identical with the L. casei factor from liver. This substance differs in microbiological activity from that of the fermentation L. casei factor used in our previously reported experiments in that the liver L. casei factor is about 17 times as active for the test organism, *Streptococcus lactis* R, at half maximum growth.

Ninety-eight mice bearing single spontaneous breast cancers were selected for present studies. In each case a definite diagnosis of malignancy was established by biopsy. The animals were kept on a normal diet (Rockland mouse pellets). Three groups were formed. The first group, 39 tumor mice, received 5 μg. of liver L. casei factor; the second group, 31 mice, received 100 μg. of liver L. casei factor; and the third group, 28 mice, received 5 μg. of the crystalline fermentation L. casei factor. All substances were injected intravenously daily for a period of 4–6 weeks. As control, the data of 71 mice of the same strain, which were observed in the laboratory during a period prior to this experiment, were used. The results are presented in the table on page 135.

31. In producing regressions of tumors, the liver L. casei factor was

(A) effective with many animals, ineffective with many others

(B) in general, effective

(C) in general, ineffective

(D) not used enough to give significant results

(E) not tested at all

Group	No. of mice	Substance and dose (ug.)	No. of mice with complete regression of tumors	No. of mice with new tumors	No. of mice with lung metastases	Mean life span in days*
1	39	Liver L. casei factor (5 ug.)	1	12	19 among 32	75 ± 6
2	31	Liver L. casei factor (100 ug.)	0	11	3 among 30	55 ± 6
3	28	Fermentation L. casei factor(5 ug.)	11	2	**	After 100 days 23 mice alive
4	71	0	0	19	13 among 61	74 ± 6.2

* Life span calculated after start of experiment.
**An evaluation cannot be given since the majority of mice in this group are alive.

32. The fermentation L. casei factor led to regressions of tumors in practically

    (A) no cases
    (B) one-fifth of the cases
    (C) one-fourteenth of the cases
    (D) one-half of the cases
    (E) one-third of the cases

33. The greatest percentage of mice showed lung metastases in group

    (A) 1
    (B) 2
    (C) 3
    (D) 4

34. Diagnosis of malignancy of the cancers was established by

    (A) examination of tissues removed from the living animal
    (B) examination of tissues removed in autopsy
    (C) palpation of the affected areas
    (D) reaction of the cancers to diagnostic pharmaceutical
    (E) none of these

The following statements are related to the information presented in the table on page 136. Select

(A) if the statement is supported by the given information
(B) if the statement is contradicted by the given information
(C) if the statement is neither supported nor contradicted by the given information

35. The average 20-year-old in Britain is likely to live longer than the average 20-year-old in the United States.

36. The present life expectancy at birth for an individual in Brazil is greater than it was for an individual in the United States in 1900.

37. There are better medical facilities in the United States than in Cambodia.

38. An individual in the United States (at birth) can expect to live about 40% longer now than he could in 1900.

39. Approximately 50% of the individuals living in Italy live past the age of 68.

LIFE EXPECTANCY AT BIRTH

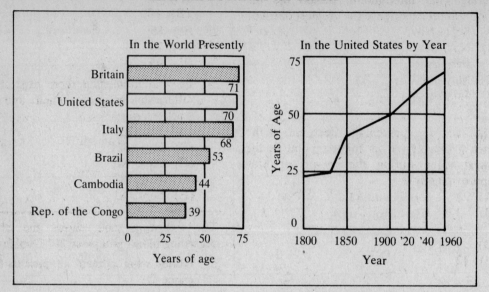

40. The life expectancy at birth in the United States is about 80% greater than it is in the Republic of the Congo.

41. At birth, a Brazilian has a greater chance of living past the age of 60 than does a Cambodian.

42. A newborn Italian could expect to live about twice as long in 1900 as he could in 1830.

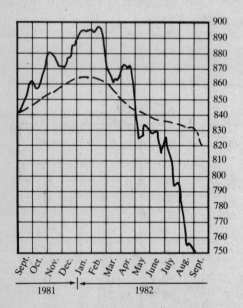

The preceding graph shows the predicted (broken line) and actual (solid line) Industrial Stock Averages over a twelve-month period.

43. In which month was the stock average highest?
    (A) December '81
    (B) January '82
    (C) February '82
    (D) October '81
    (E) April '82

44. In which month was the average lowest?
    (A) November '81
    (B) March '82
    (C) April '82
    (D) July '82
    (E) September '82

45. What is the approximate ratio of the highest stock average to the lowest?
    (A) 4:3
    (B) 5:3
    (C) 2:1
    (D) 3:2
    (E) 6:5

46. During what three-month period did the stock market experience the greatest decline?
    (A) Sept.–Nov.
    (B) Nov.–Jan.
    (C) Feb.–Apr.
    (D) May–Jul.
    (E) Jul.–Sept.

47. What was the percentage decrease in the stock average from its highest point to the lowest value during the month of May (approximately)?
    (A) 1
    (B) 3
    (C) 6
    (D) 9
    (E) 12

48. From its lowest point in Sept. '81, what was the percentage increase in the stock average up to its highest point (approximately)?
    (A) 3
    (B) 5
    (C) 7
    (D) 9
    (E) 12

49. The average at the end of the twelve-month period is approximately what percent of the average at the beginning of the twelve-month period?
    (A) 75
    (B) 80
    (C) 85
    (D) 90
    (E) 95

50. In what month did there exist the greatest difference between actual and predicted stock averages?
    (A) Jan. '82
    (B) Feb. '82
    (C) Apr. '82
    (D) Aug. '82
    (E) Sept. '82

The following table shows the observations regarding blood groups of 267 Danish families.

51. About what percent of parents had blood group O?
    (A) 30
    (B) 40
    (C) 50
    (D) 60
    (E) 80

52. What combination of blood groupings of parents produced offspring of all four blood groups?
    (A) A × AB
    (B) O × A
    (C) AB × AB
    (D) O × AB
    (E) A × B

Parents	No. of Families	Offspring			
		O	A	B	AB
O × O	41	126	1	0	0
A × A	22	10	70	0	0
O × A	68	69	102	0	0
B × B	1	1	0	1	0
O × B	13	18	0	29	0
A × B	22	13	16	13	26
O × AB	43	0	50	60	0
A × AB	42	0	59	21	33
B × AB	13	0	8	20	15
AB × AB	2	0	3	4	1
Totals	267	237	309	148	75

53. If it is true that parents, both of blood group O, can produce offspring only of blood group O, which is probably the best explanation of the one child of such parents shown in the table as being blood group A?
    (A) Faulty test sera or uncertain paternity could cause such exceptions.
    (B) Most such tables are subject to clerical errors.
    (C) The number of families sampled was too small.
    (D) The observations were made on Danish families only.
    (E) none of these

54. Children of group O were produced by how many combinations of parents neither of whom had group O blood?
    (A) 0
    (B) 10
    (C) 5
    (D) 6
    (E) 3

55. A study of 2046 offspring of Japanese families shows 691 group O, 756 A, 476 B, and 123 AB. The proportion of Japanese offspring of group AB bears what relationship to the proportion of AB offspring in the Danish sample?
    (A) equal
    (B) greater
    (C) less
    (D) non-comparable
    (E) impossible to correctly ascertain

56. The fact that there are so few families of AB × AB parentage is probably due to the fact that
    (A) personality adjustment of group AB is such that chances of marriage are decreased
    (B) such combinations of men and women do not usually occcur in the same communities
    (C) such matings tend to be sterile
    (D) there is a relatively low occurrence of blood group AB

57. The parents of what blood cross group produced the greatest number of offspring?
    (A) A × A
    (B) O × A
    (C) A × B
    (D) A × AB
    (E) B × AB

58. The parents of what blood cross group produced the greatest number of type AB offspring?
    (A) A × B
    (B) A × AB
    (C) AB × AB
    (D) B × AB

Ten judges were asked to judge the relative sweetness of five compounds (A, B, C, D, and E) by the method of paired comparisons. In judging each of the possible pairs they were required to unequivocally state which of the two compounds was the sweeter—a judgment of equality or no difference was not permitted.

The results of their judgments are summarized in the following table. In studying the table, note that each cell entry shows the number of comparisons in which the *row* compound was judged to be sweeter than the *column* compound.

	A	B	C	D	E
A		5	8	10	2
B	5		3	9	6
C	2	7		7	8
D	0	1	3		1
E	8	4	2	9	

59. How many comparisons did each judge make?
    (A) 5
    (B) 10
    (C) 15

(D) 20
(E) 25

60. Which compound was judged to be sweetest?
(A) A
(B) B
(C) C
(D) D
(E) E

61. Which compound was judged to be *least* sweet?
(A) A
(B) B
(C) C
(D) D
(E) E

62. Which one of the following statements is most nearly correct?
(A) There was almost perfect agreement among the ten judges.
(B) The clearest discrimination was between B and C.
(C) The judges were not expert in discriminating sweetnesses.
(D) Compound D was most clearly discriminated from the other four compounds.
(E) none of these

63. Between which two compounds was the discrimination least pronounced?
(A) A and D
(B) C and D
(C) C and E
(D) D and E
(E) B and A

64. Between which two compounds was the discrimination most pronounced?
(A) A and D
(B) C and D
(C) C and E
(D) D and E
(E) B and A

65. Compound A received twice as many favorable judgments when it was compared with compound B as when it was compared with compound
(A) C
(B) D
(C) E
(D) none of these

66. The sum of the judgments in favor of compound A is what percent of the sum of the judgments in favor of compound D?
(A) 20
(B) 25
(C) 125
(D) 400
(E) 500

67. What is the absolute difference between the number of judgments made in favor of compound C and the number of judgments in which compound C was found to be less sweet?
(A) 2
(B) 4
(C) 6
(D) 8
(E) 10

STOP

END OF SKILLS ANALYSIS—QUANTITATIVE QUESTIONS

ANSWER KEY FOR THE MCAT PRACTICE EXAMINATION

Section 1: Science Knowledge

1: A	26. A	51. A	76. B	101. D
2. B	27. A	52. D	77. C	102. D
3. E	28. B	53. C	78. D	103. D
4. B	29. A	54. C	79. E	104. D
5. C	30. E	55. E	80. E	105. E
6. E	31. C	56. B	81. E	106. A
7. D	32. C	57. E	82. A	107. D
8. B	33. A	58. A	83. C	108. C
9. D	34. B	59. C	84. D	109. D
10. A	35. E	60. C	85. E	110. E
11. A	36. A	61. C	86. A	111. C
12. D	37. E	62. E	87. B	112. A
13. B	38. B	63. B	88. B	113. B
14. C	39. C	64. E	89. D	114. B
15. C	40. D	65. A	90. C	115. C
16. B	41. C	66. B	91. B	116. C
17. C	42. A	67. B	92. B	117. C
18. E	43. A	68. E	93. E	118. E
19. C	44. E	69. C	94. D	119. D
20. B	45. B	70. D	95. E	120. B
21. B	46. E	71. A	96. D	121. B
22. D	47. C	72. E	97. B	122. B
23. A	48. B	73. E	98. E	123. B
24. E	49. E	74. B	99. E	124. A
25. A	50. E	75. D	100. D	125. C

Section 2: Science Problems

1. C	11. D	21. C	31. B
2. C	12. E	22. A	32. D
3. A	13. B	23. E	33. A
4. D	14. D	24. D	34. C
5. E	15. A	25. D	35. D
6. A	16. A	26. A	36. C
7. A	17. B	27. A	37. C
8. B	18. E	28. C	38. B
9. B	19. D	29. D	39. D
10. D	20. D	30. B	40. E

41. B
42. D
43. D
44. D
45. B
46. D
47. C

48. C
49. C
50. E
51. D
52. B
53. A
54. B

55. A
56. C
57. E
58. E
59. A
60. C

61. A
62. C
63. A
64. D
65. B
66. B

Section 3: Skills Analysis—Reading

1. A
2. C
3. D
4. C
5. D
6. A
7. B
8. A
9. C
10. C
11. B
12. B
13. A
14. A
15. A
16. B
17. C

18. A
19. C
20. C
21. B
22. A
23. E
24. B
25. C
26. C
27. D
28. D
29. D
30. C
31. A
32. A
33. B
34. D

35. B
36. B
37. C
38. A
39. B
40. B
41. C
42. A
43. B
44. B
45. B
46. B
47. B
48. D
49. D
50. D
51. D

52. A
53. C
54. B
55. E
56. B
57. B
58. A
59. C
60. B
61. B
62. C
63. A
64. B
65. B
66. A
67. A
68. A

Section 4: Skills Analysis—Quantitative

1. A
2. B
3. B
4. B
5. B
6. B
7. A
8. A
9. C
10. C
11. C
12. A
13. A
14. A
15. B
16. B
17. A

18. C
19. B
20. B
21. C
22. B
23. A
24. C
25. B
26. B
27. A
28. E
29. C
30. C
31. C
32. E
33. A
34. A

35. C
36. A
37. C
38. A
39. C
40. A
41. C
42. C
43. C
44. E
45. E
46. E
47. B
48. C
49. D
50. D
51. B

52. E
53. A
54. E
55. C
56. D
57. B
58. B
59. B
60. A
61. D
62. D
63. E
64. E
65. D
66. E
67. D

EXPLANATORY ANSWERS FOR
THE MCAT PRACTICE EXAMINATION

Section 1: Science Knowledge

BIOLOGY

1. **(A)** It is believed that rough E.R. ribosomes are involved in the synthesis of proteins that will leave the cell. They are conveniently situated along the walls of the E.R., the system of channels through which the proteins are transported to the Golgi apparatus. The so-called free ribosomes are complicated in steroid production.

2. **(B)** Mature red blood cells have no nuclei.

3. **(E)** The Golgi apparatus refers to a series of flattened cytoplasmic "vesicles" which function in packaging (i.e., enclosing within a membrane) the newly synthesized proteins emerging from the region of the rough endoplasmic reticulum. This packaging facilitates transport of the proteins to the cell exterior. The Golgi apparatus has also been shown to have the capacity to modify the incoming proteins by adding carbohydrate and/or sulfate moieties to them before membrane enclosure is completed.

4. **(B)** Hemophilia, an inherited disease in which the blood does not clot, is easily recognized. A tiny scratch can have lethal effects. Because of publicity and educational instruction, hemophiliacs (who are almost always male) and "carriers," or women who know they may be carriers, frequently elect not to have children. Therefore, this condition is slowly becoming eradicated from the population.

5. **(C)** Bacteriophage organisms are viruses that inject their DNA or RNA into host bacteria, eventually killing the host. Yeast cells also contain nucleic acids, but are not parasitic in nature.

6. **(E)** The most adaptable animal is the one that will tend to be "fittest" in *any* environment. The other points mentioned help, but this is the most beneficial.

7. **(D)** Diffusion of molecules from an area of high concentration to an area of low concentration is a fundamental concept in cell biology. Since the cellophane bags in this experiment are not permeable to sugar, only water molecules can diffuse. In beaker two there is a higher concentration of water in the container than in the bag. Water molecules will diffuse into the area of lower concentration in the bag.

8. **(B)** Hydrolysis means to "break with water." The reaction illustrated shows a water molecule breaking down a disaccharide into two glucose molecules.

9. **(D)** Motor neurons conduct impulses away from the central nervous system to a muscle or gland and, therefore, are involved in voluntary responses.

10. **(A)** Final cell differentiation occurs well after gastrulation and is controlled by the physical and chemical environment interacting with specific genes. Every cell, in theory at least, inherits the same sets of chromosomes. Therefore, the only correct choice is (A).

11. **(A)** A, B, and O blood genes are alleles, with A and B codominant and O recessive; therefore, the two possible crosses indicated by the wording of the problem are BB X AB or BO X AB. Working out a Punnett's square for the crosses shows that the correct answer is (A).

12. **(D)** It is now an accepted fact that base pairing is quite specific in DNA molecules. Cytosine always pairs with guanine and thymine always pairs with adenine. Uracil is only found in RNA molecules.

13. **(B)** Lysosomes are membrane-delimited cytoplasmic organelles that are generally packages of digestive enzymes (e.g., acid hydrolases). If the

contents of a lysosome were inappropriately re-leased, these enzymes would begin to digest cellular components, ultimately leading to cellular self-destruction (autolysis).

14. **(C)** Cells involved with synthesizing and secreting large quantities of protein would be expected to have all of the machinery necessary to accomplish these jobs. Mitochondria supply energy for work, ribosomes are the sites for protein synthesis, and the Golgi apparatus packages cell materials to be secreted.

15. **(C)** The isotonic fluid, known as amniotic fluid, surrounds the mammalian embryo and acts as an effective shock absorber.

16. **(B)** Several models for cell membrane structure have been proposed since the original model described by Davson and Danielli in 1941. Current-ly the model receiving the most support is the fluid mosaic model. It suggests that cell membranes are seas of lipid in which large globular proteins float about.

17. **(C)** Sensory neurons convey information from sense receptors to the central nervous system, while motor neurons convey information from the central nervous system to effector structures such as muscles and glands. Association neurons often provide an anatomical connection between sensory and motor neurons. The term "afferent" is general-ly used interchangeably with "sensory," whereas "efferent" is commonly used to indicate "motor."

18. **(E)** Mitosis, a form of cell division, can be described in four stages: prophase, metaphase, anaphase, and telophase. After paired chromo-somes separate (anaphase) and cytokinesis begins (early telophase), the two daughter nuclei form.

19. **(C)** Genes are believed to be long chains of DNA. Chromatin is a long thread composed of genes and associated proteins. Chromosomes are coiled chro-matin threads. Ribosomes are composed of pro-tein, structural RNA, and, during protein syn-thesis, messenger RNA. Of the cell organelles listed, only centrioles appear to lack any form of nucleic acid.

20. **(B)** The bile duct is a channel connecting the liver and gallbladder with the duodenum (the first part of the small intestine, in which protein, lipid, and carbohydrate digestion are completed). The bile duct provides the means by which the alkaline bile, which is produced by the liver and stored in the gallbladder, may reach the duodenum to perform its function in fat digestion. Bile is known to emulsify fats, which will prepare them for subse-quent digestion by pancreatic lipase. If the bile duct is obstructed, the bile will not easily reach the duodenum; this will directly impair fat digestion and therefore also ultimately limit the amount of dietary fat that can later be absorbed. This in turn will cause a greater amount of the dietary fat to appear in the stool.

21. **(B)** Budding is a modified mitotic cell division in which one daughter cell is larger than the other at the time of separation. Budding occurs in yeasts.

22. **(D)** The gastrocoele is the cavity in the embryonic structure known as the gastrula. The gastrula is composed of three layers: ectoderm, mesoderm, and the innermost layer, the endoderm.

23. **(A)** There are three symbiotic relationships: para-sitism is a relationship in which one species is often harmed; mutualism is a relationship in which neither species is harmed but both actually benefit; and commensalism is a relationship in which one species benefits while the other receives neither benefit nor harm. *Commensalism* literally means "eating at the same table" (*com*, together; *mensa*, table).

24. **(E)** Mutation may affect the individual but gene flow and genetic drift are factors that only affect an entire species. However, mutation, gene flow, and genetic drift all contribute to gene pool change and, therefore, ultimately to evolution.

25. **(A)** Vasopressin (also known as anti-diuretic hormone) is produced by the hypothalamus and stored in the posterior pituitary until release occurs. Its primary action of physiologic impor-tance is in controlling urine concentration; speci-fically, vasopressin promotes reabsorption of water from the urinary filtrate by the kidney tubule cells. This action results in the production of a highly concentrated urine, that is, one with a high osmolarity. A secondary effect of this hormone is to cause blood vessel constriction, leading to an elevated blood pressure because of the associated increase in resistance to blood flow. The hormone oxytocin is also produced by the hypothalamus and stored in the posterior pituitary; its major known action is to promote uterine smooth muscle contraction during labor. It is also believed to have a role in lactation, although its precise action in this process is unclear at this time.

26. **(A)** RNA would interfere with or block the normal protein synthesis occurring within the normal cell. RNA is a vital chemical necessary to the manufacture of fundamental proteins. However, they are specific from cell to cell. Receiving some from another organism would seriously impair the normal protein manufacturing reactions performed.

27. **(A)** The second meiotic division occurs with no chromosome replication and, therefore, results in the formation of haploid cells.

28. **(B)** The theory of endosymbiosis supports the idea that many cell organelles were originally independent units that invaded simple cells and established symbiotic relationships which have evolved into the complex integration recognized today as the cell ultrastructure.

29. **(A)** Skeletal, voluntary, and striated muscle are three different names for the same type of muscle. Cardiac muscle is found only in the heart; therefore, the only answer that could be correct is smooth muscle.

30. **(E)** Homologous structures exhibit a very strong evidence for common ancestry. Homologous organs are very similar in structure but adapted for widely different functions. Example: wing of bat, forearm of cat, flipper of whale, and arm of man are very similar in bone structure, but widely adapted for different uses (wing of bat for flying, forearm of cat for running, flipper of whale for swimming, and arm of man for manipulating).

31. **(C)** The villi are the specialized epithelial structures located throughout the small intestine that function to increase the absorptive surface area for lipids, carbohydrates, amino acids, vitamins, and other essential nutrients. Water, on the other hand, is predominantly reabsorbed in the large intestine, which is without villi.

32. **(C)** The only "living things" that do not contain both DNA and RNA are viruses, which always possess either DNA or RNA, but not both. Bacteriophages are types of viruses known to infect only bacteria. Inasmuch as they represent a class of viruses, they must contain only one kind of nucleic acid. The other choices given represent organisms other than viruses and therefore all contain both DNA and RNA.

33. **(A)** Pollen grains of pine must be blown by the wind to nearby ovulate cones in order to carry out fertilization. Pollen grains correspond to the sperm cells of animals.

34. **(B)** The renal portal system gathers blood from the hind fin and posterior body wall, dividing into capillaries within the kidneys. The blood is then collected by renal veins and returned to the heart. Amphibians also possess a renal portal system, which functions in much the same manner.

35. **(E)** The bronchioles terminate at the alveoli. Therefore, any blockage to these tiny air passages will prevent oxygen from reaching the air sacs and entering the capillaries which surround them.

36. **(A)** This is known as the backcross or test cross. If the black guinea pig is homozygous, then all the offspring will be hybrid black. If the black guinea pig is heterozygous, then 50% of the offspring will be hybrid black and 50% homozygous white.

37. **(E)** It is believed that RNA is the material of which memory is composed. If a planarian worm learns a maze, it, in effect, "memorizes" the solution to the problem. If the worm is then fed to an untrained planarian, it is thought that the RNA of the trained worm is transferred and assimilated. Having thus (presumably) incorporated the "solution" to the maze (i.e., RNA) within its cells, the untrained worm learns much more quickly than its predecessor.

38. **(B)** The enzymes described are employed during the process of cellular respiration. The mitochondria perform this life activity for the cell. Under the electron microscope, a much-folded inner membrane within the mitochondria is noted. The folds are called cristae. It is believed that the important cellular respiratory reactions occur within the confines of the cristae.

CHEMISTRY

39. **(C)** According to Bohr's model, the energy of the nth level, E_n, is proportional to $1/n^2$. Thus,

$$| E_{n_i} - E_{n_j} | \propto | 1/n_i^2 - 1/n_j^2 |$$

This means that as n-value increases, the difference between adjacent energy levels decreases. So we know that the transition from n = 2 to n = 1 results in a photon of the greatest energy. The photon of the greatest energy will be the photon of the highest frequency, according to the relation $E = h\nu$ where h is Planck's constant and ν is frequency.

40. **(D)** (1) $Zn + \frac{1}{2}O_1 = ZnO + 84,000$ cals
    (2) $HgO = Hg + \frac{1}{2}O_2 - 21,700$ cals
    Adding (1) and (2) and dropping the term $\frac{1}{2}O_2$ which appears on both sides of the chemical equation results in

    $$Zn + HgO = ZnO + Hg + 62,300 \text{ cals}$$

41. **(C)** Since the temperature is a measure of the kinetic energy of the gas and temperature is the only constant for all gases, the kinetic energy is the same for all gases at a particular temperature.

42. **(A)**

    $$\frac{dT_m}{dP} = \frac{MT_m}{L_m}\left(\frac{1}{p^l} - \frac{1}{p^s}\right)$$

    [Clausius-Clapeyron equation]

    If the volume of the substance increases on freezing, the density decreases so that $(1/p^l - 1/p^s) < 0$. Thus, $dT_m \propto - dP$ and therefore the melting point is lowered with an increase in external pressure.

43. **(A)**

    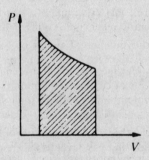

    For an adiabatic process $TV^{\gamma-1} = PV^\gamma / nR = $ constant. Therefore, we get the graph above.

44. **(E)** Water just below the freezing point (A) is denser than ice; therefore, it sinks, protecting bottom-dwelling organisms from freezing. (B) causes water to rise unnaturally high in capillary tubes, which is very important in plant physiology. High heat capacity (C) causes water to act as a thermal buffer. High heats of vaporization and fusion also help in keeping environmental temperatures stable. A high dielectric constant (D) makes water a solvent for a large variety of molecules that are essential for the chemical functioning of organisms. Since all the properties mentioned are indispensable to life, the correct answer is (E).

45. **(B)** Assume a 100 gram sample. Then

    $$\frac{77 \text{ grams}}{39 \text{ grams/mole}} = 2 \text{ moles of K}$$

    $$\frac{23 \text{ grams}}{16 \text{ grams/mole}} = 1.5 \text{ moles of O}$$

    So the elements combine in the following ratio: $K_2O_{1.5}$; thus the empirical formula K_4O_3.

46. **(E)** The total work done by or on the system will be the area enclosed by the path taken. Therefore, the area *acdga* represents the work done by the system.

47. **(C)** The minimum energy necessary would be that energy needed to move an electron from its orbit to infinity. The potential energy of the electron at the ground state is -13.6eV and at infinity is zero, so that the energy needed is 13.6 eV.

48. **(B)** The most basic substance in the group would give the water solution with the highest pH. In general, salts obtained by the neutralization of a strong acid with a strong base give neutral aqueous solutions; those obtained from weak acids and strong bases give basic solutions; and those from strong acids and weak bases give acidic solutions. With this as a guide, it can be seen that NaCl gives a neutral solution; NH_4Cl and CH_3COOH would give acidic solutions. Na_2CO_3 and $NaHCO_3$ are both derived from a strong base and a weak acid. However, the former would hydrolyze to give more NaOH than would the latter. It would, therefore, give the aqueous solution with the highest pH.

49. **(E)** The time, $t_{1/2}$, at which the original number of atoms is reduced by half, is

    $$N_{0/2} = N_0 e^{-\lambda + }{}_{1/2}$$

    which yields

    $$\text{Half life} = t_{1/2} = 1 \text{ n}(2/\lambda)$$

50. **(E)** Sp^3d hybridization consists of three orbitals in a central plane at $120°$ with one another and two equivalent orbitals perpendicular to this plane.

51. **(A)** The partial vapor pressure of a solute is a measure of the tendency of the solute to escape from the solution into the vapor phase. Hence, solubility is greatest when the partial pressure of

the solute is minimized—namely, at low temperatures (ideal gas law) and at high external pressures.

52. **(D)** Graham's Law states that the rate of diffusion is inversely proportional to the square root of the molecular weight. $U^{=235}$ is separated from natural uranium ($U^{=238}$) by a diffusion method involving the fluoride compounds $^{238}UF_6$ and $^{235}UF_6$.

53. **(C)** Without doing any calculation, it should be realized that the second ionization constant of carbonic acid, which is a weak acid, is very small and the solution will be basic, but the bicarbonate ion is not a strong base so that (C) is the only reasonable answer.

54. **(C)** The brass cylinder displaces its own weight in mercury and, since the mercury is twice as dense, half of the cylinder will be submerged.

55. **(E)** The pressure difference across a curved surface is inversely proportional to the radius of the tube. But after a capillary rise, h, this pressure difference will be ghP where P is the density of the liquid.

56. **(B)** The element whose atomic number is 7 (nitrogen) has three $2p$ electrons in its outer shell. The other elements listed all have s type outer shells with one or two electrons.

57. **(E)** Henry's Law states that the mole fraction of a component of a solution is proportional to the partial vapor pressure of that component above the solution.

58. **(A)** Air oxidation of ethyl alcohol is a common way of preparing dilute aqueous solutions of acetic acid (vinegar).

59. **(C)** Atomic species having different atomic numbers (number of protons in the nucleus) but the same mass numbers (total number of protons and neutrons in the nucleus) are called isobars.

60. **(C)**

$$3H_2O + P_2O_5 \rightarrow 2H_3PO_4$$

61. **(C)** Although the two 3s electrons form a closed shell, they lie only slightly lower in energy than the 3p electron and are readily available for bonding. The energy required to promote a 3s electron to a 3p orbital is more than offset by the energy gained in the formation of three bonds.

62. **(E)** The hydroxylated carbon is bound to four diverse groups and is, therefore, asymmetric. Hence the mirror images of this compound are not superimposable and optical isomerism exists.

63. **(B)** The atomic weight of oxygen is 16. Let the atomic weight of X be denoted by "x." Then the ratio of weights with which X combines with oxygen to form X_4O_6 is 4x/6(16). Therefore,

$$\frac{4(x)}{6(16)} = \frac{8.40}{6.50}$$

64. **(E)** In an aqueous solution, the two products remain in solution in ionized form and the reaction is reversible. In (A), (B), and (D), precipitates are formed and the reactions proceed to completion. Reaction (C) proceeds to completion as H_2 gas is given off.

65. **(A)** A faraday is the quantity of electricity capable of depositing one gram–equivalent weight of a substance in electrolysis. One faraday will supply electrons to one mole of singly charged cations, but the copper in $CuSO_4$ is bivalent, so 0.5 faraday will deposit only 0.25 moles, or 16 g of copper.

66. **(B)** Consider the dissociation of NH_4OH.

$$NH_4OH \rightleftharpoons NH_4^+ + OH^-$$

If x is the number of moles of NH_4OH which dissociates, then for a 0.1M solution the following equation holds:

$$\frac{(x)(x)}{(0.1-x)} = 1.8 \cdot 10^{-5}$$

where $0.1 - x$ is the concentration of NH_4OH after dissociation and x is equal to the concentrations of NH_4^+ and OH^- ions. Neglecting x compared to 0.1 and solving gives $x = 1.34 \cdot 10^{-3}M$.

67. **(B)** There are three equivalents of H_3PO_4 per mole and two equivalents of $Ca(OH)_2$ per mole so that the normalities of the two solutions are

$$N(H_3PO_4) = 3(0.25) = 0.75 = N_1$$
$$\text{and } N(CA(OH)_2) = \quad 2(0.30) = 0.60 = N_2$$

Using the equation $N_1V_1 = N_2V_2$ with $V_2 = 25$ ml then yields $V_1 = 20$ml.

68. **(E)** One gram of solution contains 0.8 g methanol and 0.2 g water.

$$\frac{0.8g \text{ Me OH}}{0.2g \text{ H}_2\text{O}} \cdot \frac{18g \text{ H}_2\text{O}}{1 \text{mole H}_2\text{O}} \cdot \frac{1 \text{ mole Me OH}}{32g \text{ Me OH}}$$

$$= 2.25 \frac{\text{mole Me OH}}{\text{mole H}_2\text{O}}$$

Hence the mole fraction of methanol is given by

$$\frac{2.25 \text{ moles Me OH}}{2.25 + 1.00 \text{ moles solution}} = \frac{9}{13}$$

and this ratio corresponds most closely to (**E**).

69. (**C**) Since $AgNO_3$ is readily soluble in water, the dissociation into ions must be energetically favorable and must proceed with a release of energy implying a negative hydration energy.

70. (**D**) Calcium cyanamid reacts with water (in the form of superheated steam) to yield ammonia.

$$CaCN_2 + 3H_2O \rightarrow CaCO_3 + 2NH_3 \uparrow$$

71. (**A**) In CO_2, the carbon atom is double-bonded to each of the oxygens. If the two participating oxygen atoms each contribute one electron to each of the bonds, then the electron distribution in the molecule may be represented as follows:

$$\overset{..}{O} \overset{xx}{\underset{xx}{}} C \overset{xx}{\underset{xx}{}} \overset{..}{O}$$

where "x" represents an electron participating in a bond and "·" represents an electron isolated on an atom. All but the inner shell 1s electrons are represented above and it is seen that each atom has an outer shell of eight electrons.

72. (**E**) The sulfur nucleus is identical in each of the particles and only the number of electrons differs. S^{-4} has the most electrons and hence is the heaviest.

73. (**E**) The boiling point of a compound is that temperature at which the vapor pressure reaches one atmosphere. CH_4 has the lowest boiling point of the substances listed (being a gas at room temperature) and therefore has the highest vapor pressure.

74. (**B**) One of the basic assumptions regarding an ideal gas is that there are no forces between molecules. A real gas approaches this behavior as the density is lowered and intermolecular encounters are correspondingly decreased. This calls for the conditions of (**B**).

75. (**D**) Particle accelerators operate by the action of electric and magnetic fields on the particles in question. Since these fields exert no forces on a neutral particle, a neutron cannot be accelerated by such machines.

76. (**B**) Divide the number of grams of each compound by the molecular weight of that compound (28, 32 and 44 for N_2, O_2 and CO_2, respectively) to get the number of moles of each. The results are that the mixture contains 2.5 mol N_2, 4 mol O_2 and 1 mol CO_2 so that the mole fraction of N_2 is 2.5/7.5 = 0.33.

77. (**C**) From the ideal gas law it is seen that at constant pressure, the ratio V/T is a constant.

$$V_1/T_1 = V_2/T_2$$

$$\frac{23 \text{ ml}}{283°K} = \frac{x \text{ ml}}{303°K}$$

$$x = 24.6 \text{ ml}$$

78. (**D**) The Law of Dulong and Petit states that

(specific heat per gram) (atomic wt) = 6.0

Thus, in this case,

$$\text{atomic weight} = \frac{6.0}{.166} \approx 36 \text{ grams/mole}$$

79. (**E**) For a state with azimuthal quantum number 2, the magnetic quantum number may have the values -2, -1, 0, 1 and 2.

80. (**E**) In order for hydrogen bonding to be strong, the electronegative atom must be small so that hydrogen atoms on adjacent molecules can approach close enough to form strong bonds. Since selenium is considerably larger than oxygen, the hydrogen bonding is not nearly as strong in H_2Se as in H_2O.

81. (**E**) K^+, Ca^{++}, Sc^{+++} and Ti^{++++} all have the same core of electrons ($1s^2 \, 2s^2 \, 2p^6 \, 3s^2 \, 3p^6$) around the nucleus; but Ti^{++++} has the highest nuclear charge, so that the electrons are drawn in closer to the nucleus and the atomic radius is smaller. Ti^{+++} has an extra electron in the 4s shell and naturally has a larger radius.

82. (**A**) The best way to determine relative acidity is to compare the stabilities of the anion A^- (which results from the loss of a proton by the acid HA). In this case benzenesulfonic acid's corresponding anion is the most stable, due to resonance stabilization in the aromatic ring.

83. (**C**) The sp^2 hybridization is the only one which can

provide three equivalent hydrogen atoms in a plane. The unpaired electron is in the unhybridized p orbital which lies perpendicular to the plane of the molecule.

84. **(D)** According to the equation, 8500 calories are needed to separate the ions from each other. If this energy is not provided from the environment, it will be obtained at the expense of the internal energy of the solution, leading to a lowering of its temperature.

85. **(E)** Ethanol can be oxidized in a step-wise fashion that leads ultimately to the production of CO_2. The first step in this oxidation is the production of acetaldehyde:

$$CH_3CH_2OH + [\tfrac{1}{2}O_2] \rightarrow CH_3CHO + H_2O$$
$$\text{ethanol} \qquad\qquad\qquad \text{acetaldehyde}$$

86. **(A)** A buffer solution consists of a weak acid and one of its salts, or a weak base and one of its salts, and possesses the ability to resist pH changes caused by the addition of some acid or base. On this basis, the obvious choice for a buffer solution is $HC_2H_3O_2 + NaC_2H_3O_2$.

87. **(B)** For an adiabatic process dQ is zero and it is done reversibly. Since it is done reversibly, the work done is the same for all adiabatic paths connecting the two states.

PHYSICS

88. **(B)**

For m_1 :
P.E. = K.E.
$$m_1gh_1 = \tfrac{1}{2}m_1 v_1{}^2$$
$$v_1 = \sqrt{2gh_1}$$

For m_2 :
P.E. = K.E.
$$m_2 gh_2 = \tfrac{1}{2}m_2 v_2{}^2$$
$$v_2 = \sqrt{2gh_2}$$

Since $h_2 = 4h_1$ $v_2 = \sqrt{2g\,(4h_1)} = 2\sqrt{2gh_1} = 2v_1$

89. **(D)** The index of refraction is equal to the ratio of the velocity of light in a vacuum to the velocity of light in the medium. Since the velocity of light in this medium is one-third of its velocity in a vacuum, the index of refraction of the medium is equal to 3.

90. **(C)** The force of gravitational attraction between two masses, m_1 and m_2, is equal to $Gm_1 m_2/r^2$ where G is a constant and r is the distance between the masses. If m_1, m_2, and r are doubled, the force of attraction will remain the same.

91. **(B)** The specific gravity of a liquid is a measure of its density relative to that of water. If liquids A and B have specific gravities in a ratio of 2:3, this means that liquid B is $\tfrac{3}{2}$ times as dense as liquid A, and it will therefore exert $\tfrac{3}{2}$ times as much buoyant force. If 20% of the block's volume is above the surface of liquid A, then $\tfrac{3}{2}$ of 20%, or 30%, of the volume will be above the surface in liquid B.

92. **(B)** The intensity of sound is always proportional to the term $1/R^2$, where R is the distance the sound travels from its source to some distant point. According to this inverse square relationship, the further a sound travels, that is, as R becomes larger, the smaller the intensity becomes. In this example, wave P clearly travels the greater distance in order to reach point 0 and will therefore have less intensity at that point than wave R.

93. **(E)** The force on a charge, q, is equal to qE. It is not necessary to know the distance, r, to the charge distribution or the value of the potential, v, at the given point in space. Since we are concerned only with the magnitude of the charge, its sign will not alter our calculations.

94. **(D)** Start with 100%: After one half-life elapses, there remains 50%; after another half-life, 25%; after another, 12.5%; after another, 6.25%. Thus, after four half-lives, 6.25% remains. Two days consist of 48 hours, so the half-life in this case is $48 \div$ by $4 = 12$ hrs.

95. **(E)** Since the resistors are connected in series, the current through the two must be the same. Therefore the ratio is equal to 1.

96. **(D)** Equipotential surfaces are perpendicular to the electric field that has resulted from the charge distribution.

97. **(B)**
$$F = ma \leqslant 25 \text{ nt}$$
$$25 \text{ nt} = (2\text{kg})a$$
$$a = 12.5 \text{ m/sec}^2$$

98. **(E)** The force the floor will exert upon the man will be the force due to gravity, 180 lb, minus the imaginary force due to the deceleration of the elevator.

$$F^* = F_g - ma^* \qquad m = F_g/g$$
$$g = 32 \text{ ft/sec}^2 \qquad F_g = 180 \text{ lb}$$
$$a^* = 8 \text{ ft/sec}^2$$
$$\therefore F^* = 180 \text{ lb} - [(180 \text{ lb})/(32 \text{ ft/sec}^2)]$$
$$\times (8 \text{ ft/sec}^2)$$
$$F^* = 135 \text{ lb}$$

99. **(E)** We do not know how much work is necessary to overcome air friction.

100. **(D)**

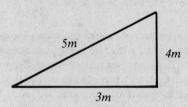

$$\begin{matrix} \text{Amount of} \\ \text{energy lost} \end{matrix} = \begin{matrix} \text{(Amount at} \\ \text{the top)} \end{matrix} - \begin{matrix} \text{(Amount to} \\ \text{the bottom)} \end{matrix}$$

$$= \text{Potential energy} - \text{kinetic energy}$$
$$= mgh - \tfrac{1}{2}mv^2$$
$$= (5 \text{ Kg})(9.8\text{m/sec})(4\text{m}) - \tfrac{1}{2}(5\text{Kg})(8 \text{ m/sec})^2$$
$$= 196 \text{ Kg} - \text{m}^2/\text{sec}^2 - 160 \text{ Kg} - \text{m}^2/\text{sec}^2$$
$$= 36 \text{ Kg} - \text{m}^2/\text{sec}^2$$

The fraction lost is 36/196 = 18/98, or about 20%.

101. **(D)** An alpha particle is a helium nucleus, and, therefore, it has atomic number 2 and mass number 4. The nuclear reaction is

$$_{88}\text{Ra}^{226} \rightarrow {}_2\text{He}^4 + {}_{86}\text{Rn}^{222}$$

102. **(D)** Power $= I^2R$. The current through the 10 r resistor is found, by using Ohm's law (V = IR), to be 8 amps. Thus,

$$P = I^2R$$
$$P = (8)^2 (10) \text{ watts} =$$
$$P = 640 \text{ watts}$$

103. **(D)** When resistors are connected in parallel, the potential across each of them is the same.

104. **(D)** Current is defined as the rate at which the charge is flowing.
Thus,
$$Q = I\triangle t.$$
$$I = 5 \text{ amp} = 5 \text{ coulomb/sec}$$
$$\triangle t = 240 \text{ sec}$$
$$\text{Therefore, } Q = 1200 \text{ C.}$$

105. **(E)** Since the plates are moved apart by the use of insulated handles, the charge on the capacitor must remain constant. For a parallel-plate, capa-

citor C is proportional to A/l, where A is the area of the plate and l is the distance between the plates. Therefore, C must decrease. By definition, $C = Q/V$. Therefore, the voltage must increase.

106. **(A)** If the original resistance of the single wire is R, each piece will have a resistance $0.1R$. If these are then connected in parallel, the total resistance is

$$1/R_t = 10(1/0.1R)$$
$$R_t = 0.01R$$
$$R_t/R = 0.01$$

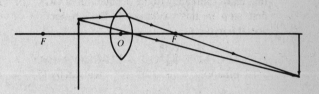

107. **(D)** As can be seen from the ray diagram above, the image is real and inverted.

108. **(C)** The magnification, $M, = -\dfrac{Di}{Do}$ where Di = distance to the image and Do = distance to the object. Thus, in this case, $M = -4$. M also equals $\dfrac{Si}{So}$. Therefore, $-4 = \dfrac{Si}{So}$ and $So = \dfrac{Si}{-4}$. Si is negative because the object is inverted.

109. **(D)** The energy stored by a capacitor is equal to ½ cv^2, where c is the capacitance and v the potential difference across the plates. In this case, $c = 2x$ and $v = 4x$.

$$E_c = \tfrac{1}{2}cv^2 = \tfrac{1}{2}(2x)(4x)^2$$
$$= \tfrac{1}{2}(2x)(16x^2)$$
$$= (x)(16x^2)$$
$$= 16x^3$$

110. **(E)** The potential difference is the work required to move a test charge from point A to B divided by the magnitude of the test charge.

$$V = 2 \text{ joules/20 coulomb}$$
$$V = 0.1 \text{ joule/coulomb}$$
$$\text{one volt} = \text{one joule/coulomb}$$
$$V = 1 \times 10^{-1} \text{ volt.}$$

111. **(C)** For a parallel plate capacitor, $C = \varepsilon\varepsilon_o A/l$, where ε is the relative dielectric constant. $\varepsilon = 1$ for air. Thus,

$$C_{air} = \varepsilon_o A/l$$
$$C_{mica} = \varepsilon_{mica}\varepsilon_o A/l = \varepsilon_{mica}\, C_{air}$$
$$= 6(15\ \mu\mu f)$$
$$C_{mica} = 90\ \mu\mu f$$

112. **(A)** $V = q/r$ for a point charge in cgs units

$$V = 4.8 \times 10^{-10} esu/0.5 \times 10^{-8} cm$$
$$V = 9.6 \times 10^{-2}\ \text{statvolts}$$
one statvolt = 300 volts
$$V = 28.8\ \text{volts}.$$

113. **(B)** The charge on the electron is 1.602×10^{-19} coulomb. The current would be the charge times the angular frequency. $I = q\omega$.

$$I = (1.602 \times 10^{-19} coulomb)\ (6.6 \times 10^{15}/sec)$$
$$I = 1.05 \times 10^{-3}\ amp.$$

114. **(B)** For series capacitors, the total capacitance is $1/C_t = 1/C_1 + 1/C_2$, where $C_1 = 0.5\ \mu f$, $C_2 = 1.0$ μf. Since the plates are connected in series and the plates of two are directly connected, each capacitor must have the same charge Q and this must be the total charge. Also, $V_1 + V_2 = 220$ volts.

$$\frac{1}{C_t} = \frac{1}{.5\ \mu f} + \frac{1}{1.0\ \mu f} \rightarrow C_t = \frac{.5}{1.5}\ \mu f$$
$$C_t = Q/V$$
$$1/3\ \mu f = Q/220\ v$$
$$Q = 7.3 \times 10^{-5}\ coulomb.$$

115. **(C)** If we start with a 100-gram sample of uranium, at the end of the first half-life, 50 grams will be left; at the end of the second half-life, 25 grams will remain; third, 12.5; fourth, 6; fifth, 3; sixth, 1.5; and finally seventh, 0.75 (less than 1 percent will remain).

116. **(C)** $I^2 R_1 = 90$ watts; $R_1 =$ resistance of lamp
$$I R_1 = 30\ \text{volts}$$
$$I = 3\ \text{amps}$$
$$120\ \text{volts} = (R + R_1)I$$
Thus, $IR = 90$ volts
$$R = 30\ \Omega$$

117. **(C)** By Snell's Law,

$$n \sin \phi = n' \sin \phi$$
$$(1.4)(.8) = \sin \phi'$$

Therefore, the ray must be internally reflected.

118. **(E)** In a nuclear reaction, the sum of the mass numbers (superscripts) on the left side of the equation must equal the corresponding sum on the right side, by the law of mass conservation. It is also true that the sums of the atomic numbers (subscripts) must be equal, by the law of charge conservation. Of the electron ($_{-1}{}^{0}e$), positron ($_{+1}{}^{0}e$), proton ($_1{}^1 H$), alpha particle ($_2{}^4 He$), and neutron ($_0{}^1 n$), only the neutron allows these requirements to be met.

119. **(D)** The parallel beam of light has an energy density U, and the parallel beam reflected must also have energy density U to conserve energy. This means that there has been a change in momentum of $2\,U \times A$, where A is the area of the surface. Therefore,
$$F = 2UA$$
$$p = F/A = 2\,U.$$

120. **(B)** Before the release, the two men were supporting the plank equally, so the man we are interested in feels a force of $\frac{1}{2}\,W$, initially. Immediately after the collision we may consider the rod to be falling and rotating about its center of mass.

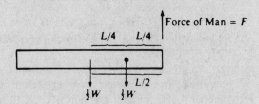

$$F\left(\frac{L}{2}\right) - \left(\frac{W}{2}\right)\left(\frac{L}{4}\right) + \left(\frac{W}{2}\right)\left(\frac{L}{2}\right)$$
$$F = \frac{3W}{4}$$

So the change in force the man feels is

$$\frac{1}{4}(3\,W - 2\,W) = \frac{1}{4}\,W.$$

121. **(B)** The resistance of a metallic element is dependent upon the disorder of the free electrons in it. The disorder increases with the thermal energy of the bar. Therefore, when the temperature is lowered, so is the resistance.

122. **(B)** When the ball is at its zenith it is momentarily motionless. As such it has no *kinetic* energy (since this energy is related to movement) but has a great deal of *potential* energy (since it is an unstable situation—i.e., it is about to fall). The only option that correctly describes this situation is (B).

123. **(B)** The velocity at which these two objects will roll depends upon how much of the potential energy will be transformed into rotational energy and how much into translational.

$$\tfrac{1}{2} Mv^2 + \tfrac{1}{2} Iw^2 = Mgh$$

where h is the height the bodies have dropped and v is the angular velocity of the object. For both $\omega = v/R$, where R is the radius.

Sphere: $\tfrac{1}{2} Mv^2 + \tfrac{1}{2} (\tfrac{2}{5} MR^2)(v/R)^2 = Mgh$

$$v = \sqrt{\tfrac{10}{7} gh}$$

Cylinder: $\tfrac{1}{2} Mv^2 + \tfrac{1}{2} (\tfrac{1}{2} MR^2)(v/R)^2 = Mgh$
$$v = \sqrt{\tfrac{4}{3} gh}$$

Therefore, the sphere is rolling faster than the cylinder and will reach the bottom first independent of the mass and radius.

124. **(A)** By definition, a conservative field is one in which energy is conserved. That is, if you return to the same point you have the same energy at that point. This implies that the work done must be independent of the paths and dependent only upon the end points.

125. **(C)** Since the capacitors are connected in series, they must have the same charge, Q.

$$120\ V = V_1 + V_2$$
$$C_1 = Q/V_1 \qquad C_2 = Q/V_2$$
$$Q = C_1 V_1$$
$$V_2 = C_1 V_1 / C_2$$
$$120\ V = V_1(1 + C_1/C_2)$$
$$120\ V = 3V_1/2$$
$$V_1 = 80\ \text{volts}$$

Section 2: Science Problems

1. **(C)** The equation

$$\text{rate} = K\,([A\ (g)])^n$$

where K is the rate constant and n is some unknown power, holds for any rate-concentration pair. Take, for example, measurements 1 and 4.

Measurement 1: .030 moles/liter-sec $= K$ (.10 moles/liter)^n

Measurement 4: .480 moles/liter-sec $= K$ (.40 moles/liter)^n

Dividing the second equation by the first equation, we arrive at

$$16 = (\tfrac{.4}{.1})^n$$
$$16 = (4)^n$$
$$n = 2$$

Therefore, the reaction is second order with respect to $[A\ (g)]$.

2. **(C)** To find the rate constant of the reaction, look at the information given for measurement 1, for example.

$$\text{rate} = K\,([A\ (g)])^n$$
$$.030\ \text{moles/liter-second} = K\,(.1\ \text{moles/liter})^2$$
$$K = 3\ \text{liters/mole-sec}$$

3. **(A)** When a reaction is called zero-order with respect to a particular substance, this means that the rate of reaction is essentially unaffected by changes in the concentration of that substance. Therefore, a plot of reaction rate versus $[A\ (g)]$ should be linear.

4. **(D)**

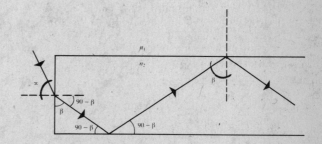

According to Snell's law, $n_1 \sin \alpha = n_2 \sin (90 - \beta)$. Since $\sin (90 - \beta) = \cos \beta$, $n_1 = n_2 \cos \beta / \sin \alpha$.

5. **(E)** When light enters a medium with a different optical density, its velocity changes according to the relation $n_2 v_2 = n_1 v_1$, where in media 1 and 2, $n_{1,2}$ and $v_{1,2}$ are the respective indices of refraction and velocities of light. Since the index of refraction

of the optical fiber is greater than that of the tissue, the velocity of the light must decrease upon entering the fiber. Since its frequency never changes when light enters a new medium, its wavelength must decrease, along with the velocity, to maintain equality in the relation $v = f\lambda$ where v = velocity, f = frequency, and λ = wave length. The period of light is equal to the reciprocal of its frequency. In this case, since the frequency remains the same, the period must also remain unchanged.

6. **(A)** Shorter-wavelength (blue) light is refracted more than longer-wavelength (red) light. Thus, the angle of refraction $(90 - \beta$: see answer 4) would decrease. Therefore, angle β would increase.

7. **(A)** The aldehyde at C1 reacts with the alcoholic group at C5.

8. **(B)** The β anomer is more stable than the α anomer. It is more stable because the –OH group is in the equatorial position. In the α anomer, the OH group is in the axial position (where the steric hindrance is more pronounced).

9. **(B)** Generally, furanoses are more reactive because there is more strain in a five-membered ring.

10. **(D)** Mitochondria contain some DNA. Cytosine is a nitrogenous base found in DNA. Mitochondria contain many of the respiratory enzymes. Glucose is the "fuel" for respiration.

11. **(D)** Golgi bodies and rough endoplasmic reticulum are concerned with the packaging and transport of proteins (which are made up of amino acids). The smooth endoplasmic reticulum is not concerned with proteins. It is involved in the processing of steroids and glycogen.

12. **(E)** Since RNA, DNA, respiration, and protein synthesis are involved in the life of bacteria, I, II, III, and IV, respectively, could have been responsible for the labeling.

13. **(B)** The heat gained by the added water in going from 10°C to 30°C must equal the heat lost by the 100 Kilograms of water in going from 40°C to 30°C. The specific heat of water is 1 calorie 1 gm = °C. Let x equal the number of grams of added water. Thus,

(mass) (temperature change) (specific heat) =
            (mass) (temperature change) (specific heat)

100×10^3 grams (10°C) 1 cal/gm – °C =
            x grams (20°C). 1 cal/gm – °C
1000×10^3 calories = 20 X calories
$50 \times 10^3 = X$

Therefore, 50 Kilograms (50,000 grams) must be added.

14. **(D)** The heat needed to melt the ice must equal the heat lost by the 100 Kilograms of water at 30°C. Thus,

(80 cal/gm) 10×10^3 gm = 100×10^3 gm (X)
            1 cal/gm = °C
            $8 \times 10^5 = 10^5 (X)$/°C
            $X = 8°C$

15. **(A)** In any closed system, entropy increases.

16. **(A)** After 10 seconds, there remain 100×10^{10} radioactive nuclei. Since there were originally 200×10^{10}, 10 seconds is the half-life (the time it takes for one half of the nuclei to decay).

17. **(B)** 40 seconds equals 4 half-lives (see answer 16). So the number of radioactive nuclei that remain has been divided in half four times; from 100% to 50% to 25% to 12.5% to 6.25%. Thus, 6.25% $(6\frac{1}{4}\%)$ remains.

18. **(E)** It is impossible for all of the nuclei to decay.

19. **(D)** Conservation of mass requires that the same volume of fluid pass each cross section during any given time interval. The volume of water which passes a given cross section is equal to the velocity times the cross sectional area. (This is Bernouilli's Law.) Thus,

$$(\text{Vol})_A = (\pi r_A{}^2)\,(\text{Vel})_A$$
$$(\text{Vol})_B = (\pi r_B{}^2)\,(\text{Vel})_B$$
$$\pi(r_A{}^2)\,(\text{Vel})_A = \pi(r_B{}^2)\,(\text{Vel})_B$$
$$(\text{Vel})_B = (\text{Vel})_A \left(\frac{r_A{}^2}{r_B{}^2}\right)$$

$$= 30\,\frac{\text{ft}}{\text{sec}} \left(\frac{100\text{mm}^2}{25\text{mm}^2}\right) = 120\,\frac{\text{ft}}{\text{sec}}$$

20. **(D)** The buoyant force $F_b = \rho V g$ where ρ = density, V = volume, and g = acceleration due to gravity. Thus, $F_b \propto \rho$. Since the same platelet was allowed to submerge in the water and in the blood plasma,

$$\frac{F_b\,(\text{plasma})}{F_b\,(\text{water})} = \frac{\rho\,(\text{plasma})}{\rho(\text{water})} = \text{specific gravity}$$
$$(\text{plasma})$$

Therefore, specific gravity (plasma)

$$= \frac{2 \times 10^- \text{ dynes}}{1 \times 10^{-3} \text{ dynes}} = 2.$$

21. **(C)** The pressure depends on the weight of the column of blood above the given point. The weight of such a column is given by $\rho g h A$ where ρ = the density of the blood, g = the acceleration due to gravity, h = the height of the column, and A = the area over which the force is applied. Since Force = (Pressure) (Area), Pressure = $\rho g h$. Thus, pressure depends on the density and depth.

22. **(A)** Two separate characteristics (genes) are involved in this problem: color of cattle and presence or absence of horns. The offspring exhibit the polled trait. Therefore, this is a dominant gene according to Mendel's first law (Law of Dominance). The offspring also display the roan color. This is an exception to Mendel's first law because red or white should be prominent. However, an intermediate shade is noted, which exhibits blending or an example of lack of domination by either gene.

23. **(E)** According to Mendel's third law (Law of Unit Characters or Independent Assortment), each gene should separate independently of one another following a 9:3:3:1 ratio. This means that 9/16 of the offspring should exhibit both dominant characteristics, 6/16 should exhibit one dominant and one recessive trait, and only 1/16 should show the double recessive character.

24. **(D)** The genes for red and white color (configuration for hybrid trait roan) independently separate to appear in the F_2 generation according to Mendel's third law.

25. **(D)** According to Le Châtelier's principle, if the pressure on a system at equilibrium is increased, the reaction will be driven in such a direction as to relieve the pressure (i.e., in the direction that will produce fewer molecules). Since there is no indication as to whether A, B, and C are solid, liquid, or gas, we cannot apply the principle and therefore cannot answer the question.

26. **(A)** Addition of heat displaces the reaction so that heat is absorbed. Thus, raising the temperature would drive the reaction to the left as written.

27. **(A)** A system in equilibrium that is perturbed will shift in such a direction so as to relieve the perturbation. Thus, the addition of A would drive the reaction to the right. The removal of B or the addition of C would drive the reaction to the left.

28. **(C)** This is a series circuit, so that its net resistance will equal the sum of the resistance of the motor, R_2, and R_1. The current in a series circuit is the same at every point. Therefore, when the ammeter reads 1 amp, this must represent the current for the entire circuit. According to Ohm's Law, the current in amperes will be equal to the total voltage divided by the total resistance—that is,

$$1 \text{ amp} = \frac{16 \text{ volts}}{4 \text{ ohms} + R_2 + R_1}$$

$$4 \text{ ohms} + R_2 + R_1 = 16$$
$$R_2 + R_1 = 12 \text{ ohms}$$

29. **(D)** The power dissipated by the motor will be equal to $i^2 R$, where $i = 1$ amp and $R = 4$ ohms. The units of power will be expressed as joules/second, or watts—in this case, our answer will be $(1)^2(4)$, or 4 watts.

30. **(B)** One ampere is an amount of current represented by one coulomb of charge passing a given point in the circuit per second. This relationship can be expressed as

$$\text{current} = \frac{\text{charge}}{\text{time}}. \text{ Here } 0.5 \text{ amps} = \frac{x \text{ coulombs}}{10 \text{ seconds}}.$$

$$x = (0.5)(10)$$
$$x = 5 \text{ coulombs}$$

31. **(B)** According to Dalton's Law of Partial Pressures, the mole fraction of a gas is its partial pressure divided by the total pressure of the gas sample. In this case, the mole fraction of gas B equals $\frac{300}{1520}$, which is approximately $\frac{1}{5}$.

32. **(D)** The pressure of the gas mixture is $500 + 300 + 720$, or 1520 mm Hg. Since 1 atmosphere of pressure equals 760 mm Hg, 1520 mm Hg must equal 2 atmospheres.

33. **(A)** 1 mole of an ideal gas occupies 22.4 liters at STP. $\frac{11 \text{ liters/minute}}{22.4 \text{ liters/mole}}$ will give us the number of moles of the gas mixture administered per minute. The value is approximately .5 moles/minute. Of this amount, 12% will be gas C. Therefore, $(.5)(.12) = .06$ moles/minute of gas C.

34. **(C)** In human embryonic development, it charac-

teristically takes 30 hours from the time of fertilization to reach the 2-cell stage. Forty hours are required for the fertilized egg to reach the 4-cell stage, whereas 48 hours are needed for the zygote to reach the 8-cell stage.

35. **(D)** If the mitotic disturbance always occurs during metaphase, then we may conclude that some event, process, etc., unique to metaphase is being disrupted by colchicine. Of the choices, the formation of the spindle apparatus is the only one exclusively associated with metaphase. Note that synapsis, (C), refers to the pairing of homologous chromosomes during meiosis.

36. **(C)** Colchicine will be expected to have an effect on any cells that are either mitotically active or that may become mitotically active under certain conditions. Of the choices, the red blood cell precursors and intestinal lining cells normally demonstrate an ongoing level of mitotic activity. Liver cells are not generally mitotically active, but may become so if damaged or destroyed liver cells require replacement. Mature nerve cells, however, have permanently lost all of their mitotic capabilities.

37. **(C)** After one half-life, $\frac{1}{2}$ of a radioactive sample will remain. After two half-lives, $(\frac{1}{2})(\frac{1}{2})$, or $\frac{1}{4}$, of the original sample will remain. This means that $\frac{3}{4}$ of the original sample will have decayed. In this question, two half-lives will be equal to 2(9 seconds), or 18 seconds.

38. **(B)** Any nucleus has a smaller mass than the combined mass of the neutrons and protons of which it is composed. The difference is converted into an energy known as the binding energy.

39. **(D)** A positron is represented by the symbol $_{+1}^{0}e$, indicating an atomic number of +1 and

an atomic mass of 0. Here, $\frac{131}{54}y + _{+1}^{0}e$ will

yield an element with an atomic number of 54 + 1, or 55, and an atomic mass of 131 + 0, or 131.

40. **(E)** We do not know the eye color of F and we are not sure of C's eye color. Thus, the eye color of H cannot be determined.

41. **(B)** E is a carrier female, possessing one color-blind gene and one "normal" gene. If she marries a color-blind male, the following Punnett Square applies, c = color-blind gene:

	X^c	Y
X^c	X^cX^c	X^cY
X	XX^c	XY

Results: 25% normal male
25% color-blind male
25% carrier female
25% color-blind female

Thus, all of the daughters possess at least one gene for color blindness.

42. **(D)** There will always be a 50% chance (or extremely close to 50% chance) that the next child will be male. Each new birth is an independent event.

43. **(D)**

$$Ka = \frac{[H^+][A^-]}{[HA]}$$

$$1 \times 10^{-5} = \frac{[H^+] \cdot .22 \text{ moles/liter}}{.22 \text{ moles/liter}}$$

$$[H^+] = 1 \times 10^{-5}$$
$$pH = -\log[H^+]$$
$$pH = -(-5) = 5$$

44. **(D)** The addition of HCl will increase the weak acid concentration by .18 moles/liter and decrease the anion concentration by the same amount.

$$K_a = \frac{[H^+][A^-]}{[HA]}$$

$$[H^+] = 1 \times 10^{-5} \frac{.04}{.40} = 10^{-6}$$

$$pH = -\log[H^+] = -(-6) = 6$$

45. **(B)** There is one equivalent in 36.5 grams because HCl gives up only one mole of protons per mole of HCl. Since 12 grams equals about one-third of a mole, there is about one-third of one equivalent in 12 grams.

46. **(D)** A concave mirror normally acts to converge incoming light rays. In the case of incoming *parallel* rays, the mirror will bring these to a focus at the focal point on the opposite side of the mirror.

47. **(C)** A concave mirror and a convex lens have very

similar optical effects in that both act to converge incoming rays of light and generally produce real images.

48. **(C)** The parasympathetic division of the autonomic nervous system acts to produce pupillary constriction, whereas the sympathetic division promotes pupillary dilation. More than 80% of the refraction of incoming light rays is achieved by the cornea, with the lens normally making some additional adjustments to allow the incoming light to be brought into sharp focus on the surface of the retina. The optic nerve serves only a sensory function—that is, it receives visual information from the environment and transmits it toward the central nervous system for processing.

49. **(C)** $x = 0$ °C only if this phase change was carried out at 1 atm. pressure. Since this is not indicated, the statement is neither supported nor contradicted.

50. **(E)** Point E is in the gaseous state where there is the most disorder and therefore the greatest entropy.

51. **(D)** Between points B and C the temperature of liquid water is increasing.

52. **(B)** If there is no external torque on the system, there must be conservation of angular momentum.

$$m\omega_1 r_1^2 = m\omega_2 r_2^2$$
$$\omega_2 = \omega_1 (r_1/r_2)^2$$

53. **(A)** The kinetic energy of a body moving in a circle is

$$T = \tfrac{1}{2} mr^2 \omega^2$$

$$T_1 = \tfrac{1}{2} mr^2_1 \omega^2_1$$

$$T_2 = \tfrac{1}{2} mr^2_2 \omega^2_2$$

$$\frac{T_2}{T_1} = \frac{r^2_2 \omega^2_2}{r^2_1 \omega^2_1} = \frac{r^2_2 [\omega_1 (r_1/r_2)^2]^2}{r^2_1}$$

$$T_2/T_1 = (r_1/r_2)^2$$

54. **(B)** The acceleration is given by

$$\vec{a_1} = \frac{\vec{v}^1_1}{r_1}$$ where $\vec{v_1}$ is the linear velocity,

a vector. The direction of the velocity is everchanging. The magnitude (given by the scalar quantity, speed = s_1), is constant. Since the radius, r_1, is a

(constant) scalar quantity, the acceleration varies in direction but not in magnitude.

55. **(A)** All sex cells receive the haploid number of chromosomes. One member from each chromosome pair in cell X, through reduction division, was passed on to the sperm nucleus of the pollen grain.

56. **(C)** If reduction division had not accompanied gametogenesis, the pollen grain and ovule would both have contained the diploid number of chromosomes as shown in cell X. If the two gametes unite, the resulting zygote would contain 12 chromosomes, or double the normal amount, as shown in diagram 3.

57. **(E)** The rod chromosome in diagram 1 is half black and half white, a fine example of crossing-over.

58. **(E)** By inhibiting the enzyme that deactivates cyclic AMP, theophylline will act to prolong the action of cyclic AMP. This will tend to potentiate the action of any hormones that use cyclic AMP as a "second messenger." In this case, theophylline will act to amplify the effects of thyroxine. Since thyroxine normally tends to increase basal metabolic rate, deep tendon reflexes, and heart and breathing rates, these will all be increased further in the presence of theophylline overdose.

59. **(A)** This question tells us that cyclic AMP acts as a second messenger for epinephrine, glucagon, vasopressin, and parathyroid hormone. Cyclic AMP must therefore be important in promoting an increased rate of glycogen degradation and subsequent conversion to glucose, since this is a primary effect of both epinephrine and glucagon. Epinephrine and glucagon also ordinarily produce an increased rate of fat breakdown (lipolysis) by tissues. Vasopressin (via cyclic AMP) promotes the reabsorption of water from the urinary filtrate by the kidney collecting tubules. This promotes formation of a more concentrated urine (one with a higher osmolarity). Parathyroid hormone (via cyclic AMP) promotes the resorption of calcium from bone, which produces an increase in serum calcium concentration.

60. **(C)** The sign of the $\triangle G°$ (Gibbs free energy) can be used to evaluate how likely it is that a given reaction will proceed spontaneously. A negative value of $\triangle G°$ (which we have on this example) suggests that the reaction as written will proceed spontaneously. A positive value of $\triangle G°$ suggests that the reaction will not proceed spontaneously. $\triangle S$ is the symbol used to represent changes in

entropy—a negative value of $\triangle S$ would, for example, suggest that the entropy of the system has decreased in converting reactants to products. $\triangle H$ (enthalpy) values can be used to compare the energy of the products with that of the reactants. A negative $\triangle H$ suggests that the products contain less energy than the reactants, which implies an exothermic process. A positive $\triangle H$ generally signifies an endothermic process.

61. **(A)** Individual A is a female possessing only normal genes for blood clotting. Individual B is a male possessing a gene for hemophilia inherited from his mother. It is impossible for individual D to be a hemophiliac female, as shown by the following Punnett Square (h = hemophiliac gene).

	X^h	Y
X	$X^h X$	XY
X	$X^h X$	XY

Only carrier females are produced. These females have normal blood clotting factors, but can transmit this gene to their male offspring.

62. **(C)** As explained before, individual D must be a hemophiliac carrier. Her mother (individual A) possesses only genes for blue eyes (recessive trait). Her father (individual B) is heterozygous for eye color, possessing one gene for blue eyes and one gene for dark eyes. If Aa times aa are then crossed, there is a 50–50 chance of having a blue-eyed or dark-eyed child.

63. **(A)** Individual E is the sister of the aforementioned individual D. They have the same parents, so that the same reasoning employed for question 62 (above) holds true here.

64. **(D)** The work done by friction (W_f) will equal the change in mechanical energy experienced by the system as the box descends the plane. The change in mechanical energy, in turn, will represent the difference between the initial potential energy (the box starts from rest) and the final kinetic energy. Here,

$$
\begin{aligned}
W_f &= mgh - \tfrac{1}{2}mv^2 \\
&= (20)(9.8)(10) - \tfrac{1}{2}(20)(10)^2 \\
&= 1960 - 1000 \\
&= 960 \text{ joules}
\end{aligned}
$$

65. **(B)** The force of friction will be equal to the product of the coefficient of sliding friction and the normal force, where the normal force represents the component of the box's weight perpendicular to the incline. This normal force can be mathematically expressed as $mg \cos \theta$, where θ = angle of inclination of the inclined plane. The component of the box's weight parallel to the incline is given as $mg \sin \theta$.

$$F_f = M_f N = M_f mg \cos \theta$$

Therefore,

$$M_f = \frac{F_f}{mg \cos 30°}$$

66. **(B)** If friction does not act, then mechanical energy must be conserved. This means that the initial potential energy must be equal to the final kinetic energy.

$$
\begin{aligned}
mgh &= \tfrac{1}{2}mv^2 \\
(20)(9.8)(10) &= (\tfrac{1}{2})(20)(v^2) \\
1960 &= 10\,v^2 \\
196 &= v^2 \\
v &= 14 \text{ meters/second}
\end{aligned}
$$

Section 3: Skills Analysis—Reading

1. **(A)** It is stated in paragraph two that the inhibitory component disappears more quickly with the passage of time than does the excitatory component. In experiment B, the conditioning trials are distributed, i.e., performed over a period of time. Therefore, the latency of the response in A will be longer.

2. **(C)** When the animal is more inhibited than excited, it will not respond.

3. **(D)** In experiment D, the inhibitory component disappears more rapidly (because the trials are distributed). So more trials are needed to extinguish the conditioned response in D.

4. **(C)** The last sentence of the passages states that the inhibitory component is more readily destroyed upon the occurrence of some novel stimulus than is the excitatory component. Since there was no response, the sound must have dissipated both components.

5. **(D)** Comparisons of hungry to satiated animals are not given in the passage.

6. **(A)** It is stated that the inhibitory component disappears more rapidly with the passage of time than does the excitatory component. Thus, the longer one waits, the less the latency.

7. **(B)** It is stated in the first paragraph that with repeated trials, the latency decreases.

8. **(B)** This is contradicted in the final sentence of the passage, and also, by implication, in paragraph two.

9. **(C)** Salt- to freshwater plants are not mentioned in the passage.

10. **(C)** The methods are only listed in the passage; they are not compared.

11. **(B)** This is contradicted in the first sentence of the passage.

12. **(B)** It is stated in paragraph four that the distribution of water varies with time.

13. **(A)** The author makes this statement in paragraph two.

14. **(A)** Paragraph six mentions that storage projects increase total evaporation and thus actually reduce the total water supply available.

15. **(A)** The first sentence of paragraph three states that continuous fermentation is an improvement on the batch process.

16. **(B)** This is contradicted by the first sentence of paragraph four.

17. **(C)** The various carbohydrates are listed in paragraph five. They are not compared.

18. **(A)** This is implied in the final paragraph.

19. **(C)** Although the two processes are outlined in the passage, no mention is made of such a search.

20. **(C)** The specifics of the biochemical processes that take place within the cells are not discussed in the passage.

21. **(B)** Paragraph four discusses the intermediate products in terms of *chemical* synthesis only. *Biological* conversion processes begin with substance *a* and end with product *e* without intervention by the chemist.

22. **(A)** The effect of British rule on the economy of Hong Kong is outlined in paragraph four.

23. **(E)** In the fifth paragraph, Hong Kong is said to have saved itself when it switched its business concentration from trading to manufacture.

24. **(B)** According to paragraph four, Hong Kong's economy prospered until the island fell to the Japanese in 1941.

25. **(C)** If Hong Kong's population (4.33 million) is divided by China's population (850 million), Hong Kong's population can be determined to be 1/200 that of China.

26. **(C)** These countries are listed in the final paragraph as countries that import goods manufactured in Hong Kong.

27. **(D)** The first paragraph states that Hong Kong came under Chinese rule in 200 B.C.

28. **(D)** Choice D is the only factor not mentioned as having either a direct or an indirect influence on Hong Kong's shift from a trading to a manufacturing economy.

29. **(D)** This is outlined as a remedy for unemployment in the final paragraph.

30. **(C)** The author is obviously impressed with Keynesian economic theory (see, for example, the first sentence of the passage).

31. **(A)** According to the final paragraph, Keynes favors the employment of all willing workers.

32. **(A)** The purpose of the passage is to describe Keynesian theory, which requires government intervention to assure economic stability.

33. **(B)** The easiest way to answer this question is to notice that I must follow IV immediately: If people are saving more and the rate of interest drops, then they are likely to invest their money instead of saving it at a low return.

34. **(D)** Paragraph two explains how, according to classical economics, interest rates and investments would balance one another to keep total spending stable and unemployment low.

35. **(B)** This is contradicted by the final sentence of the third paragraph.

36. **(B)** According to paragraph three, not a single biosynthetic pathway leading to an antibiotic has been determined.

37. **(C)** The method of inducing the mutations is not mentioned in the passage.

38. **(A)** The harmful result (as stated in paragraph four) is the presence of chromosomal aberrations.

39. **(B)** This is contradicted in paragraph six, where the example of *Cephalosporium acremonium* is considered.

40. **(B)** The problem of inherited instability will still remain.

41. **(C)** This point of comparison is not discussed in the passage.

42. **(A)** This statement can be found in the first sentence of the fourth paragraph.

43. **(B)** According to paragraph four, the author expects foreign and domestic consumption of U.S. soybeans to grow seventy-three percent over the next few years.

44. **(B)** The final paragraph indicates that this is not likely to occur.

45. **(B)** Paragraph three discusses factors that have limited development of SCP as a major source of protein for human and animal consumption.

46. **(B)** As stated in paragraph two, living agents are characterized by their ability to grow or reproduce. When viruses exhibited this ability, many people were convinced that viruses were small living organisms. The other choices either do not necessarily imply life or are not characteristic of viruses.

47. **(B)** This is stated explicitly in paragraph one, besides being the only choice that makes sense.

48. **(D)** It is stated in paragraph three that the smallest living things were about 200 millimicra in size. Choices (A), (B), and (C) were not affected by the discovery of viruses.

49. **(D)** Choices (A), (B), and (C) are contradicted by the passage. It is stated in paragraph three that some viruses are smaller than some protein molecules; it is implied that viruses are larger than most nucleoproteins.

50. **(D)** It is stated in the second sentence of paragraph four that both genes and viruses are made of nucleoproteins.

51. **(D)** It is stated in paragraph five that basic biological phenomena do not vary strikingly from species to species and that cancer is not unique to man.

52. **(A)** It is stated in paragraph six that the fact that viruses can mutate increases the likelihood that they may cause human cancer.

53. **(C)** The passage is divided equally between viruses, cancer, genes, and life and touches on the interrelationship of the four.

54. **(B)** The entire passage deals with life along the seashore.

55. **(E)** In paragraph five, these two adaptations are mentioned as contributing to an animal's ability to live in sandy regions comfortably.

56. **(B)** In paragraph eight, it is stated that aquatic animals are supported largely by materials washed into the sea.

57. **(B)** Because of the morphological adaptations necessary for life on a sandy beach, there is more variety on a rocky shore. The morphological adaptations are necessary because of the fact that the sandy areas are continually being washed by the surf.

58. **(A)** Organisms living at the high-tide mark must maintain themselves in air between high tides.

59. **(C)** This is stated in paragraph eight.

60. **(B)** As has been established in the above questions, the greatest variety of living things can be found on a rocky seashore.

61. **(B)** It is stated in the first paragraph that the sea has been the scene of the greatest stability and that this has contributed to life in the sea remaining virtually unchanged over a long period of time.

62. **(C)** The causes are enumerated in the first paragraph. They are not compared.

63. **(A)** The final sentence of the second paragraph makes this assertion.

64. **(B)** Epidemics are likely to appear in the early

post-attack period, according to paragraph two; the most serious immediate problem, however, will be treating injuries resulting directly from the blast.

65. **(B)** The author states that only forty percent of the survivors of Hiroshima sustained multiple injuries and implies that this number indicates what is likely to occur.

66. **(A)** Paragraph three develops this idea at length.

67. **(A)** The relation between resistance to infection and radiation exposure is discussed in the fifth paragraph.

68. **(A)** These diseases, usually rare, will be likely to spread, due to the increased vulnerability of survivors.

Section 4: Skills Analysis—Quantitative

1. **(A)** Since the number of telephones per person was smallest in Los Angeles in 1930, the number of people per telephone was greatest.

2. **(B)** Boston's went from .2 to 2.0, an increase of 1.8. Chicago's went from .4 to 3.5, an increase of 3.1.

3. **(B)** Boston had 2 telephones per person in 1970 while Los Angeles had 3. If there were two-thirds as many people living in Boston as in Los Angeles, there would be $\frac{2}{3} \times \frac{2}{3} = \frac{4}{9}$ as many telephones in Boston.

4. **(B)** There were .4 telephones per person in Chicago in 1930. Thus, there were $1/.4 = 2.5$ people per telephone. In Los Angeles, there were $1/.1 = 10$ people per telephone. Thus, there were one-fourth as many people per telephone in Chicago in 1930 as in Los Angeles in 1930.

5. **(B)** As can be seen from the table, the projected number of telephones per person in Chicago does not change (regardless of any changes in population).

6. **(B)** The change in Boston was from .2 to 1.0. The difference, which is .8, constitutes only a 400% increase.

7. **(A)** In each successive ten-year period, there was an increase of .5 telephones per person.

8. **(A)** Slope is the change in the vertical coordinate

divided by the change in the horizontal coordinate. All of the cities had the same change (50 years) in the horizontal coordinate. Since Los Angeles had the greatest change in the "Number of Telephones per Person," it would have the greatest slope.

9. **(C)** We cannot answer this because we are not supplied with the relevant data regarding population changes in Los Angeles.

10. **(C)** Since the 1990 data is projected, we cannot determine whether or not there was an increase in the number of telephones per person in Chicago from 1970 to 1990.

11. **(C)** We are not presented with data for "females only." We cannot combine the information in the two graphs because we do not know the relative numbers of males and females. For example, if there are far fewer females than males but their average life span is greater than 100 years, it is possible that those few women bring the average for "males and females" up to 82 years. However, if there are the same number of males as females, the average for females would have to be 86 to bring the "males and females" average up to 82.

12. **(A)** The average life expectancy for 20-year-old males is 73.

13. **(A)** The average life span of 20-year-old females must be 73 because 20-year-old "males only" and 20-year-old "males and females" have an average life expectancy of 73 years. This is true regardless of the relative numbers of males and females.

14. **(A)** Since "males and females" increases at a higher rate than "males only" (with increased age), "females only" would increase at a greater rate than "males only."

15. **(B)** The average 40-year-old male has 34 more years to live. The average male who has just been born has 70 more years to live.

16. **(B)** The life expectancy for "males only" and for "males and females" at birth is 70 years. Therefore, the life expectancy for "females only" at birth is 70 years. Females and males therefore have equal life expectancies at birth.

17. **(A)** In the graph on the right, as "Years of Age" increases, so does "average expected life span."

18. **(C)** We cannot determine the percentage of individuals who live longer than 80 years in either

the "40-year-old-males" or "60-year-old-males" categories. Both could have zero percent reaching the age of 80 and both could have quite a large percent reaching the age of 80.

19. **(B)** Five students were denied acceptance anywhere. Two students were accepted to at least one school. Five is only 150% more than two.

20. **(B)** $2/12$ (or $1/6$) of the biology undergraduates were not accepted anywhere. $1/7$ of the students from the Department of Economics were not accepted anywhere. $1/6$ is greater than $1/7$.

21. **(C)** There is nothing presented which correlates intelligence with getting into medical school.

22. **(B)** $1/3$ of the history undergraduates were not accepted at any school.

23. **(A)** No literature graduates applied to medical school. 19 physics undergraduates were accepted by at least one school.

24. **(C)** We are not told at how many schools each of the 15 accepted chemistry undergraduates was accepted. So the total could be less than, equal to, or greater than the 16 political science applicants.

25. **(B)** $4/14$ (much less than 40%) of the School of Humanities graduates were not accepted at any school.

26. **(B)** Thirty-one of 89 (much less than half) of the School of Humanities applicants were not accepted at any school.

27. **(A)** It is apparent from the data that certain chemicals will cause the flies to be attracted and they will show a preference for a sugar cube so treated.

28. **(E)** The boiling point of chemical E is lower than that of B, but B attracts more flies. The boiling point of E is higher than D, but D attracts more flies. Therefore, there is no ironclad relationship between boiling point and chemical attractancy.

29. **(C)** The melting points of the chemicals were not given.

30. **(C)** There is only information on how long it took each fly to reach one of the cubes. There is no information given as to which cubes were visited after the flies landed for the first time.

31. **(C)** In producing regressions of tumors, the liver L. casei factor was, in general, ineffective.

32. **(E)** The fermentation of L. casei factor led to regressions of tumors in practically one-third of the cases.

33. **(A)** The greatest percentage of mice showed lung metastases in group 1.

34. **(A)** Diagnosis of malignancy of the cancers was established by examination of tissues removed from the living animal.

35. **(C)** The data are presented as life expectancies at birth. The expectancies may change after an individual reaches a certain age.

36. **(A)** The present life expectancy at birth for a Brazilian is 53; for an individual in the United States in 1900, it was about 50.

37. **(C)** There is no data presented which compares the quality of medical facilities among the countries. This cannot be deduced from life expectancy data because there are many factors other than the quality of medical facilities which affect the duration of one's life (for example dietary and environmental factors).

38. **(A)** The life expectancy at birth is now 70 years. In 1900 it was 50 years; 70 is 40% more than 50.

39. **(C)** We are not given any data concerning the percent of the population that is alive past any certain age.

40. **(A)** The life expectancy at birth is 70 years in the United States. It is 39 years in the Congo Republic; 70 is about 80% greater than 39.

41. **(C)** There is no data concerning the percents of the populations in the two countries that live past the age of 60. Even though the average in Brazil is 53, no one may live past 55, for example. Whereas in Cambodia, with an average life expectancy of 44, there may be diseases that kill infants, while many of the survivors of the diseases may live past 80.

42. **(C)** The data presented in the graph on the right applies only to the United States.

43. **(C)** The solid line reaches its highest point in February of '82.

44. **(E)** The solid line reaches its lowest point in September of '82.

45. **(E)** 900/750 = 6/5

46. **(E)** There was a tremendous decline (approximately 70 points) from July to September '82. This is far greater than the decline experienced in any of the other three-month periods listed.

47. **(B)** The stock average went from 850 to 825 in May. This is a 25/850 = 1/34 = approximately 3% decrease.

48. **(C)** The stock average went from 840 to 900. The increase is 60/840 = 1/4 = approximately 7%.

49. **(D)** The average at the end is 750. At the beginning it was 840; 750 is approximately 90% of 840.

50. **(D)** In August of '82, the difference was 833 − 755 = 78, greater than the difference in any other period.

51. **(B)** There are four parental places on the chart listing blood type O. Parents $O \times O = 41$; $O \times A = 34$; $O \times B = 6.5$; $O \times AB = 21.5$. This totals 103 possible parents possessing this genotype. There are 267 families involved in this study. Dividing 267 into 103, the figure of approximately 40 percent is arrived at.

52. **(E)** Only $A \times B$ results in all four blood types appearing in the offspring.

53. **(A)** According to all known laws of genetics, $O \times O$ should only result in O offspring. There must have been either faulty test sera or uncertain paternity responsible for the tabulation of one blood type A as reported in the chart.

54. **(E)** The chart lists O offspring produced by $A \times A$, $B \times B$, and $A \times B$ (three different combinations).

55. **(C)** There were a total of 767 Danish offspring included in the study. The proportion of Danish offspring that were type AB is 75/767, or 9.8%. The proportion of Japanese offspring of type AB is 123/2046, or 6.0%.

56. **(D)** The small percentage of people having AB blood has established very high odds against the frequency of marriage among those who possess this increasingly rare blood type.

57. **(B)** It is necessary to total the entries of each row opposite the respective parental blood type crosses. Upon comparing the results, it is found that $O \times A$ group parents produced 172 offspring. No other blood cross group produced more.

58. **(B)** Upon comparing the entries in the column labeled "AB Offspring," it is found that $A \times AB$ parents produced 33 such children. No other blood cross group produced more.

59. **(B)** Since the total of all the cells in the table is 100 and we are told that there were 10 judges, each judge made 10 comparisons.

60. **(A)** The sum of the row in which compound A is included is greater than the sum of any other row.

61. **(D)** The sum of the row in which compound D is included is less than the sum of any other row.

62. **(D)** There was very little disagreement by the judges in the case of comparisons involving compound D. For example, there was no disagreement at all when the judges compared A and D: All ten judged A sweeter. Clearly, however, there was not perfect agreement among the judges in all cases. This makes choice (A) incorrect. No information supports choice (C).

63. **(E)** The discrimination was least pronounced in the case of A versus B comparisons; the judges were deadlocked at 5 in favor of each.

64. **(E)** As mentioned above, there was perfect discrimination between A and D.

65. **(D)** A received 5 favorable judgments when compared with B. This is twice as many as $2\frac{1}{2}$, which is not included in the table.

66. **(E)** There were 25 judgments in favor of A and 5 in favor of D; 25 is 500% of 5.

67. **(D)** 24 judgments were made in favor of C. C was judged less sweet in 16 comparisons. The difference is 8.

Part Four

GRADUATE RECORD
EXAMINATION
(GRE)

GRADUATE RECORD
EXAMINATION
(GRE)

The Graduate Record Examination (GRE) has the primary function of assisting admissions officers of graduate schools in appraising the academic abilities of applicants for graduate studies. Certain highly competitive graduate schools in Veterinary Medicine require their applicants to take the GRE, and sometimes also a GRE Advanced (subject) test. Refer to the chart on page 17 for the requirements of the schools to which you are thinking of applying. If a school of your choice requires the GRE, check with them to see if you should take the examination on or by a given date. You'll need to register for this test (as for many other advanced standardized examinations) well in advance of the test date.

The GRE now consists of seven 30-minute sections divided among three categories: Verbal Ability, Quantitative Ability, and Analytical Reasoning. Six of the seven sections will be used to determine your scores, two of each category. The seventh section is experimental and is used by the Educational Testing Service (ETS) to help them develop future tests. You will not be told which of your seven sections is experimental. If your form of the test has three Verbal sections, two Quantitative (math) sections, and two Analytical sections, you'll know that one of the Verbal sections is experimental, but not which one—ETS takes pains to obscure this information. If one section of your examination contains questions totally unlike those in the other sections, you'll know this to be the experimental section. More often, the experimental section will blend in with the others of its type. The seven sections may be given in any order.

GRE ANALYSIS AND TIMETABLE

Test Category	Total Number of Questions Used to Calculate Your Score	Time Allowed
Verbal (two sections)	38	30 minutes
	38	30 minutes
Quantitative (two sections)	30	30 minutes
	30	30 minutes
Analytical Reasoning (two sections)	25	30 minutes
	25	30 minutes
A seventh section of any one of the above categories	?	30 minutes

A 10- or 15-minute break is given at some time during the examination, logically after section 3 or section 4. Total testing time, allowing for this break, comes to $3\frac{3}{4}$ hours. Administration procedures can be expected to take up another $\frac{1}{2}$ hour or so.

Three scores will be reported for your GRE: one for each category of question, as given in the chart above. You will also be given percentile rankings for each of your three scores; percentiles show how your scores compared with those earned by all other candidates taking the test. The *Bulletin* provided by ETS has more information about scores, score reports, and all other matters pertaining to the examination.

Important: You are no longer penalized for incorrect answers on the GRE (though you still are for the advanced subject tests).

ANSWER SHEET FOR THE GRE PRACTICE EXAMINATION

Section I

1 Ⓐ Ⓑ Ⓒ Ⓓ Ⓔ	8 Ⓐ Ⓑ Ⓒ Ⓓ Ⓔ	15 Ⓐ Ⓑ Ⓒ Ⓓ Ⓔ	22 Ⓐ Ⓑ Ⓒ Ⓓ Ⓔ	29 Ⓐ Ⓑ Ⓒ Ⓓ Ⓔ	36 Ⓐ Ⓑ Ⓒ Ⓓ Ⓔ
2 Ⓐ Ⓑ Ⓒ Ⓓ Ⓔ	9 Ⓐ Ⓑ Ⓒ Ⓓ Ⓔ	16 Ⓐ Ⓑ Ⓒ Ⓓ Ⓔ	23 Ⓐ Ⓑ Ⓒ Ⓓ Ⓔ	30 Ⓐ Ⓑ Ⓒ Ⓓ Ⓔ	37 Ⓐ Ⓑ Ⓒ Ⓓ Ⓔ
3 Ⓐ Ⓑ Ⓒ Ⓓ Ⓔ	10 Ⓐ Ⓑ Ⓒ Ⓓ Ⓔ	17 Ⓐ Ⓑ Ⓒ Ⓓ Ⓔ	24 Ⓐ Ⓑ Ⓒ Ⓓ Ⓔ	31 Ⓐ Ⓑ Ⓒ Ⓓ Ⓔ	38 Ⓐ Ⓑ Ⓒ Ⓓ Ⓔ
4 Ⓐ Ⓑ Ⓒ Ⓓ Ⓔ	11 Ⓐ Ⓑ Ⓒ Ⓓ Ⓔ	18 Ⓐ Ⓑ Ⓒ Ⓓ Ⓔ	25 Ⓐ Ⓑ Ⓒ Ⓓ Ⓔ	32 Ⓐ Ⓑ Ⓒ Ⓓ Ⓔ	
5 Ⓐ Ⓑ Ⓒ Ⓓ Ⓔ	12 Ⓐ Ⓑ Ⓒ Ⓓ Ⓔ	19 Ⓐ Ⓑ Ⓒ Ⓓ Ⓔ	26 Ⓐ Ⓑ Ⓒ Ⓓ Ⓔ	33 Ⓐ Ⓑ Ⓒ Ⓓ Ⓔ	
6 Ⓐ Ⓑ Ⓒ Ⓓ Ⓔ	13 Ⓐ Ⓑ Ⓒ Ⓓ Ⓔ	20 Ⓐ Ⓑ Ⓒ Ⓓ Ⓔ	27 Ⓐ Ⓑ Ⓒ Ⓓ Ⓔ	34 Ⓐ Ⓑ Ⓒ Ⓓ Ⓔ	
7 Ⓐ Ⓑ Ⓒ Ⓓ Ⓔ	14 Ⓐ Ⓑ Ⓒ Ⓓ Ⓔ	21 Ⓐ Ⓑ Ⓒ Ⓓ Ⓔ	28 Ⓐ Ⓑ Ⓒ Ⓓ Ⓔ	35 Ⓐ Ⓑ Ⓒ Ⓓ Ⓔ	

Section II

1 Ⓐ Ⓑ Ⓒ Ⓓ Ⓔ	8 Ⓐ Ⓑ Ⓒ Ⓓ Ⓔ	15 Ⓐ Ⓑ Ⓒ Ⓓ Ⓔ	22 Ⓐ Ⓑ Ⓒ Ⓓ Ⓔ	29 Ⓐ Ⓑ Ⓒ Ⓓ Ⓔ	36 Ⓐ Ⓑ Ⓒ Ⓓ Ⓔ
2 Ⓐ Ⓑ Ⓒ Ⓓ Ⓔ	9 Ⓐ Ⓑ Ⓒ Ⓓ Ⓔ	16 Ⓐ Ⓑ Ⓒ Ⓓ Ⓔ	23 Ⓐ Ⓑ Ⓒ Ⓓ Ⓔ	30 Ⓐ Ⓑ Ⓒ Ⓓ Ⓔ	37 Ⓐ Ⓑ Ⓒ Ⓓ Ⓔ
3 Ⓐ Ⓑ Ⓒ Ⓓ Ⓔ	10 Ⓐ Ⓑ Ⓒ Ⓓ Ⓔ	17 Ⓐ Ⓑ Ⓒ Ⓓ Ⓔ	24 Ⓐ Ⓑ Ⓒ Ⓓ Ⓔ	31 Ⓐ Ⓑ Ⓒ Ⓓ Ⓔ	38 Ⓐ Ⓑ Ⓒ Ⓓ Ⓔ
4 Ⓐ Ⓑ Ⓒ Ⓓ Ⓔ	11 Ⓐ Ⓑ Ⓒ Ⓓ Ⓔ	18 Ⓐ Ⓑ Ⓒ Ⓓ Ⓔ	25 Ⓐ Ⓑ Ⓒ Ⓓ Ⓔ	32 Ⓐ Ⓑ Ⓒ Ⓓ Ⓔ	
5 Ⓐ Ⓑ Ⓒ Ⓓ Ⓔ	12 Ⓐ Ⓑ Ⓒ Ⓓ Ⓔ	19 Ⓐ Ⓑ Ⓒ Ⓓ Ⓔ	26 Ⓐ Ⓑ Ⓒ Ⓓ Ⓔ	33 Ⓐ Ⓑ Ⓒ Ⓓ Ⓔ	
6 Ⓐ Ⓑ Ⓒ Ⓓ Ⓔ	13 Ⓐ Ⓑ Ⓒ Ⓓ Ⓔ	20 Ⓐ Ⓑ Ⓒ Ⓓ Ⓔ	27 Ⓐ Ⓑ Ⓒ Ⓓ Ⓔ	34 Ⓐ Ⓑ Ⓒ Ⓓ Ⓔ	
7 Ⓐ Ⓑ Ⓒ Ⓓ Ⓔ	14 Ⓐ Ⓑ Ⓒ Ⓓ Ⓔ	21 Ⓐ Ⓑ Ⓒ Ⓓ Ⓔ	28 Ⓐ Ⓑ Ⓒ Ⓓ Ⓔ	35 Ⓐ Ⓑ Ⓒ Ⓓ Ⓔ	

Section III

1 Ⓐ Ⓑ Ⓒ Ⓓ Ⓔ	6 Ⓐ Ⓑ Ⓒ Ⓓ Ⓔ	11 Ⓐ Ⓑ Ⓒ Ⓓ Ⓔ	16 Ⓐ Ⓑ Ⓒ Ⓓ Ⓔ	21 Ⓐ Ⓑ Ⓒ Ⓓ Ⓔ	26 Ⓐ Ⓑ Ⓒ Ⓓ Ⓔ
2 Ⓐ Ⓑ Ⓒ Ⓓ Ⓔ	7 Ⓐ Ⓑ Ⓒ Ⓓ Ⓔ	12 Ⓐ Ⓑ Ⓒ Ⓓ Ⓔ	17 Ⓐ Ⓑ Ⓒ Ⓓ Ⓔ	22 Ⓐ Ⓑ Ⓒ Ⓓ Ⓔ	27 Ⓐ Ⓑ Ⓒ Ⓓ Ⓔ
3 Ⓐ Ⓑ Ⓒ Ⓓ Ⓔ	8 Ⓐ Ⓑ Ⓒ Ⓓ Ⓔ	13 Ⓐ Ⓑ Ⓒ Ⓓ Ⓔ	18 Ⓐ Ⓑ Ⓒ Ⓓ Ⓔ	23 Ⓐ Ⓑ Ⓒ Ⓓ Ⓔ	28 Ⓐ Ⓑ Ⓒ Ⓓ Ⓔ
4 Ⓐ Ⓑ Ⓒ Ⓓ Ⓔ	9 Ⓐ Ⓑ Ⓒ Ⓓ Ⓔ	14 Ⓐ Ⓑ Ⓒ Ⓓ Ⓔ	19 Ⓐ Ⓑ Ⓒ Ⓓ Ⓔ	24 Ⓐ Ⓑ Ⓒ Ⓓ Ⓔ	29 Ⓐ Ⓑ Ⓒ Ⓓ Ⓔ
5 Ⓐ Ⓑ Ⓒ Ⓓ Ⓔ	10 Ⓐ Ⓑ Ⓒ Ⓓ Ⓔ	15 Ⓐ Ⓑ Ⓒ Ⓓ Ⓔ	20 Ⓐ Ⓑ Ⓒ Ⓓ Ⓔ	25 Ⓐ Ⓑ Ⓒ Ⓓ Ⓔ	30 Ⓐ Ⓑ Ⓒ Ⓓ Ⓔ

Section IV

1 Ⓐ Ⓑ Ⓒ Ⓓ Ⓔ   6 Ⓐ Ⓑ Ⓒ Ⓓ Ⓔ   11 Ⓐ Ⓑ Ⓒ Ⓓ Ⓔ   16 Ⓐ Ⓑ Ⓒ Ⓓ Ⓔ   21 Ⓐ Ⓑ Ⓒ Ⓓ Ⓔ   26 Ⓐ Ⓑ Ⓒ Ⓓ Ⓔ

2 Ⓐ Ⓑ Ⓒ Ⓓ Ⓔ   7 Ⓐ Ⓑ Ⓒ Ⓓ Ⓔ   12 Ⓐ Ⓑ Ⓒ Ⓓ Ⓔ   17 Ⓐ Ⓑ Ⓒ Ⓓ Ⓔ   22 Ⓐ Ⓑ Ⓒ Ⓓ Ⓔ   27 Ⓐ Ⓑ Ⓒ Ⓓ Ⓔ

3 Ⓐ Ⓑ Ⓒ Ⓓ Ⓔ   8 Ⓐ Ⓑ Ⓒ Ⓓ Ⓔ   13 Ⓐ Ⓑ Ⓒ Ⓓ Ⓔ   18 Ⓐ Ⓑ Ⓒ Ⓓ Ⓔ   23 Ⓐ Ⓑ Ⓒ Ⓓ Ⓔ   28 Ⓐ Ⓑ Ⓒ Ⓓ Ⓔ

4 Ⓐ Ⓑ Ⓒ Ⓓ Ⓔ   9 Ⓐ Ⓑ Ⓒ Ⓓ Ⓔ   14 Ⓐ Ⓑ Ⓒ Ⓓ Ⓔ   19 Ⓐ Ⓑ Ⓒ Ⓓ Ⓔ   24 Ⓐ Ⓑ Ⓒ Ⓓ Ⓔ   29 Ⓐ Ⓑ Ⓒ Ⓓ Ⓔ

5 Ⓐ Ⓑ Ⓒ Ⓓ Ⓔ   10 Ⓐ Ⓑ Ⓒ Ⓓ Ⓔ   15 Ⓐ Ⓑ Ⓒ Ⓓ Ⓔ   20 Ⓐ Ⓑ Ⓒ Ⓓ Ⓔ   25 Ⓐ Ⓑ Ⓒ Ⓓ Ⓔ   30 Ⓐ Ⓑ Ⓒ Ⓓ Ⓔ

Section V

1 Ⓐ Ⓑ Ⓒ Ⓓ Ⓔ   6 Ⓐ Ⓑ Ⓒ Ⓓ Ⓔ   11 Ⓐ Ⓑ Ⓒ Ⓓ Ⓔ   16 Ⓐ Ⓑ Ⓒ Ⓓ Ⓔ   21 Ⓐ Ⓑ Ⓒ Ⓓ Ⓔ

2 Ⓐ Ⓑ Ⓒ Ⓓ Ⓔ   7 Ⓐ Ⓑ Ⓒ Ⓓ Ⓔ   12 Ⓐ Ⓑ Ⓒ Ⓓ Ⓔ   17 Ⓐ Ⓑ Ⓒ Ⓓ Ⓔ   22 Ⓐ Ⓑ Ⓒ Ⓓ Ⓔ

3 Ⓐ Ⓑ Ⓒ Ⓓ Ⓔ   8 Ⓐ Ⓑ Ⓒ Ⓓ Ⓔ   13 Ⓐ Ⓑ Ⓒ Ⓓ Ⓔ   18 Ⓐ Ⓑ Ⓒ Ⓓ Ⓔ   23 Ⓐ Ⓑ Ⓒ Ⓓ Ⓔ

4 Ⓐ Ⓑ Ⓒ Ⓓ Ⓔ   9 Ⓐ Ⓑ Ⓒ Ⓓ Ⓔ   14 Ⓐ Ⓑ Ⓒ Ⓓ Ⓔ   19 Ⓐ Ⓑ Ⓒ Ⓓ Ⓔ   24 Ⓐ Ⓑ Ⓒ Ⓓ Ⓔ

5 Ⓐ Ⓑ Ⓒ Ⓓ Ⓔ   10 Ⓐ Ⓑ Ⓒ Ⓓ Ⓔ   15 Ⓐ Ⓑ Ⓒ Ⓓ Ⓔ   20 Ⓐ Ⓑ Ⓒ Ⓓ Ⓔ   25 Ⓐ Ⓑ Ⓒ Ⓓ Ⓔ

Section VI

1 Ⓐ Ⓑ Ⓒ Ⓓ Ⓔ   6 Ⓐ Ⓑ Ⓒ Ⓓ Ⓔ   11 Ⓐ Ⓑ Ⓒ Ⓓ Ⓔ   16 Ⓐ Ⓑ Ⓒ Ⓓ Ⓔ   21 Ⓐ Ⓑ Ⓒ Ⓓ Ⓔ

2 Ⓐ Ⓑ Ⓒ Ⓓ Ⓔ   7 Ⓐ Ⓑ Ⓒ Ⓓ Ⓔ   12 Ⓐ Ⓑ Ⓒ Ⓓ Ⓔ   17 Ⓐ Ⓑ Ⓒ Ⓓ Ⓔ   22 Ⓐ Ⓑ Ⓒ Ⓓ Ⓔ

3 Ⓐ Ⓑ Ⓒ Ⓓ Ⓔ   8 Ⓐ Ⓑ Ⓒ Ⓓ Ⓔ   13 Ⓐ Ⓑ Ⓒ Ⓓ Ⓔ   18 Ⓐ Ⓑ Ⓒ Ⓓ Ⓔ   23 Ⓐ Ⓑ Ⓒ Ⓓ Ⓔ

4 Ⓐ Ⓑ Ⓒ Ⓓ Ⓔ   9 Ⓐ Ⓑ Ⓒ Ⓓ Ⓔ   14 Ⓐ Ⓑ Ⓒ Ⓓ Ⓔ   19 Ⓐ Ⓑ Ⓒ Ⓓ Ⓔ   24 Ⓐ Ⓑ Ⓒ Ⓓ Ⓔ

5 Ⓐ Ⓑ Ⓒ Ⓓ Ⓔ   10 Ⓐ Ⓑ Ⓒ Ⓓ Ⓔ   15 Ⓐ Ⓑ Ⓒ Ⓓ Ⓔ   20 Ⓐ Ⓑ Ⓒ Ⓓ Ⓔ   25 Ⓐ Ⓑ Ⓒ Ⓓ Ⓔ

Section VII

1 Ⓐ Ⓑ Ⓒ Ⓓ Ⓔ   6 Ⓐ Ⓑ Ⓒ Ⓓ Ⓔ   11 Ⓐ Ⓑ Ⓒ Ⓓ Ⓔ   16 Ⓐ Ⓑ Ⓒ Ⓓ Ⓔ   21 Ⓐ Ⓑ Ⓒ Ⓓ Ⓔ

2 Ⓐ Ⓑ Ⓒ Ⓓ Ⓔ   7 Ⓐ Ⓑ Ⓒ Ⓓ Ⓔ   12 Ⓐ Ⓑ Ⓒ Ⓓ Ⓔ   17 Ⓐ Ⓑ Ⓒ Ⓓ Ⓔ   22 Ⓐ Ⓑ Ⓒ Ⓓ Ⓔ

3 Ⓐ Ⓑ Ⓒ Ⓓ Ⓔ   8 Ⓐ Ⓑ Ⓒ Ⓓ Ⓔ   13 Ⓐ Ⓑ Ⓒ Ⓓ Ⓔ   18 Ⓐ Ⓑ Ⓒ Ⓓ Ⓔ   23 Ⓐ Ⓑ Ⓒ Ⓓ Ⓔ

4 Ⓐ Ⓑ Ⓒ Ⓓ Ⓔ   9 Ⓐ Ⓑ Ⓒ Ⓓ Ⓔ   14 Ⓐ Ⓑ Ⓒ Ⓓ Ⓔ   19 Ⓐ Ⓑ Ⓒ Ⓓ Ⓔ   24 Ⓐ Ⓑ Ⓒ Ⓓ Ⓔ

5 Ⓐ Ⓑ Ⓒ Ⓓ Ⓔ   10 Ⓐ Ⓑ Ⓒ Ⓓ Ⓔ   15 Ⓐ Ⓑ Ⓒ Ⓓ Ⓔ   20 Ⓐ Ⓑ Ⓒ Ⓓ Ⓔ   25 Ⓐ Ⓑ Ⓒ Ⓓ Ⓔ

GRE PRACTICE EXAMINATION

SECTION I

30 minutes
38 questions

Directions: Each of the questions below contains one or more blank spaces, each blank indicating an omitted word. Each sentence is followed by five (5) lettered words or sets of words. Read and determine the general sense of each sentence. Then choose the word or set of words which, when inserted in the sentence, best fits the meaning of the sentence.

1. We should have _____ trouble ahead when the road _____ into a gravel path.
   (A) interrogated—shrank
   (B) anticipated—dwindled
   (C) expected—grew
   (D) enjoyed—transformed
   (E) seen—collapsed

2. The _____ of the waiter, fresh lobster, was all gone, so we _____ ourselves with crab.
   (A) suggestion—resolved
   (B) embarrassment—consoled
   (C) recommendation—contented
   (D) specialty—pelted
   (E) regrets—relieved

3. The _____ workroom had not been used in years.
   (A) derelict
   (B) bustling
   (C) bereft
   (D) bereaved
   (E) stricken

4. Tempers ran hot among the old-timers, who _____ the young mayor and his _____ city council.

   (A) despised—attractive
   (B) admired—elite
   (C) resented—reform
   (D) forgave—activist
   (E) feared—apathetic

5. With the discovery of _____ alternative fuel source, oil prices dropped significantly.
   (A) a potential
   (B) a feasible
   (C) a possible
   (D) a variant
   (E) an inexpensive

6. The masters of the world are the bacteria and viruses. They _____ all other life and all other life lives and reproduces merely to provide them with _____.
   (A) dominate—companionship
   (B) outnumber—room and board
   (C) infest—opportunity
   (D) serve—shelter
   (E) are symbiotic with—partners

7. He could understand that his prisoners would _____ him at first, but he had hoped that after all this time his fairness would inspire _____ rather than trepidation at his arrival.
   (A) misunderstand—love
   (B) escape—cordiality
   (C) abhor—loyalty
   (D) dislike—cameraderie
   (E) fear—trust

171

Directions: In each of the following questions, you are given a related pair of words or phrases in capital letters. Each capitalized pair is followed by five (5) lettered pairs of words or phrases. Choose the pair which best expresses a relationship similar to that expressed by the original pair.

8. CAT : MOUSE ::
    (A) bird : worm
    (B) dog : tail
    (C) trap : cheese
    (D) hide : seek
    (E) lion : snake

9. VANILLA : BEAN ::
    (A) tabasco : stem
    (B) chili : seed
    (C) mint : flower
    (D) ginger : root
    (E) sage : berry

10. ENERGY : DISSIPATE ::
    (A) battery : recharge
    (B) atom : split
    (C) food : eat
    (D) money : squander
    (E) gas : generate

11. NOSE : FACE ::
    (A) ring : finger
    (B) stem : root
    (C) knob : door
    (D) shoe : foot
    (E) vine : building

12. RIFLE : SOLDIER ::
    (A) bow : arrow
    (B) sword : knight
    (C) horse : cowboy
    (D) marine: tank
    (E) lock : robber

13. DEER : VENISON ::
    (A) pig : hog
    (B) sheep : mutton
    (C) lamb : veal
    (D) steer : stew
    (E) beef : stew

14. INEFFABLE : KNOWLEDGE ::
    (A) genial : interesting
    (B) puzzling : trick

    (C) frustrating : release
    (D) baffling : solution
    (E) controllable : rage

15. ICING : CAKE ::
    (A) veneer : table
    (B) ice : pond
    (C) pastry : bake
    (D) apple : pie
    (E) printing : page

16. CHALK : BLACKBOARD ::
    (A) door : handle
    (B) table : chair
    (C) ink : paper
    (D) pencil : writing
    (E) paint : wall

Directions: Below each of the following passages, you will find questions or incomplete statements about the passage. Each statement or question is followed by lettered words or expressions. Select the word or expression that most satisfactorily completes each statement or answers each question in accordance with the meaning of the passage. After you choose the best answer, blacken the corresponding space on the answer sheet.

There is a confused notion in the minds of many persons, that the gathering of the property of the poor into the hands of the rich does no ultimate harm, since in whosesoever hands it may be, it must be spent at last, and thus, they think, return to the poor again. This fallacy has been again and again exposed; but granting the plea true, the same apology may, of course, be made for blackmail, or any other form of robbery. It might be (though practically it never is) as advantageous for the nation that the robber should have the spending of the money he extorts, as that the person robbed should have spent it. But this is no excuse for the theft. If I were to put a turnpike on the road where it passes my own gate, and endeavor to exact a shilling from every passenger, the public would soon do away with my gate, without listening to any pleas on my part that it was as advantageous to them, in the end, that I should spend their shillings, as that they themselves should. But if, instead of outfacing them with a turnpike, I can only persuade them to come in and buy stones, or old iron, or any other useless thing, out of my ground, I may rob them to the same extent, and be moreover, thanked as a public benefactor and promoter of commercial prosperity. And this main question for the poor of England—for the poor of all countries—is wholly omitted in every treatise on the subject of wealth. Even by the laborers themselves, the operation of capital is regarded only in its effect on their immediate interests, never in the far more terrific power of its appointment of the kind and the object of labor. It matters little, ultimately, how much a laborer is paid for making anything; but it matters fearfully what the thing is, which he is compelled to make. If his labor is so ordered as to produce food, fresh air, and fresh water, no matter that his wages are low;—the food and the fresh air and water will be at last there, and he will at last get them. But if he is paid to destroy food and fresh air, or to produce iron bars instead of them,—the food and air will finally *not* be there, and he will *not* get them, to his great and final inconvenience. So that, conclusively, in political as in household economy, the great question is, not so much what money you have in your pocket, as what you will buy with it and do with it.

17. We may infer that the author probably lived in the
    (A) 1960's in the United States
    (B) early days of British industrialization
    (C) 18th-century France
    (D) Golden Age of Greece
    (E) England of King Arthur

18. It can be inferred that the author probably favors
    (A) capitalism
    (B) totalitarianism
    (C) socialism
    (D) anarchism
    (E) theocracy

19. According to the passage, the individual should be particularly concerned with
    (A) how much wealth he can accumulate
    (B) the acquisition of land property rather than money
    (C) charging the customer a fair price
    (D) the quality of goods which he purchases with his funds
    (E) working as hard as possible

20. The passage implies that
    (A) "A stitch in time saves nine."
    (B) "It is better late than never."
    (C) "He who steals my purse steals trash."
    (D) "None but the brave deserve the fair"
    (E) "All's well that ends well."

21. It can be inferred that in regard to the accumulation of wealth the author
    (A) equates the rich with the thief
    (B) indicates that there are few honest businessmen
    (C) condones some dishonesty in business dealings
    (D) believes destruction of property is good because it creates consumer demand
    (E) says that the robber is a benefactor

22. What is the "main question for the poor" referred to by the author in the passages?
    (A) the use to which the laborer can put his money
    (B) the methods by which capital may be accumulated
    (C) the results of their work and their lack of authority to determine to what ends their work shall be put
    (D) whether full measure of recompense shall be accorded to the laboring person for the investment of his time in worthy work
    (E) the extent to which a man can call his life his own

23. According to the views expressed in the passage, people should be happiest doing which of the following?
    (A) mining ore for the manufacture of weapons
    (B) cleaning sewage ponds at a treatment plant
    (C) waiting tables for a rich man
    (D) helping a poor man do his job
    (E) studying economic theory

24. The author of the above passage would probably react to an energy shortage by
    (A) blaming the rich for the problem
    (B) urging that energy be used more efficiently and effectively
    (C) supporting the search for more oil,

coal, and other energy-producing mineral deposits
(D) denying that there is really any shortage at all
(E) fomenting revolution by the poor

Man, said Aristotle, is a social animal. This sociability requires peaceful congregation, and the history of mankind is mainly a movement through time of human collectivities that range from migrant tribal bands to large and complex civilizations. Survival has been due to the ability to create the means by which men in groups retain their unity and allegiance to one another.

Order was caused by the need and desire to survive the challenge of the environment. This orderly condition came to be called the "state," and the rules that maintained it, the "law." With time the partner to this tranquillity, man marched across the centuries of his evolution to the brink of exploring the boundaries of his own galaxy. Of all living organisms, only man has the capacity to interpret his own evolution as progress. As social life changed, the worth and rights of each member in the larger group, of which he was a part, increased. As the groups grew from clans to civilizations, the value of the individual did not diminish, but became instead a guide to the rules that govern all men.

25. The best expression of the main idea of this article is
    (A) oppression and society
    (B) the evolution of man
    (C) man's animal instincts
    (D) the basis for social order
    (E) a history of violence and strife

26. The author would expect the greatest attention to individual rights and values to be found in
    (A) farming communities
    (B) small villages
    (C) prehistoric families
    (D) nomadic tribes
    (E) modern cities

27. According to the article, man's uniqueness is attributed to the fact that he is
    (A) evolving from a simpler to a more complex being

(B) a social animal
(C) capable of noting his own progress
(D) capable of inflicting injury and causing violence
(E) able to survive by forming groups with allegiance to one another

Directions: Each of the following questions consists of a word printed in capital letters, followed by five (5) lettered words or phrases. Select the word or phrase which is most nearly *opposite* to the capitalized word in meaning.

28. REFRACTORY:
    (A) refreshing
    (B) burdensome
    (C) privileged
    (D) manageable
    (E) upright

29. ADROIT:
    (A) deterred
    (B) skillful
    (C) foolish
    (D) sinister
    (E) awkward

30. PALLIATE:
    (A) apologize
    (B) hesitate
    (C) wait impatiently
    (D) decide finally
    (E) worsen

31. VILIFY:
    (A) sing the praises of
    (B) show satisfaction with
    (C) regard with distrust
    (D) welcome with glee
    (E) accept halfheartedly

32. IRASCIBLE:
    (A) placid
    (B) fortuitous
    (C) shameless
    (D) entrancing
    (E) yielding

33. GELID:
    (A) chilly

(B) solid
(C) mature
(D) pallid
(E) boiling

34. CONDIGN:
(A) unavoidable
(B) unsatisfactory
(C) unguarded
(D) undeserved
(E) uninitiated

35. PUNCTILIOUS:
(A) tardy
(B) correct
(C) careless
(D) apathetic
(E) repulsive

36. FECKLESS:
(A) spotted
(B) fatuous
(C) fawning
(D) strong
(E) calm

37. INSOLENT:
(A) sullen
(B) rich
(C) determined
(D) kind
(E) affable

38. SERENDIPITOUS:
(A) calm
(B) planned
(C) flat
(D) evil
(E) regulated

STOP

END OF SECTION. IF YOU HAVE ANY TIME LEFT, GO
OVER YOUR WORK IN THIS SECTION ONLY. DO NOT
WORK IN ANY OTHER SECTION OF THE TEST.

SECTION II

30 minutes
38 questions

Directions: Each of the questions below contains one or more blank spaces, each blank indicating an omitted word. Each sentence is followed by five (5) lettered words or sets of words. Read and determine the general sense of the sentence. Then choose the word or set of words which, when inserted in the sentence, best fits the meaning of the sentence.

1. The product of a _____ religious home, he often found _____ in prayer.
(A) zealously—distraction
(B) devoutly—solace
(C) vigorously—comfort

(D) fanatically—misgivings
(E) pious—answers

2. Our _____ objections finally got us thrown out of the stadium.
(A) hurled
(B) modest
(C) wary
(D) vocal
(E) pliant

3. Only a single wall still stood in mute _____ to Nature's force.
(A) evidence

(B)   tribute
(C)   remainder
(D)   memory
(E)   testimony

4. After completing her usual morning chores, Linda found herself _____ tired.
    (A)   surprisingly
    (B)   erratically
    (C)   buoyantly
    (D)   forcibly
    (E)   unceasingly

5. The current spirit of _____ among the various departments of the university have led to a number of _____ publications which might not otherwise have been written.
    (A)   competition—angry
    (B)   futility—significant
    (C)   cooperation—interdisciplinary
    (D)   patriotism—American
    (E)   machoism—pugilistic

6. Human senses are designed to ____ specific stimuli, and after a focus is achieved, other sensory data is _____.
    (A)   look for—heightened
    (B)   respond to—insulated
    (C)   concentrate on—discounted
    (D)   favor—added up
    (E)   create—born

7. Immigrants arriving in a new country have the special problem of _____ their established behaviors and learning new habits whose results are _____.
    (A)   abandoning—uncertain
    (B)   strengthening—different
    (C)   controlling—guaranteed
    (D)   loosening—definite
    (E)   maintaining—simpler

Directions: In each of the following questions, you are given a related pair of words or phrases in capital letters. Each capitalized pair is followed by five (5) lettered pairs of words or phrases. Choose the pair which best expresses a relationship similar to that expressed by the original pair.

8. MONEY : EMBEZZLEMENT ::
    (A)   bank : cashier
    (B)   writing : plagiarism
    (C)   remarks : insult
    (D)   radiation : bomb
    (E)   death : murder

9. FOIL : FENCE ::
    (A)   pencil : mark
    (B)   road : run
    (C)   gloves : box
    (D)   train : travel
    (E)   bow : bend

10. CLIMB : TREE ::
    (A)   row : canoe
    (B)   ascend : cliff
    (C)   throw : balloon
    (D)   file : nail
    (E)   float : loan

11. LION : CUB ::
    (A)   duck : drake
    (B)   rooster : chicken
    (C)   human : child
    (D)   mother : daughter
    (E)   fox : vixen

12. ROOM : HOUSE ::
    (A)   refrigerator : kitchen
    (B)   chair : room
    (C)   cabin : ship
    (D)   wheel : car
    (E)   cockpit : plane

13. ACORN : OAK ::
    (A)   fig : bush
    (B)   flower : stalk
    (C)   nut : plant
    (D)   bulb : tulip
    (E)   branch : leaf

14. SORROW : DEATH ::
    (A)   laugh : cry
    (B)   plum : peach
    (C)   happiness : birth
    (D)   fear : hate
    (E)   confusion : anger

15. EXPLOSION : DEBRIS ::
    (A) fire : ashes
    (B) flood : water
    (C) famine : war
    (D) disease : germ
    (E) heat : burn

16. SOLECISM : GRAMMAR ::
    (A) divorce : marriage
    (B) foul : rules
    (C) incest : family
    (D) stumble : running
    (E) apostasy : dogma

Directions: Below each of the following passages, you will find questions or incomplete statements about the passage. Each statement or question is followed by lettered words or expressions. Select the word or expression that most satisfactorily completes each statement, or answers each question in accordance with the meaning of the passage. After you have chosen the best answer, blacken the corresponding space on the answer sheet.

The deliberate violation of constituted law (civil disobedience) is never morally justified if the law being violated is not the prime target or focal point of the protest. While our government maintains the principle of the Constitution by providing methods for and protection of those engaged in individual or group dissent, the violation of law simply as a technique of demonstration constitutes rebellion.

Civil disobedience is by definition a violation of the law. The theory of civil disobedience recognizes that its actions, regardless of their justification, must be punished. However, disobedience of laws not the subject of dissent, but merely used to dramatize dissent, is regarded as morally as well as legally unacceptable. It is only with respect to those laws which offend the fundamental values of human life that moral defense of civil disobedience can be rationally supported.

For a just society to exist, the principle of tolerance must be accepted, both by the government in regard to properly expressed individual dissent and by the individual toward legally established majority verdicts. No individual has a monopoly on freedom and all must tolerate opposition. Dissenters must accept dissent from their dissent, giving it all the respect they claim for themselves. To disregard this principle is to

make civil disobedience not only legally wrong but morally unjustifiable.

17. The author's attitude toward civil disobedience is one of
    (A) indifference
    (B) admiration
    (C) hostility
    (D) respect
    (E) contempt

18. What would the author most likely feel about a demonstration against apartheid which resulted in the disruption of businesses not associated with the problem in any way?
    (A) profound antipathy toward the goal of the demonstration
    (B) severe condemnation of the location of the businesses
    (C) tolerant acceptance of the demonstration's results
    (D) amused indifference toward the demonstrator's goals
    (E) regretful disapproval of the methods of protest

19. It can be inferred from the passage that
    (A) a just society cannot accept illegal civil disobedience
    (B) a just society cannot accept immoral actions of any sort
    (C) dissenters who use civil disobedience cannot use it merely to dramatize their cause
    (D) civil disobedience is sometimes the right thing to do
    (E) many authorities respect dissent as necessary to the functioning of a free society

The Planning Commission asserts that the needed reduction in acute care hospital beds can best be accomplished by closing the smaller hospitals, mainly voluntary and proprietary. This strategy follows from the argument that closing entire institutions saves more money than closing the equivalent number of beds scattered throughout the health system.

The issue is not that simple. Larger hospitals generally are designed to provide more complex care. Routine care at large hospitals costs more than the same care given at smaller hospitals. Therefore, closure of all the small hospitals would commit the city to paying considerably more for inpatient care delivered at acute care hospitals than would be the case with a mixture of large and small institutions. Since reimbursement rates at the large hospitals are now based on total costs, paying the large institutions a lower rate for routine care would simply raise the rates for complex care by a comparable amount. Such a reimbursement rate adjustment might make the charges for each individual case more accurately reflect the actual costs, but there would be no reduction in total costs.

There is some evidence that giant hospitals are not the most efficient. Service organizations—and medical care remains largely a service industry—frequently find that savings of scale have an upper limit. Similarly, the quality of routine care in the very largest hospitals appears to be less than optimum. Also, the concentration of all hospital beds in a few locations may affect the access to care.

Thus, simply closing the smaller hospitals will not necessarily save money or improve the quality of care.

Since the fact remains that there are too many acute care hospital beds in the city, the problem is to devise a proper strategy for selecting and urging the closure of the excess beds, however many it may turn out to be.

The closing of whole buildings within large medical centers has many of the cost advantages of closing the whole of smaller institutions, because the fixed costs can also be reduced in such cases. Unfortunately, many of the separate buildings at medical centers are special use facilities, the relocation of which is extremely costly. Still, a search should be made for such opportunities.

The current lack of adequate ambulatory care facilities raises another possibility. Some floors or other large compact areas of hospitals could be transferred from inpatient to ambulatory uses. Reimbursement of ambulatory services is chaotic, but the problem is being addressed. The overhead associated with the entire hospital should not be charged even *pro rata* to the ambulatory facilities. Even if it were, the total cost would probably be less than that of building a new facility. Many other issues would also need study, especially the potential overcentralization of ambulatory services.

The Planning Commission language seems to imply that one reason for closing smaller hospitals is that they are "mainly voluntary and proprietary," thus, preserving the public hospital system by making the rest of the hospital system absorb the needed cuts. It is · important to preserve the public hospital system for many reasons, but the issue should be faced directly and not hidden behind arguments about hosptial size. If indeed that was the meaning.

20. The best title for the passage would be
    (A) Maintaining Adequate Hospital Facilities
    (B) Defending the Public Hospitals
    (C) Methods of Selecting Hospital Beds to be Closed
    (D) Protecting the Proprietary and Voluntary Hospitals
    (E) Economic Efficiency in Hospital Bed Closings

21. The Planning Commission is accused by the author of being
    (A) unfair
    (B) racist
    (C) foolish
    (D) shortsighted
    (E) ignorant

22. On the subject of the number of hospital beds the author
    (A) is in complete agreement with the Planning Commission
    (B) wishes to see large numbers of beds closed
    (C) wishes to forestall the closing of any more hospital beds
    (D) is unsure of the number of excess beds there really are
    (E) wishes to avoid exchanging quantity for quality

23. All of the following are reasons the author opposes the Planning Commision's Recommendation EXCEPT
    (A) service industries have an upper limit for savings of scale
    (B) single buildings of large centers may be closable instead of smaller hospitals

(C) public hospitals have a unique contribution to make and should not be closed

(D) the smaller hospitals recommended for closure provide services more cheaply than larger hospitals

(E) hospitals are service organizations

24. With which of the following would the author probably NOT agree?
(A) Large medical centers provide better and more complex care than do smaller hospitals.
(B) Reimbursement rates do not necessarily reflect the actual costs of providing medical care to a given patient.
(C) Patients needing only routine medical care can often be distinguished from those requiring complex care prior to hospitalization.
(D) Too much centralization of ambulatory care is possible.
(E) Access to medical care is an important issue.

25. The author's purpose in discussing ambulatory care is to
(A) discuss alternatives to closing hospital beds
(B) present a method of reducing the fiscal disadvantages of closing only parts of larger hospitals
(C) show another opportunity for saving money
(D) help preserve the public hospital system
(E) attack the inefficient use of space in larger hospitals

26. With which of the following is the author LEAST likely to agree?
(A) a proposal to save costs in a prison system by building only very large prison complexes
(B) a plan to stop the closing of any beds whatsoever in the city, until the costs of various alternatives can be fully considered
(C) an order by the Planning Commission mandating that no public hospitals be closed
(D) a proposal by an architecture firm that

new hospital buildings have centralized record systems

(E) a mayoral commission being formed to study the plight of the elderly

27. How does the author feel that his suggestions for closing inpatient beds could impact on the ambulatory care system?
(A) Ambulatory care costs will probably be reduced.
(B) A reduction of hospital beds will increase the demand for ambulatory services.
(C) Smaller hospitals will have to cut back ambulatory services to stay fiscally viable.
(D) The Planning Commission would order the opening of new ambulatory services.
(E) The use as ambulatory facilities of the space made available in large hospitals by bed closings might result in having too many ambulatory services based in large hospitals.

Directions: Each of the following questions consists of a word printed in capital letters, followed by five (5) lettered words or phrases. Select the word or phrase which is most nearly *opposite* to the capitalized word in meaning.

28. FETID:
(A) in an embryonic state
(B) easily enraged
(C) acclaimed by peers
(D) reduced to skin and bones
(E) having a pleasant odor

29. ILLUSORY:
(A) nimble
(B) realistic
(C) powerful
(D) underrated
(E) remarkable

30. DOUR:
(A) gay
(B) sweet
(C) wealthy

(D) responsive
(E) noiseless

31. MENDACIOUS:
   (A) broken
   (B) efficacious
   (C) truthful
   (D) destructive
   (E) brilliant

32. ENERVATE:
   (A) debilitate
   (B) fortify
   (C) introduce
   (D) conclude
   (E) escalate

33. DISCRETE:
   (A) loud
   (B) combined
   (C) loose
   (D) circle
   (E) major

34. PRIMITIVE:
   (A) polite
   (B) naive
   (C) weak
   (D) sophisticated
   (E) knowledgeable

35. PARTITION:
   (A) solidify
   (B) unify
   (C) parse
   (D) enjoin
   (E) maintain

36. CLANDESTINE:
   (A) aboveground
   (B) public
   (C) outside
   (D) burnt out
   (E) physical

37. PHLEGMATIC:
   (A) hoarse
   (B) voluntary
   (C) oral
   (D) effusive
   (E) impulsive

38. MANUMIT:
   (A) throw
   (B) lock
   (C) promise
   (D) uncountable
   (E) enslave

STOP

END OF SECTION. IF YOU HAVE ANY TIME LEFT, GO
OVER YOUR WORK IN THIS SECTION ONLY. DO NOT
WORK IN ANY OTHER SECTION OF THE TEST.

SECTION III

30 minutes
30 questions

Directions: For each of the following questions two quantities are given, one in Column A and one in Column B. Compare the two quantities and mark your answer sheet with the correct lettered conclusion. These are your options:
   A: If the quantity in Column A is the greater;

B: if the quantity in Column B is the greater;
C: if the two quantities are equal;
D: if the relationship cannot be determined from the information given.

Common Information: In any question, information applying to both columns is centered between the columns and above the quantities in columns A and B. The common information applies to both columns. Any symbol that appears in both columns represents the same idea or quantity in both columns.

Numbers: All numbers used are real numbers.

Figures: Assume that the position of points, angles, regions and so forth are in the order shown. Figures are assumed to lie in a plane unless otherwise indicated. Figures accompanying questions are intended to provide information you can use in answering the questions. However, unless a note states that a figure is drawn to scale, you should solve the problems by using your knowledge of mathematics and *not* by estimating sizes by sight or measurement.

Lines: Assume that lines shown as straight are indeed straight.

COLUMN A	COLUMN B
1. the distance travelled by a car with an average speed of 30 miles per hour	the distance travelled by a car with an average speed of 40 miles per hour
2. The number of tens in 46	The number of thousands in 3612
3. 7.6351123	7.636

4.

AD	DC

5.

$$\frac{12}{10-8}$$

$$\frac{12}{10-6}$$

6.

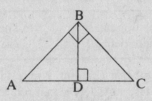

$z° + y°$	$x°$

7. the area of a square with side 30 inches | the area of a square with side two feet six inches |

COLUMN A	COLUMN B

8.

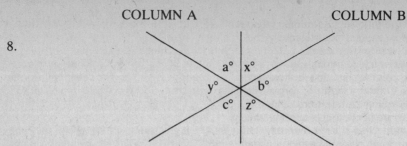

x + y + z	a + b + c

Questions 9 and 10 refer to the following figure:

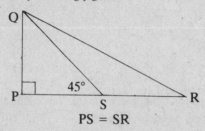

PS = SR

9.	PS	QP
10.	the area of PQS	the area of SQR
11.	The fraction of a day represented by 16 hours	The fraction of an hour represented by 45 minutes
12.	The sum of the 3 greatest odd integers less than 20	The sum of the 3 greatest even integers less than 20

13. Roberta can run a mile in 7.2 minutes, and Debbie can run 7.2 miles in an hour.

Roberta's average rate per hour	Debbie's average rate per hour

14. The relationships among the grades of 5 students are as follows:
   A's grade is higher than that of B.
   E's grade is less than that of D.
   D's grade is less than that of C.
   B's grade is higher than that of C.

E's grade	A's grade

15.
$$x = \frac{1}{4}(3x + \frac{8}{x^2})$$

x	2

Directions: For each of the following questions, select the best of the answer choices and blacken the corresponding space on your answer sheet.
Numbers: All numbers used are real numbers.
Figures: The diagrams and figures that accompany these questions are for the purpose of providing information useful in answering the questions. Unless it is stated that a specific figure is not drawn to scale, the diagrams and figures are drawn as accurately as possible. All figures are in a plane unless otherwise indicated.

16. Of the following which is LEAST?
    (A) $\frac{3}{5}$
    (B) $\frac{2}{3}$
    (C) $\frac{17}{29}$
    (D) $\frac{3}{7}$
    (E) $\frac{4}{5}$

17. If a square MNOP has an area of 16, then its perimeter is
    (A) 4
    (B) 8
    (C) 16
    (D) 32
    (E) 64

18. John has more money than Mary but less than Bill. If the amounts held by John, Mary and Bill are x, y, and z, respectively, which of the following is true?
    (A) $z < x < y$
    (B) $x < z < y$
    (C) $y < x < z$
    (D) $y < z < x$
    (E) $x < y < z$

19. If $x = 3$ and $(x - y)^2 = 4$, then y could be
    (A) -5
    (B) -1
    (C) 0
    (D) 5
    (E) 9

20. 10% of 360 is how much more than 5% of 360?
    (A) 5
    (B) 9
    (C) 18
    (D) 36
    (E) 48

21. If $x^2 + 3x + 10 = 1 + x^2$, then $x^2 =$
    (A) 0
    (B) 1
    (C) 4
    (D) 7
    (E) 9

Questions 22–25 refer to the information in the graph on page 184:

22. In the year 1971, approximately how many vehicles that were purchased were imported?
    (A) 2.25 million
    (B) 6 million
    (C) 8.25 million
    (D) 14.25 million
    (E) 21 million

23. The percent increase in the average purchase price of a vehicle from 1950 to 1970 was approximately
    (A) 75%
    (B) 150%
    (C) 225%
    (D) 275%
    (E) 340%

24. In which of the following time periods was there the greatest increase in the total number of family-owned vehicles purchased?
    (A) 1950–1951
    (B) 1959–1960
    (C) 1960–1962
    (D) 1964–1966
    (E) 1971–1974

25. Between 1950 and 1974, the average number of vehicles owned per household increased by approximately what percent?
    (A) 1.1%
    (B) 2.2%
    (C) 50%
    (D) 100%
    (E) 220%

26. Which of the following must be true?

    I. Any two lines which are parallel to a third line are also parallel to each other.

PURCHASES OF FAMILY-OWNED VEHICLES IN COUNTRY X
(in millions of units)

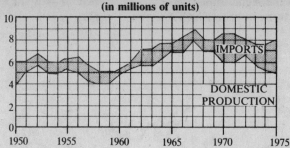

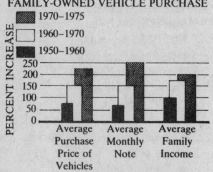

FINANCIAL FACTORS OF
FAMILY-OWNED VEHICLE PURCHASE

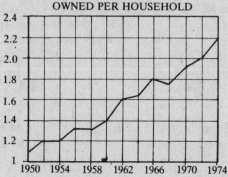

AVERAGE NUMBER OF VEHICLES
OWNED PER HOUSEHOLD

II.   Any two planes which are parallel to a third plane are parallel to each other.

III. Any two lines which are parallel to the same plane are parallel to each other.

(A) I only
(B) II only
(C) I and II only
(D) II and III only
(E) I, II, and III

27. An item costs 90% of its original price. If 90¢ is added to the discount price, the cost of the item will be equal to its original price. What is the original price of the item?
(A) $.09
(B) $.90
(C) $9.00
(D) $9.90
(E) $9.99

28. In the figure below, the coordinates of the vertices A and B are $(2,0)$ and $(0,2)$, respectively. What is the area of the square ABCD?
(A) 2
(B) 4
(C) $4\sqrt{2}$
(D) 8
(E) $8\sqrt{2}$

29. If $mx + ny = 12my$, and $my \neq 0$, then $\frac{x}{y} + \frac{n}{m} =$
(A) 12
(B) 12mn
(C) 12m + 12y
(D) 0
(E) mx + ny

30. In circle O shown to the right, MN > NO.
    All of the following must be true EXCEPT
    (A) MN < 2MO
    (B) x > y

    (C) z = y
    (D) x = y + z
    (E) x > 60°

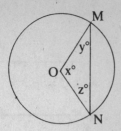

STOP

END OF SECTION. IF YOU HAVE ANY TIME LEFT, GO
OVER YOUR WORK IN THIS SECTION ONLY. DO NOT
WORK IN ANY OTHER SECTION OF THE TEST.

SECTION IV

30 minutes
30 questions

Directions: For each of the following questions two quantities are given, one in Column A
and one in Column B. Compare the two quantities and mark your answer sheet with the
correct lettered conclusion. These are your options:
   A: If the quantity in Column A is the greater;
   B: if the quantity in Column B is the greater;
   C: if the two quantities are equal;
   D: if the relationship cannot be determined from the information given.
Common Information: In any question, information applying to both columns is centered
between the columns and above the quantities in columns A and B. The common information applies to both columns. Any symbol that appears in both columns represents the
same idea or quantity in both columns.
Numbers: All numbers used are real numbers.
Figures: Assume that the position of points, angles, regions and so forth are in the order
shown. Figures are assumed to lie in a plane unless otherwise indicated. Figures accompanying questions are intended to provide information you can use in answering the questions. However, unless a note states that a figure is drawn to scale, you should solve the
problems by using your knowledge of mathematics and *not* by estimating sizes by sight or
measurement.
Lines: Assume that lines shown as straight are indeed straight.

COLUMN A	COLUMN B
1. $\qquad$ 10	$\dfrac{1}{0.1} + \dfrac{0.1}{10}$

2.

$l_1 \parallel l_2$

x° (right angle) l_1, y° l_2

| x | y |

COLUMN A	COLUMN B

3. $\quad 3 \times \frac{1}{3} \times 6 \times \frac{1}{6}$ $\qquad\qquad$ $4 \times \frac{1}{4} \times 7 \times \frac{1}{7}$

---

4. $\qquad\qquad$ $3x + 2 = 11$

$\qquad$ x $\qquad\qquad\qquad\qquad\qquad$ 2

---

5. $\qquad\qquad$ $x > 0$ and $y > 0$

$\qquad$ 5% of x $\qquad\qquad\qquad\qquad$ 5% of y

6.

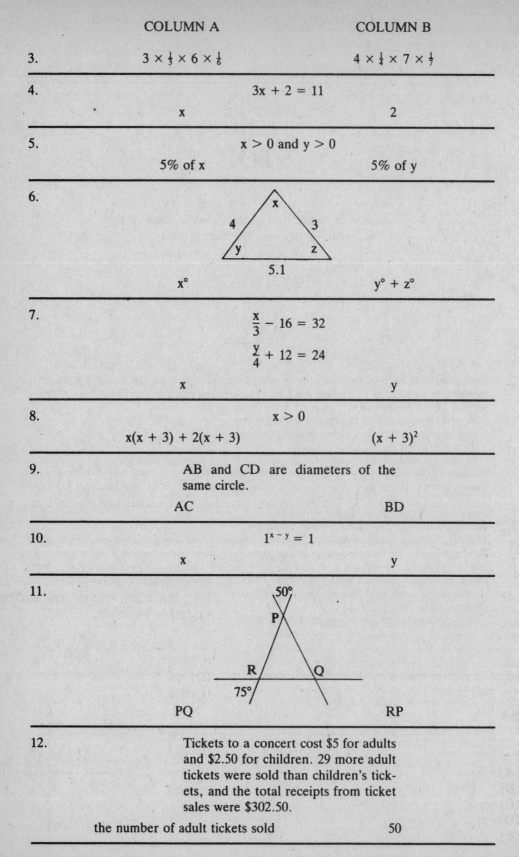

5.1

$\qquad$ $x°$ $\qquad\qquad\qquad\qquad\qquad$ $y° + z°$

---

7. $\qquad\qquad$ $\dfrac{x}{3} - 16 = 32$

$\qquad\qquad$ $\dfrac{y}{4} + 12 = 24$

$\qquad$ x $\qquad\qquad\qquad\qquad\qquad$ y

---

8. $\qquad\qquad$ $x > 0$

$\quad x(x + 3) + 2(x + 3)$ $\qquad\qquad$ $(x + 3)^2$

---

9. $\qquad$ AB and CD are diameters of the same circle.

$\qquad$ AC $\qquad\qquad\qquad\qquad\qquad$ BD

---

10. $\qquad\qquad$ $1^{x - y} = 1$

$\qquad$ x $\qquad\qquad\qquad\qquad\qquad$ y

11.

$\qquad$ PQ $\qquad\qquad\qquad\qquad\qquad$ RP

---

12. $\qquad$ Tickets to a concert cost $5 for adults and $2.50 for children. 29 more adult tickets were sold than children's tickets, and the total receipts from ticket sales were $302.50.

the number of adult tickets sold $\qquad\qquad$ 50

COLUMN A	COLUMN B

13. the number of integer multiples of 4 between 281 and 301 | the number of integer multiples of 5 between 2401 and 2419

14.

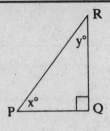

$$\frac{x°}{y°} = \frac{2}{1}$$

$\dfrac{PQ}{PR}$ $\dfrac{1}{2}$

15.

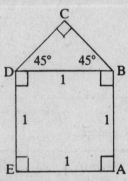

the area enclosed by polygon ABCDE   1.25

Directions: For each of the following questions, select the best of the answer choices and blacken the corresponding space on your answer sheet.

Numbers: All numbers used are real numbers.

Figures: The diagrams and figures that accompany these questions are for the purpose of providing information useful in answering the questions. Unless it is stated that a specific figure is not drawn to scale, the diagrams and figures are drawn as accurately as possible. All figures are in a plane unless otherwise indicated.

16. $\frac{4}{5} - \frac{3}{4} =$
  (A) $-\frac{7}{9}$
  (B) $-\frac{3}{5}$
  (C) $-\frac{1}{20}$
  (D) $\frac{1}{20}$
  (E) $\frac{3}{5}$

17. Into how many line segments, each 2 inches long, can a line segment one and one-half yards long be divided?
  (A) 9
  (B) 18
  (C) 27
  (D) 36
  (E) 48

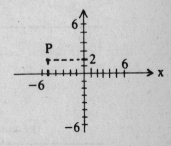

18. In the figure on the preceding page, the coordinates of point P are
    (A) (−5,−2)
    (B) (−5,2)
    (C) (−2,5)
    (D) (2,−5)
    (E) (5,2)

19. If circle O has a radius of 4, and if P and Q are points on circle O, then the maximum length of arc which could separate P and Q is
    (A) 8π
    (B) 4π
    (C) 4
    (D) 2π
    (E) 2

20. All of the following are prime numbers EXCEPT
    (A) 13
    (B) 17
    (C) 41
    (D) 79
    (E) 91

21. A girl at point X walks 1 mile east, then 2 miles north, then 1 mile east, then 1 mile north, than 1 mile east, then 1 mile north to arrive at point Y. From point Y, what is the shortest distance to point X?
    (A) 7 miles
    (B) 6 miles
    (C) 5 miles
    (D) 2.5 miles
    (E) 1 mile

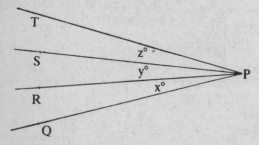

22. In the figure above, the measure of ∠QPS is equal to the measure of ∠TPR. Which of the following must be true?
    (A) x = y
    (B) y = z
    (C) x = z

    (D) x = y = z
    (E) none of the above

Questions 23–27 refer to the following graph:

QUARTERLY ANNUAL PROFIT RATES* FOR DEPARTMENT STORE X

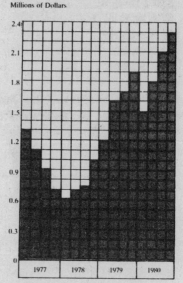

*ANNUAL PROFIT RATE = 4× THE ACTUAL PROFITS MADE IN THAT QUARTER

23. Approximately what was the actual profit made by Department Store X in the second quarter of 1979?
    (A) $6.4 million
    (B) $1.6 million
    (C) $1.2 million
    (D) $0.4 million
    (E) $0.3 million

24. For the time period shown on the graph, in which of the following quarters did Department Store X make the least amount of profits?
    (A) third quarter of 1980
    (B) second quarter of 1979
    (C) first quarter of 1979
    (D) third quarter of 1978
    (E) second quarter of 1977

25. During the period 1978–1980, inclusive, how many quarters exceeded an annual profit rate of $1.5 million?
    (A) 6
    (B) 5

(C) 4
(D) 3
(E) 2

26. In the year 1980, total profit made by Department Store X was approximately
(A) $30.2 million
(B) $7.6 million
(C) $1.9 million
(D) $1.2 million
(E) $.75 million

27. The total annual profit made by Department Store X increased by approximately what percent from 1977 to 1980 inclusive?
(A) 40%
(B) 50%
(C) 90%
(D) 120%
(E) 150%

28. $4 - 3(2 + 1(3 - (2 + 3) + 2) + 2) + 4 =$
(A) −4
(B) 0
(C) 2
(D) 8
(E) 12

29. Newtown is due north of Oscarville. Highway L runs 31° south of east from Newtown and Highway M runs 44° north of east from Oscarville. If L and M are straight, what is the measure of the acute angle they form at their intersection?
(A) 105°
(B) 89°
(C) 75°
(D) 59°
(E) 46°

30. If a sum of money is divided equally among n children, each child will receive $60. If another child is added to the group, then when the sum is divided equally among all the children, each child will receive a $50 share. What is the sum of money?
(A) $3000
(B) $300
(C) $110
(D) $10
(E) Cannot be determined from the information given.

STOP

END OF SECTION. IF YOU HAVE ANY TIME LEFT, GO
OVER YOUR WORK IN THIS SECTION ONLY. DO NOT
WORK IN ANY OTHER SECTION OF THE TEST.

SECTION V

30 minutes
25 questions

Directions: Each of the following questions or groups of questions is based on a short passage or a set of propositions. In answering these questions it may sometimes be helpful to draw a simple picture or chart. When you have selected the best answer to each question, darken the corresponding circle on your answer sheet.

Questions 1–4

To apply for a Dark Days Fellowship, a student must see the Dean of Students, fill out a financial statement, and obtain a thesis approval from either Professor Fansler or Professor Cross.

A student must see the Dean of Students before filling out the financial statement in order to make sure that it is filled out correctly.

The Dean of Students has office hours for students only on Thursday and Friday mornings, and Monday and Tuesday afternoons.

The Financial Aid Office, where the financial statement has to be filed in person, is open only Monday and Tuesday mornings, Wednesday afternoons, and Friday mornings.

Professor Fansler is in her office only on Monday and Tuesday mornings.

Professor Cross is in his office only on Tuesday and Friday mornings.

1. A student has already seen the Dean of Students and wishes to complete the rest of the application process in one day. If he must obtain his approval from Professor Fansler, when should he come to the campus?
   (A) Monday morning only
   (B) Tuesday morning only
   (C) Friday morning only
   (D) either Monday or Tuesday morning
   (E) either Monday, Tuesday, or Friday morning

2. If a student completed her application process in one visit, which of the following must be false?
   I. She got her thesis approved by Professor Cross.
   II. She got her thesis approved by Professor Fansler.
   III. She completed everything in the afternoon.

   (A) I only
   (B) II only
   (C) III only
   (D) I and III only
   (E) II and III only

3. If a student wanting to apply for a Dark Days Fellowship has classes only on Tuesdays and Thursdays and doesn't want to make an extra trip to the campus, which of the following is true?
   I. The thesis approval must be obtained from Professor Fansler.

II. The thesis approval must be obtained from Professor Cross.
III. The entire application process can be completed in one day.
IV. The entire application process can be completed within the same school week.

(A) I and II only
(C) II and III only
(C) I, II, and III only
(D) None of the statements are true.
(E) All of the statements are true.

4. A student has already obtained thesis approval from Professor Fansler. She wishes to complete the application process in only one more visit. When can she do this?
   (A) Monday or Tuesday only
   (B) Monday, Tuesday, or Friday only
   (C) Friday morning only
   (D) any morning except Wednesday
   (E) any morning except Wednesday or Thursday.

5. PROFESSOR: Under the rule of primogeniture, the first male child born to a man's first wife is always first in line to inherit the family estate.
   STUDENT: That can't be true; the Duchess of Warburton was her father's only surviving child by his only wife and she inherited his entire estate.

   The student has misinterpreted the professor's remark to mean which of the following
   (A) Only men can father male children.
   (B) A daughter cannot be a first-born child.
   (C) Only sons can inherit the family estate.
   (D) Illegitimate children cannot inherit their fathers' property.
   (E) A woman cannot inherit her mother's property.

6. As dietician for this 300-person school I am concerned about the sudden shortage of beef. It seems that we will have to begin to serve fish as our main source of protein. Even though beef costs more per pound

than fish, I expect that the cost I pay for protein will rise if I continue to serve the same amount of protein using fish as I did with beef.

The speaker makes which of the following assumptions?
(A) Fish is more expensive per pound than beef.
(B) Students will soon be paying more for their meals.
(C) Cattle ranchers make greater profits than fishermen.
(D) Per measure of protein, fish is more expensive than beef.
(E) Cattle are more costly to raise than fish.

Questions 7–9

The detective is following a subject who goes into a new seven-story office building. The detective doesn't want to risk sharing the elevator with the subject. Fortunately the building has a modern elevator panel which shows the location of the elevator and exactly to which up and down calls it is responding.

The subject got on the elevator with two other persons.

Each floor of the building has only one office, and it is not possible to use the stairway to go from floor to floor.

The elevator stopped on the third, fourth, fifth, and seventh floors. There were no calls for the elevator at those floors.

The elevator returned directly to the lobby from the seventh floor and was empty when it arrived.

7. If the detective assumes that the subject did not push more than one floor button or do anything suspicious in front of any witnesses, which of the following is the detective's safest conclusion?
(A) The subject got off at either the fifth or the seventh floor.
(B) The subject got off at the fourth, fifth, or seventh floor.
(C) The subject got off at the fifth floor.
(D) The subject got off at the fourth or fifth floor.
(E) The subject got off at the third or fourth floor.

8. If, on the next trip, the elevator stops at the second, third, and seventh floors going up, and the sixth floor coming down, on how many different floors must the detective consider checking for the subject?
(A) 6
(B) 5
(C) 4
(D) 3
(E) 2

9. The detective learns that one of the persons riding the elevator with the subject got out on the fourth floor, and someone else got in on that floor. On which floor(s) is(are) the subject(s) most likely to have gotten out?

I. the third floor
II. the fourth floor
III. the fifth floor
IV. the seventh floor

(A) I and II only
(B) I, II and III only
(C) I, II, and IV only
(D) III and IV only
(E) I, II, III, and IV

Questions 10–11

I. All wheeled conveyances which travel on the highway are polluters.
II. Bicycles are not polluters.
III. Whenever I drive my car on the highway, it rains.
IV. It is raining.

10. If the above statements are all true, which of the following statements must also be true?
(A) Bicycles do not travel on the highway.
(B) Bicycles travel on the highway only if it is raining.
(C) If my car is not polluting, then it is not raining.
(D) I am now driving my car on the highway.
(E) My car is not a polluter.

11. The conclusion "my car is not polluting" could be logically deduced from statements I–IV if statement
(A) II were changed to: "Bicycles are polluters."

(B) II were changed to: "My car is a polluter."

(C) III were changed to: "If bicycles were polluters, I would be driving my car on the highway."

(D) IV were changed to: "Rainwater is polluted."

(E) IV were changed to: "It is not raining."

Questions 12–16

I. Some Z are not Y.
II. Some Y are not X.
III. Some X are not Z.
IV. All X are not Y.

12. Which of the following can be deduced from conditions I, II, and III?
(A) There are no X that are both Y and Z.
(B) Some X are not Y.
(C) Some Z are not X.
(D) Some Y are not Z.
(E) None of the above.

13. Which of the following must be false, given conditions I, II, III, and IV?
(A) There are no X that are neither Y nor Z.
(B) There are no Z that are not X.
(C) There are no X that are Z.
(D) There are no Y that are Z.
(E) None of the above.

14. Given the above conditions, which of the following conditions adds no new information?

I. No Z are both X and Y.
II. Some X are neither Z nor Y.
III. Some Y are neither X nor Z.

(A) I only
(B) II only
(C) III only
(D) I and II only
(E) I and III only

15. Which of the following are inconsistent with the given information?
(A) Some Z are not X.
(B) Some Y are not Z.
(C) No X are not Z.

(D) No Y are not Z.

(E) All of the above are inconsistent with the given information.

16. If no Z are Y and no X are Z, which of the following must be false?
(A) Some Z are neither X nor Y.
(B) Some Y are neither X nor Z.
(C) Some X are neither Y nor Z.
(D) No Z are never X.
(E) No Z are never non-Y.

Questions 17–22

The National Zoo has a very active panda bear colony. One day six of the pandas broke out of their compound and visited the seals. After they were returned to their compound, they were examined by the Panda-keeper. The following facts were recorded.

Bin-bin is fatter than Ging-ging and drier than Eena.
Col-col is slimmer than Fan-fan and wetter than Ging-ging.
Dan-dan is fatter than Bin-bin and wetter than Ging-ging.
Eena is slimmer than Ging-ging and drier than Col-col.
Fan-fan is slimmer than Eena and drier than Bin-bin.
Ging-ging is fatter than Fan-fan and wetter than Bin-bin.

17. Which of the pandas is (are) fatter than Eena and drier than Ging-ging?
(A) Dan-dan only
(B) Fan-fan only
(C) Bin-bin only
(D) both Fan-fan and Col-col
(E) both Dan-dan and Bin-bin

18. Which of the pandas is both slimmer and wetter than Eena?
(A) Ging-ging
(B) Fan-fan
(C) Dan-dan
(D) Col-col
(E) Bin-bin

19. Which of the following is (are) both fatter and wetter than Ging-ging?
(A) Fan-fan

(B) Dan-dan
(C) Col-col
(D) Fan-fan and Col-col
(E) Eena and Dan-dan

20. Which of the following is the driest?
(A) Col-col
(B) Dan-dan
(C) Eena
(D) Fan-fan
(E) Ging-ging

21. Which of the following statements must be false?

   I. Dan-dan is drier than Col-col.
   II. Fan-fan is wetter than Dan-dan.
   III. Dan-dan is three inches fatter than Ging-ging.

   (A) I only
   (B) II only
   (C) III only
   (D) I and II only
   (E) II and III only

22. A new panda, Yin-yin, is purchased from the Peking Zoo. If dominance in panda bears is determined by fatness, then what will Yin-yin's rank be if he is fatter than Fan-fan and slimmer than Bin-bin?
   (A) second from the top
   (B) third from the top
   (C) fourth from the top
   (D) next to the bottom
   (E) Cannot be determined from the information given.

23. In *The Adventure of the Bruce-Partington Plans,* Sherlock Holmes explained to Dr. Watson that the body had been placed on top of the train while the train paused at a signal.

   "It seems most improbable," remarked Watson.

   "We must fall back upon the old axiom," continued Holmes, "that when all other contingencies fail, whatever remains, however improbable, must be the truth."

   Which of the following is the most effective criticism of the logic contained in Holmes' response to Watson?

(A) You will never be able to obtain a conviction in a court of law.
(B) You can never be sure you have accounted for all other contingencies.
(C) You will need further evidence to satisfy the police.
(D) The very idea of putting a dead body on top of a train seems preposterous.
(E) You still have to find the person responsible for putting the body on top of the train.

24. Rousseau assumed that human beings in the state of nature are characterized by a feeling of sympathy toward their fellow humans and other living creatures. In order to explain the existence of social ills, such as the exploitation of man by man, Rousseau maintained that our natural feelings are crushed under the weight of unsympathetic social institutions.

   Rousseau's argument described above would be most strengthened if it could be explained how
   (A) creatures naturally characterized by feelings of sympathy for all living creatures could create unsympathetic social institutions
   (B) we can restructure our social institutions so that they will foster our natural sympathies for one another
   (C) modern reformers might lead the way to a life which is not inconsistent with the ideals of the state of nature
   (D) non-exploitative conduct could arise in conditions of the state of nature
   (E) a return to the state of nature from modern society might be accomplished

25. Judging by the architecture, I would say that the chapel dates from the early eighteenth century. Furthermore, the marble threshold to the refectory is worn to a depth of one and three-eighths inches at the middle. Since the facilities were designed to accommodate approximately forty monks, I estimate that the monastery was occupied for approximately seventy-five years before it was abandoned, and that date would coincide with the violent civil and religious wars of the first decade of the 1800's.

Which of the following is NOT an assumption made by the author in describing the dates of the buildings?

(A) The marble threshold he studied is the same one originally included in the building.

(B) Architectural features can be associated with certain historical periods.

(C) The monastery he is investigating was nearly fully occupied during the time span in question.

(D) There is a correlation between usage and wear of marble flooring.

(E) Religious organizations have often abandoned outlying monasteries during times of political strife.

STOP

END OF SECTION. IF YOU HAVE ANY TIME LEFT, GO OVER YOUR WORK IN THIS SECTION ONLY. DO NOT WORK IN ANY OTHER SECTION OF THE TEST.

SECTION VI

30 minutes
25 questions

Directions: Each of the following questions or groups of questions is based on a short passage or a set of propositions. In answering these questions it may sometimes be helpful to draw a simple picture or chart. When you have selected the best answer to each question, darken the corresponding circle on your answer sheet.

Questions 1–3:

Five cats, F, G, H, J, and K, are being tested for three parts in a cat-food commercial. The on-camera cats must eat heartily and avoid fighting with each other. F is the best eater, but the most likely to fight. G and H eat best only when they are together, but fight with K.

1. If J is sick and cannot perform, which of the following can be inferred about an attempt to film the commercial?

   I. F, G, and H will do the commercial.
   II. G and H will fight with each other.
   III. The cats will likely fight during the filming.

(A) I only
(B) II only
(C) III only
(D) I and III only
(E) I, II, and III

2. If G and J go home, how many additional peaceful cats will be needed to fill out the cast?

(A) 0
(B) 1
(C) 2
(D) 3
(E) The commercial cannot be successfully filmed.

3. If F calms down and will no longer fight, how many different casts of cats are available?

(A) 1
(B) 2
(C) 3
(D) 4
(E) 5

4. Which of the following activities would depend upon an assumption which is inconsistent with the judgment that you cannot argue with taste?

(A) a special exhibition at a museum

(B) a beauty contest

(C) a system of garbage collection and disposal

(D) a cookbook filled with old New England recipes

(E) a movie festival

Questions 5–6

Stock market analysts always attribute a sudden drop in the market to some domestic or international political crisis. I maintain, however, that these declines are attributable to the phases of the moon, which also cause periodic political upheavals and increases in tension in world affairs.

5. Which of the following best describes the author's method of questioning the claim of market analysts?

(A) He presents a counter-example.

(B) He presents statistical evidence.

(C) He suggests an alternative causal linkage.

(D) He appeals to generally accepted beliefs.

(E) He demonstrates that market analysts' reports are unreliable.

6. It can be inferred that the author is critical of the stock analysts because he

(A) believes that they have oversimplified the connection between political crisis and fluctuations of the market

(B) knows that the stock market generally shows more gains than losses

(C) suspects that stock analysts have a vested interest in the stock market, and are therefore likely to distort their explanations

(D) anticipates making large profits in the market himself

(E) is worried that if the connection between political events and stock market prices becomes well known, unscrupulous investors will take advantage of the information.

Questions 7–11

Farmer Brown has a large square field divided into nine smaller squares, all equal, arranged in three rows of three fields each. One side of the field runs exactly east-west.

The middle square must be planted with rice because it is wet.

The wheat and barley should be contiguous so that they can be harvested all at once by the mechanical harvester.

Two of the fields should be planted with soybeans.

The northwesternmost field should be planted with peanuts, and the southern third of the field is suitable only for vegetables.

Questions 7–9 refer to the following squares:

(A) the square immediately north of the rice

(B) the square immediately east of the rice

(C) the square immediately west of the rice

(D) the square immediately east of the peanuts

(E) the square immediate northeast of the rice

7. Which square cannot be planted with soybeans?

8. Which square cannot be planted with wheat?

9. If Farmer Brown decides to plant the wheat next to the peanuts, in which square will the barley be?

10. If the three southern squares are planted, from west to east, with squash, tomatoes, and potatoes, which vegetables could be planted next to soybeans?

   I.   Squash
   II. Tomatoes
   III. Potatoes

(A) I only

(B) II only

(C) III only

(D) I and III only

(E) I, II, and III

11. If Farmer Brown decides not to plant any peanuts or wheat, what is the maximum number of fields of vegetables that he could plant?

(A) 3

(B) 5
(C) 6
(D) 7
(E) 8

Questions 12–15

   I.   L, M, Z, and P are all possible.
  II.   All M are L.
 III.   All L are Z.
 IV.   No M are Z.
  V.   Some Z are L.
 VI.   No P are both M and L but not Z.

12. Which of the above statements contradicts previous ones?
  (A) III
  (B) IV
  (C) V
  (D) VI
  (E) None of the statements contradicts previous statements.

13. If statements II and III are true, which of the other statements must also be true?
  (A) IV only
  (B) V only
  (C) VI only
  (D) IV and V only
  (E) V and VI only

14. If X is an L, it must also be a(n)
  (A) M only
  (B) P only
  (C) Z only
  (D) L and Z only
  (E) L, P, and Z

15. Given the above statements, which of the following must be false?
  (A) There are some L's.
  (B) Some Z are not L.
  (C) There are some P's which are Z's but not M or L.
  (D) There cannot be any Z's that are not L or M.
  (E) None of the above are necessarily false.

Questions 16–22

Captain Mulhouse is choosing the last part of his crew for the sailboat *Fearsome*, with which he hopes to earn the right to defend the America's Cup. He needs four more crew members, of whom at least two must be grinders for the winches, with the others being sail trimmers.

The candidates for grinder are David, Erica, and Francis.
The candidates for trimmer are Larry, Mary, Nancy, and Paul.
Nancy will not crew with Paul.
Erica will not crew with Larry.
David will not crew with Nancy.

16. If Nancy is chosen, which of the following must be other members of the crew?
  (A) David, Erica, and Mary
  (B) Erica, Francis, and Larry
  (C) Erica, Francis, and Mary
  (D) Erica, Francis, and Paul
  (E) Francis, Larry, and Mary

17. If Paul is chosen, which candidates will NOT be chosen to be on the crew?
  (A) David, Erica, and Francis
  (B) David, Erica, and Mary
  (C) David, Francis, and Larry
  (D) David, Francis, and Mary
  (E) Erica, Francis, and Larry

18. Given the above statements about the relationships among the potential crew members, which of the following must be true?

   I.   If David is rejected, then Mary must be chosen.
  II.   If David is rejected, then Francis must be chosen.
 III.   If David is chosen, then Paul must also be chosen.

  (A) II only
  (B) III only
  (C) I and II only
  (D) I and III only
  (E) II and III only

19. If Larry is chosen as a trimmer, which of the following could be the other members of crew?

   I.   David, Francis, and Mary
  II.   David, Francis, and Nancy
 III.   David, Francis, and Paul

(A) I only
(B) II only
(C) III only
(D) I and II only
(E) I and III only

20. Which of the following statements must be true?

    I. If Captain Mulhouse chooses Larry, then Francis must also be chosen.
    II. If Captain Mulhouse chooses Mary, then Nancy must also be chosen.
    III. If Larry is chosen, Nancy cannot be chosen.

(A) I only
(B) I and II only
(C) I and III only
(D) II and III only
(E) I, II, and III

21. If Paul is chosen to be part of the *Fearsome*'s crew and David is not, who must be the other members of the crew?
(A) Erica, Francis, and Larry
(B) Erica, Francis, and Mary
(C) Erica, Francis, and Nancy
(D) Erica, Mary, and Nancy
(E) Francis, Larry, and Mary

22. If Erica makes the crew and Francis does not, which of the following statements must be true?

    I. Paul will be a member of the crew.
    II. Mary will be a member of the crew.

(A) both I and II
(B) neither I nor II
(C) I only
(D) II only
(E) either I or II, but not both

23. Since Ronnie's range is so narrow, he will never be an outstanding vocalist.

The statement above is based on which of the following assumptions?

    I. A person's range is an important indicator of his probable success or failure as a professional musician.

II. Vocalizing requires a range of at least two and one-half octaves.
III. Physical characteristics can affect how well one sings.

(A) I only
(B) II only
(B) I and III
(D) III only
(E) I, II, and III

24. MARY: All of the graduates from Midland High School go to State College.
ANN: I don't know. Some of the students at State College come from North Hills High School.

Ann's response shows that she has interpreted Mary's remark to mean that
(A) most of the students from North Hills High School attend State College
(B) none of the students at State College are from Midland High School
(C) only students from Midland High School attend State College
(D) Midland High School is a better school than North Hills High School
(E) some Midland High School graduates do not attend college

25. All Burrahobbits are Trollbeaters, and some Burrahobbits are Greeblegrabbers.

If these statements are true, which of the following must also be true?

    I. If something is neither a Trollbeater nor a Greeblegrabber, it cannot be a Burrahobbit.
    II. It is not possible not to be a Trollbeater without being a Greeblegrabber.
    III. Any given thing either is a Trollbeater or it is not a Burrahobbit.

(A) I only
(B) II only
(C) I and II only
(D) III only
(E) I, II, and III

STOP

END OF SECTION. IF YOU HAVE ANY TIME LEFT, GO
OVER YOUR WORK IN THIS SECTION ONLY. DO NOT
WORK IN ANY OTHER SECTION OF THE TEST.

SECTION VII

30 minutes
25 questions

Directions: For each of the following questions two quantities are given, one in Column A and one in Column B. Compare the two quantities and mark your answer sheet with the correct lettered conclusion. These are your options:

A: If the quantity in Column A is the greater;
B: if the quantity in Column B is the greater;
C: if the two quantitices are equal;
D: if the relationship cannot be determined from the information given.

Common Information: In any question, information applying to both columns is centered between the columns and above the quantities in columns A and B. The common information applies to both columns. Any symbol that appears in both columns represents the same idea or quantity in both columns.

Numbers: All numbers used are real numbers.

Figures: Assume that the position of points, angles, regions, and so forth are in the order shown. Figures are assumed to lie in a plane unless otherwise indicated. Figures accompanying questions are intended to provide information you can use in answering the questions. However, unless a note states that a figure is drawn to scale, you should solve the problems by using your knowledge of mathematics and *not* by estimating sizes by sight or measurement.

Lines: Assume that lines shown as straight are indeed straight.

COLUMN A	COLUMN B

1. $\sqrt{9}$ $\sqrt{5} + \sqrt{4}$

---

2. $\frac{1}{6}$ 16%

---

3. $$x^- - 4 = 0$$

   x   2

---

4.   the cost of three pounds of grapes   the cost of four pounds of bananas

---

5. $0.17 + 6.01 + 5.27832$ 12

6.

$\dfrac{\text{area of sector P}}{\text{area of sector Q}}$ $\dfrac{\text{area of sector R}}{\text{area of sector S}}$

7.

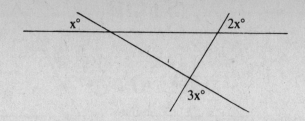

| x | 30 |

8.

$$x > 0 \text{ and } y < 0$$

| $x^2 + y^2$ | $(x + y)^2$ |

9.

$$x \text{ is } 150\% \text{ of } y \text{ and } y > 0$$

| x | y |

COLUMN A   COLUMN B

10.

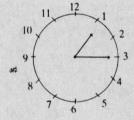

| The number the minute hand points to after turning 480° clockwise. | The number the minute hand points to after turning 720° clockwise. |

11.

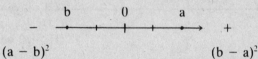

| $(a - b)^2$ | $(b - a)^2$ |

12.

$$2^m = 64$$
$$3^n = 81$$

| m | n |

13.   *Room P*   *Room Q*

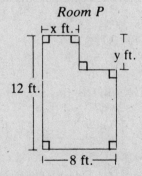   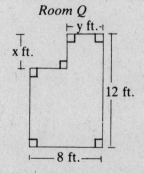

| perimeter of room P | perimeter of room Q |

14.

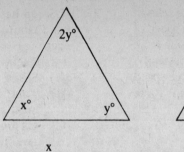

x   2y

---

15.   Total weight of x cartons each   Total weight of y cartons each
        weighing y pounds   weighing x pounds

Directions: For each of the following questions, select the best of the answer choices and blacken the corresponding space on your answer sheet.

Numbers: All numbers used are real numbers.

Figures: The diagrams and figures that accompany these questions are for the purpose of providing information useful in answering the questions. Unless it is stated that a specific figure is not drawn to scale, the diagrams and figures are drawn as accurately as possible. All figures are in a plane unless otherwise indicated.

16. If w, x, y, and z are real numbers, each of the following equals w(x + y + z) EXCEPT
    (A) wx + wy + wz
    (B) (x + y + z)w
    (C) wx + w(y + z)
    (D) 3w + x + y + z
    (E) w(x + y) + wz

17. .1% of 10 =
    (A) 1
    (B) .1
    (C) .01
    (D) .001
    (E) .0001

18. If x = +4, then (x − 7)(x + 2) =
    (A) −66
    (B) −18
    (C) 0
    (D) 3
    (E) 17

19. If 2x + y = 7 and x − y = 2, then x + y =
    (A) 6
    (B) 4
    (C) $\frac{3}{2}$
    (D) 0
    (E) −5

20. In the square below with side 4, the ratio $\dfrac{\text{area of shaded region}}{\text{area of unshaded region}}$ =
    (A) $\dfrac{2 + x}{4}$
    (B) $\dfrac{4 - x}{8}$
    (C) 2
    (D) $\dfrac{4 + x}{4 - x}$
    (E) 2x

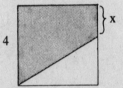

21. Ned is two years older than Mike, who is twice as old as Linda. If the ages of the three total 27 years, how old is Mike?
    (A) 5 years
    (B) 8 years
    (C) 9 years
    (D) 10 years
    (E) 12 years

22. A taxicab charges $1.00 for the first one-fifth mile of a trip and 20¢ for each following one-fifth mile or part thereof. If a trip is $2\frac{1}{2}$ miles long, what will be the fare?
    (A) $2.60
    (B) $3.10
    (C) $3.20
    (D) $3.40
    (E) $3.60

23. What is the side of a square if its area is $36x^2$?
    (A) 9
    (B) 9x
    (C) $6x^2$
    (D) 6
    (E) 6x

24. A girl rode her bicycle from home to school, a distance of 15 miles, at an average speed of 15 miles per hour. She returned home from school by walking at an average speed of 5 miles per hour. What was her average speed for the round trip if she took the same route in both directions?
    (A) 7.5 miles per hour
    (B) 10 miles per hour
    (C) 12.5 miles per hour
    (D) 13 miles per hour
    (E) 25 miles per hour

25. If Susan has $5 more than Tom, and if Tom has $2 more than Ed, which of the following exchanges will ensure that each of the three has an equal amount of money?
    (A) Susan must give Ed $3 and Tom $1.
    (B) Tom must give Susan $4 and Susan must give Ed $5.
    (C) Ed must give Susan $1 and Susan must give Tom $1.
    (D) Susan must give Ed $4 and Tom must give Ed $5.
    (E) Either Susan or Ed must give Tom $7.

STOP

END OF SECTION. IF YOU HAVE ANY TIME LEFT, GO OVER YOUR WORK IN THIS SECTION ONLY. DO NOT WORK IN ANY OTHER SECTION OF THE TEST.

ANSWER KEY FOR THE GRE PRACTICE EXAMINATION

Section I

1. B	10. D	19. D	28. D	37. E
2. C	11. C	20. E	29. E	38. B
3. A	12. B	21. A	30. E	
4. C	13. B	22. C	31. A	
5. E	14. D	23. B	32. A	
6. B	15. A	24. B	33. E	
7. E	16. C	25. D	34. D	
8. A	17. B	26. E	35. C	
9. D	18. C	27. C	36. D	

Section II

1. B	10. B	19. D	28. E	37. D
2. D	11. C	20. E	29. B	38. E
3. E	12. C	21. D	30. A	
4. A	13. D	22. D	31. C	
5. C	14. C	23. C	32. B	
6. C	15. A	24. A	33. B	
7. A	16. B	25. B	34. D	
8. B	17. D	26. A	35. B	
9. C	18. E	27. E	36. B	

Section III

1. B	7. C	13. C	19. B	25. A
2. A	8. A	14. B	20. A	26. C
3. D	9. A	15. C	21. D	27. A
4. D	10. A	16. D	22. D	28. B
5. B	11. C	17. C	23. D	29. D
6. A	12. A	18. B	24. E	30. A

Section IV

1. B	7. A	13. A	19. B	25. A
2. C	8. B	14. C	20. E	26. C
3. C	9. C	15. C	21. C	27. C
4. A	10. D	16. D	22. C	28. A
5. D	11. A	17. C	23. D	29. C
6. A	12. C	18. B	24. D	30. B

Section V

1. D	6. D	11. E	16. D	21. B
2. E	7. B	12. E	17. C	22. E
3. D	8. B	13. A	18. D	23. B
4. C	9. E	14. D	19. B	24. A
5. C	10. A	15. C	20. D	25. E

Section VI

1. C	6. A	11. B	16. C	21. B
2. C	7. E	12. B	17. E	22. A
3. C	8. C	13. C	18. C	23. D
4. B	9. E	14. D	19. E	24. C
5. C	10. D	15. D	20. A	25. A

Section VII

1. B	6. C	11. D	16. E	21. A
2. D	7. D	12. E	17. D	22. C
3. A	8. C	13. E	18. A	23. B
4. D	9. E	14. E	19. B	24. D
5. E	10. C	15. D	20. D	25. D

EXPLANATORY ANSWERS FOR THE GRE PRACTICE EXAMINATION

SECTION I

1. **(B)** As most people do not enjoy trouble, and as you can't interrogate it, we may logically conclude that they foresaw, or anticipated, trouble. A road doesn't grow into a path, nor does it collapse into one.

2. **(C)** The word waiter makes it clear that it is a dining situation that is being described. Thus, the crab will not be used to pelt, throw at, or resolve ourselves. This eliminates (A) and (D). (E) would also be a rather peculiar usage and should be eliminated. Between (B) and (C), the decision can be made by noting the structure of the sentence. The lobster is clearly the result of some act of the waiter. It is possible that the lobster is the embarrassment of the waiter, but more reasonable that it was his recommendation, especially since its being gone resulted in the eating of crab. Thus, (C) is the best choice.

3. **(A)** Derelict in this sense means empty, abandoned. Only people are bereaved or bereft. Bustling means busy and is thus incompatible with disuse.

4. **(C)** This sentence implies discord between the old-timers and the young mayor. Old-timers are likely to resent those officials who are trying to change, or reform, things.

5. **(E)** There may be many possible alternative fuel sources, but unless they are inexpensive, they won't affect the price of gas.

6. **(B)** Since the burden of the sentence is that the bacteria and viruses are the masters, (D) and (E) do not work because they do not describe a situation of virus mastery in the first blank. For the second blank, the idea that viruses and bacteria live off all other life, (B), is a good carrying through of the idea of mastery. (A) fails since companionship is not required by bacteria or provided them by humans or birds. (C) is second-best, but opportunity is rather general, and (B) describes just which opportunity is being offered and taken, thus (B) is the best answer choice.

7. **(E)** Since the author of the sentence is clearly a guard or something like that of the prisoners, he would expect some negative reaction from them. The word trepidation after the second blank is a contrast to the second blank and also describes the kind of feeling which was expected at first, but which the author finds disappointing now. Trepidation is alarm, or mild fear or unease; thus (E), fear, is best for the first blank. The second blank can be approached as either being the opposite of trepidation, which could be trust, again (E), or by asking what would best describe the result of a guard treating his prisoners with fairness. It is unlikely that a prisoner would ever love his guard or be loyal to him, though (B), (D), and (E) are all acceptable.

8. **(A)** The relationship between cat and mouse is predator to prey. (A) shows this same relationship between bird and worm. A dog may chase its tail, but not as a predator. A lion may on occasion kill a snake, but it is not its typical prey. (D) has the merit of evoking the idea of a cat-and-mouse game being hide and seek. Of course, it is the mouse (second element) which hides and the cat which seeks. A purely verbal relationship such as would be needed to justify cat and mouse is absent from the GRE. Trap and cheese has no merit aside from the alleged fact that mice like cheese.

9. **(D)** A vanilla bean is the source of the flavoring vanilla. We thus have a product and a source, or original form. Ginger is a root. None of the other choices correctly state the source or form of the flavoring cited. Tabasco comes from peppers, as does chili. Mint and sage are leaves.

10. **(D)** Energy is something that is dissipated. Money is squandered. The linkage is strengthened by noting that dissipated has the idea that there was no beneficial result from the expenditure of energy. The same holds true for squander. (A) has no merit since recharging a battery is just the opposite of dissipating energy; it is collecting it and making it useful. (B) has some merit in that the result of splitting an atom is certainly the release and dissipation of a great deal of energy, but it is a process of splitting, which itself is not dissipating. (C) has a little real merit since eating food certainly results in the food being broken down and changed, but it is not intrinsically wasteful or lacking in purpose. (E)'s only merit is that a gas will likely dissipate after it is generated. This is totally inadequate.

11. (C) A nose is a part of a face that sticks out. A knob is a part of a door that also sticks out. The first guess at an analogy might say that a nose goes

on the face. This would fit all five of the answer choices and thus be good, but would need refinement. The next thing would be to look at the answer choices and see the different ways that the first item goes onto the second item. (A) and (D) have the first item go over and around the second item. (B) merely has the first item as an extension of the second. (E) has the first item as something that is on the surface of the second item, but does not particularly stick out, but rather clings closely to the surfaces. (C) is the relationship that relates to the original pair in the best way.

12. **(B)** A rifle is the typical weapon of a soldier, at least as a soldier would be understood today. A sword is a typical weapon of a knight. In approaching this problem it is clear that weapons are an issue, or at least tools. (E) is not a tool of the robber, but rather a tool against him, so that's out. (A) has a weapon in the first slot, but instead of the user of the weapon in the second slot, we find another weapon. This fails. (C) has a tool of the cowboy, but it is not the same as a rifle. It may be true that a horse is the cowboy's best friend and the rifle is the soldier's best friend, but that is no basis for an analogy question on the GRE. Marine and tank in (D) would be very nice, except that it is backward. This does not happen often, but it happens.

13. **(B)** Venison is the name for meat from a deer. Mutton is the name for meat from a sheep. (C) is simply wrong since veal is meat from a young cow, not a lamb, which is a young sheep. (E) is very weak since a stew can be made with any meat. (A) fails because both of the words are names for the same group of animals and not the name for the meat from those animals, which is pork. (D) is the second-best answer, since when you order a steak in a restaurant, you will get the meat of a steer. However, that is not the name of the meat of a steer, but of a particular cut of meat. Steer meat also comes in many other cuts. Thus, steak is not the name of a type of meat from a particular animal, and (B) is correct.

14. **(D)** Something that is ineffable cannot be known. Something that is baffling cannot be solved. (C) has some merit since one might say of a certain situation that it is frustrating because there is no release from it, but that is an awkward way of putting it and not really what frustrating means. In (B), one finds that a trick is puzzling, but that is positive in its connection, while the original analogy is negative. (E) has no real connection since the essence of a rage is not whether or not it is controllable. Similarly for genial and interesting. Thus, (D) is the answer.

15. **(A)** The first idea of the analogy between icing and cake would be either that the icing goes on the cake or that it is a part of the cake. All of the

answer choices meet one of these criteria or both. (C) and (D) do not have any special merit because they are baking terms. On the contrary, if they were to work, they would have to be even tighter than some other, non-overlapping answer choice. (C) fails because baking is the process of making pastry, and cake is not a process here. Ice might cake up on some exposed part of a house or plane or something, but what is meant here is plain old icing on the cake. (D) fails because the apple is only in the pie and not on it. (E) would fail with the additional idea that the icing is a significant layer on top of the cake and the thickness of the print on the page is not something that is significant enough to come to our attention. No other answer choice but (A) has the idea of decoration and beauty that is implicit in the stem pair. One speaks of the icing on the cake as the last touch to making something just right. A veneer is a thin layer of beautiful wood that is laid over another material to make a beautiful finish or outside appearance. Unlike the ice in the pond, it is applied by people for a particular purpose. Thus, (A) is the best answer.

16. **(C)** Chalk is used to make marks on a blackboard. They are associated through the process of writing. (A) can be eliminated since a door and a handle are separate parts of the same operation or mechanism, but there is nothing that has one of them making a mark on the other. (C), (D), and (E) do have that marking idea. (B), like (A), is only a physical relationship and no process is invoked. (D) can be eliminated since its second item is the name of the process rather than the thing that is written upon. In contrasting (C) and (E), the major difference is the typical use of ink and paper for writing. While it is true that paper and ink are used for things other than writing, and paint can be used to write on a wall, these are not the typical uses which first come to mind. Thus, (C) is better than (E). One slight difficulty is that chalk is solid and thus is both the material deposited on the surface and the implement that is held. Pen and brush might do as well as ink and paint.

17. **(B)** The passage makes only one geographic reference, and that is to England, with the use of "this is the question" for England. Thus, (A), (C), and (D) are out. Since the author is doing a fairly modern analysis of the problems of distributing wealth, it is not likely that he lived in King Arthur's time. Hence, (B) rather than (E).

18. **(C)** (B), (D), and (E) are eliminated on the simple grounds that there is nothing in the passage on which to base them. The preference for (C) over (A) is not great, but can be arrived at by considering that what the author is advocating is paying less attention to the wages and the money part of the economy and more towards its ultimate ends. The denial of the virtue of money and the

implication that the rich are robbers (by analogy) also tend away from capitalism at least, if not toward socialism.

19. **(D)** (D) is included in the concluding sentence of the passage. (A) and (E) are specifically disputed in the passage, since it is the entire process that matters and not merely the pay rate or effort. (C) is not disputed, but is not emphasized either, while (B) is simply absent.

20. **(E)** The passage emphasizes that it is the ends of the productive process that are critical, thus, giving some support to (E). (C) has some appeal since money as such is not too important to the author, but its uses are important. (A), (B), and (D) derive any attractiveness they may have solely from the relative obscurity of (E).

21. **(A)** While the author stops short of outright accusation of the rich as robbers, they are treated in much the same manner in the passage, which creates the analogy desired.

    (E) is untrue. The author says that one might as well say the robber is a benefactor, or at least does no harm, but this is a way of disputing a statement, not agreeing with it.

    (D) fails since the passage is generally opposed to waste, while (B) and (C) are incorrect because only dishonesty is mentioned in relation to business.

22. **(C)** The choice is between (A) and (C). (B) is of no interest to the author, while (D) is only acceptable for the last three words. (E) is relevant but far too general.

    (A) refers to the last sentence and (C) refers to the sentences immediately after the posing of the great question. The distinction here is that (A) describes the great question for ALL members of society, while (C) describes the plight of the poor specifically.

23. **(B)** (B) is preferable because it is something that helps to provide the necessities of life—clean air and water, etc. (D) fails since it does not specify the job. (A) is not strong since weapons are generally destructive, though this is not impossible. (C) is less attractive than (B) since it has no stated positive value. The dislike of the rich would also enter into it. (E) is attractive since it is clear that this is something of which the author has done a great deed. It is clearly the second-best choice, but is not as good as (B) since there is no clear message in the passage as to the value of studying theory. If (E) specifically were the arousal of the laborer to his best interests, that might be even better than (B) since it would mean all would do good work and not just the one.

24. **(B)** (A) is attractive since the author certainly is not in favor of the rich or most of their works. However, his main point—the "main question for the poor"—is the use to which the resources of society are to be put. He will definitely see that it is waste and poor use of resources which lead to such problems as an energy shortage, since he has claimed that there will be enough of the good things if only everyone would work at the right things in the right way.

    While (C) has the advantage of being a very simple and direct response to an energy shortage, we are looking for something in the passage to link to our answer, and there is really nothing to support the idea that the author wishes to see more mineral exploitation. On the contrary, he denigrates such activities.

    (D) has no basis in the passage, but might appear to have the connection that the author does believe that there are enough resources to go around. Thus it might be mistakenly inferred that he would deny the shortage altogether. This is mistaken because the author says in the passage that all sorts of shortages and a despoiling of the environment are perfectly possible—even likely— if nothing is changed.

    (E), like (A), is something the author might well like to do on general principles, but there is no immediate link to the question, especially not in preference to (B).

25. **(D)** Choices (A) and (E) are incorrect because neither oppression nor violence are mentioned or implied in the passage. Choices (B) and (C) are also incorrect; evolution and instinct are mentioned in the passage, but as supporting ideas rather than as the central theme. We are left with choice (D), which does relate the main idea—the concept of social order—which is mentioned or at least implied in almost every sentence.

26. **(E)** The author states in the second paragraph that "as social life changed, the worth and rights of each member in the larger group, of which he was a part, increased." Since the social groups grew from clans to civilizations, the largest social group mentioned in the choices was "modern cities." It can therefore be assumed that the greatest attention to rights and values will be found there.

27. **(C)** It is stated very clearly that "of all living creatures, only man has the capacity to interpret his own evolution as progress." Choices (A), (B), (D), and (E) are all characteristics of many living organisms and therefore would not be unique to man.

28. **(D)** Refractory means stubborn or unmanageable. (D) is a perfect opposite to that meaning of refractory. None of the other answer choices connects to this meaning.

29. **(E)** Adroit means expert in something, particularly manual or mental tasks. Awkward is a good

opposite to the manual dexterity meaning of adroit. Skillful is close to being a synonym. Sinister comes from the Latin root meaning left, and although adroit comes from the Latin root meaning right, they are not opposites in English.

30. **(E)** Palliate means to make less severe or bad. Worsen is a perfect opposite.

31. **(A)** Vilify means to heap insults on. (A), (B), and (D) all have some merit. (A) is better since insult and praise are perfect opposites. The use of the word sing might be somewhat confusing since it is an idiomatic usage and one would not sing insults, but one does sing praises. Presumably one would not do (B) or (D) if one was vilifying someone, but they are not direct opposites. (E) would be opposite something that meant accept totally, not vilify.

32. **(A)** Irascible means irritable, and sounds like it, too. Placid is a very good opposite since a placid person is not easily disturbed. Fortuitous means fortunate; entrancing means able to put one into a trance, presumably a trance of delight. Shameless is the only word, other than placid, which is a personality characteristic, but it is not the same sort of thing at all.

33. **(E)** Gelid means frozen. Boiling is a good opposite since these are the two normal extremes of water. Chilly means mildly cold and has a connection to gelid, but a good antonym will be the same thing in an opposite way and mildly cold (chilly) is not as good an opposite to very cold (gelid) as is very hot (boiling).

34. **(D)** Condign means deserved or fitting, particularly of a punishment. Undeserved is a rather precise opposite. Unguarded might echo the use of condign with punishments, but it is not correct.

35. **(C)** A punctilious person takes extreme care over all aspects of his duties. Careless is taking no care or even extremely poor care. Tardy, meaning late, tries to reach for the word punctual, but that means on the dot (punct-) in terms of time, while punctilious means up to the dot or mark in terms of care and completeness. Correct has no merit since it describes something that is done consciensciously or scrupulously, and thus is not opposite at all.

36. **(D)** Feckless means weak, ineffective, feeble, or worthless. Strong is opposite to one of the meanings (feeble). Fatuous means foolish and ineffective; fawning is to seek favor by servile behavior. Calm might have some appeal, but the connection is to the word reckless, not feckless.

37. **(E)** Insolent means boldly rude. Affable means polite. This is a good opposite, though a word

meaning extremely polite would be even better. Sullen is more of a synonym than an antonym. Kind is a positive personality trait and insolence is a negative one, but that is never enough for an antonym. More precision is required.

38. **(B)** A serendipitous discovery is a desirable but unsought result. The degree of desirability is not the issue so much as the unplanned nature of the discovery. Thus, planned is an acceptable opposite, while evil is not. There is no moral connotation to serendipity. Regulated is probably the second-best answer choice and has real merit. However, regulated applies more to control than specifically to planning, and thus is not quite to the point.

SECTION II

1. **(B)** To say a pious religious home is redundant. Only (B) completes the thought and intent of the sentence.

2. **(D)** The objections mentioned must have been vocal to get them thrown out.

3. **(E)** A single wall implies that, formerly, there were other walls. That only one wall still stood is testimony, not tribute, to Nature's power. Evidence to is poor diction.

4. **(A)** Assuming that routine activity is not exhausting, it would be surprising to find yourself exhausted by it one day.

5. **(C)** (E) fails since pugilistic, in the second blank, is not the way to describe articles unless they are about boxing. (D) is also poor since we have no particular indication that the university is in the United States or the Americas. In considering the first blank, we might discount (B) on the grounds that among is hinting at a relationship between the various departments and futility is not a relationship word, while cooperation and competition are precisely that. In choosing between (A) and (C), we would have to ask whether competition would be more likely to breed angry articles or if cooperation would lead to interdisciplinary ones. Since we are talking about the departments of a university, interdisciplinary is very apt, while competition in a university need not yield angry articles. Thus, (C) is the best answer choice.

6. **(C)** The first blank is something that leads up to having a focus on specific stimuli. (E) is rather a poor lead-in to focus, but the others are all possible. For the second blank, (B) and (D) are inadequate since the other data would not be insulated without some statement of what they were insulated from, if indeed sensory data being

insulated makes any sense at all. Isolated would have worked, perhaps, but that is not present. Added up is also inadequate, though added might have been acceptable. In choosing between (A) and (C), we have to take the workings of the pair of words into account. In (A) the situation would be that the focus starts in one place and then other things are somehow increased by the focus being in one place. This is a little strange, but (C) is a perfectly reasonable situation. If the senses are designed for specific stimuli, then it would be most reasonable that other stimuli would fade. Hence, (C) is the best answer.

7. **(A)** If new behaviors are learned, then the likelihood is that the old behaviors are changed. Also, the situation of being in a new country would mean changes are needed. Thus, (A) and (D) are the best ways of filling in the first blank. The difference between (A) and (D) for the second blank could not be sharper. (A) says uncertain and (D) says definite. If one is learning new habits in a new country, it is more reasonable to speak of uncertainties presenting a problem than of definite results presenting a problem. Thus, (A) is the better answer choice.

8. **(B)** Embezzlement is the unlawful taking of money. Plagiarism is the unlawful taking of a writing. The idea of lawful and unlawful uses of things can create a number of special words, which make interesting analogy problems. (E) is the only other choice to have an unlawful idea, and murder is certainly unlawful death, but it is the giving of death, if you will, rather than the taking of it and thus does not conform to the original pair as well as (B). (A) links only to the idea of money and does not replicate any relationship from the original. (C) and (D) have no idea of unlawfulness. Thus, (B) is the best answer.

9. **(C)** A foil is a type of sword used in fencing. Gloves are a type of equipment used in boxing. (A) has merit since a pencil is used to mark, but (C) is just as good on that level and also carries the idea of sporting equipment. Likewise, (B) and (D) have some idea of the first word being a way of performing the second, but it is not as good as (C). (E) does have an idea of sporting equipment, but the activity referred to in the second word, bending, is done to the bow and not with it and is not the sport itself.

10. **(B)** Climb is what one does to a tree in order to get to the top of it. Ascend is the word that is used to describe the climbing of a cliff. Scale could also be used, but it isn't here. The other answer choices, except (C), are also fairly typical actions performed with or to the objects mentioned in the second position. However, they lack the additional idea of being a way of getting to the top of

the item mentioned. (C) lacks even that and hence fails totally. Thus, (B) is the best answer.

11. **(C)** Cub is the name given to a young lion. Child is the name given to a young human. A drake is a male duck, and a vixen is a female fox. Rooster is a male chicken. Mother and daughter are only different in age, but have the similarity of belonging to the same family, which a lion and cub do not necessarily do.

12. **(C)** A room is a part of a house and in particular it is usually a living unit of the house. A cabin is a living unit of a ship. (A), (B), and (D) all have the idea of the first item being in the second one, but they are not constituent parts in the way a house is made up of a number of rooms. (C) and (E) both have the idea of the first item's being spaces inside the second item. However, a cabin is a living space and a cockpit is not; thus, (C) is the best answer.

13. **(D)** "Great oaks from little acorns grow," and tulips grow from bulbs. (A) and (C), while relationships between living things, are not the seed to the final plant. (B) and (E) also lack the idea of the seed, though they do have the merit of having the leaf or flower grow out of the stalk or branch. (B) and (E) would make a reasonable analogy with each other, but not with the given stem pair. Thus, (D) is the best answer.

14. **(C)** Sorrow is the appropriate and typical feeling accompanying a death. Happiness is the appropriate and typical feeling accompanying a birth. In each case the feeling is felt by others than the dead or new-born person, of course. None of the other answer choices has a feeling and an event appropriate to the feeling. Indeed, none of the others has any event at all.

15. **(A)** The leftovers after an explosion is debris. The leftovers after a fire are ashes. As a first approximation, one might have tried the idea of the first item leading to or causing the second item. (C) does not fit this concept and is eliminated. (D) does but is backward. The leftovers from a flood, (B), are more properly the flotsam and jetsam deposited about the landscape rather than the water itself, which *is* the flood. In distinguishing (A) from (E), the decisive issue is that in the original pair and in (A), the second item is a waste product, while in (E) the burn is a resulting hurt. One would throw out debris and ashes, but one would not throw out the burn.

16. **(B)** A solecism is a violation of the rules of good speech, including the rules of grammar. A foul is a violation of the rules of a game. (A) refers to the end of a marriage, not a mistake or a violation of the rules, and so is not adequate. In (E), apostasy is the total desertion of some dogma, but not an error under the rules of the dogma; or if it is an

error, it is so severe as to be in a different class than solecism. In (C), incest is certainly a violation of the normal rules of how a family should operate, but the word family does not refer to the *rules* of family life. Mores might have worked, but it is not present. (B) and (D) are both clearly errors. However, the difference between them is that the stumble is an error in doing the act of running, while a foul is an error in following the rules of something. Since a solecism can be an error in following the rules of grammar, (B) is the better answer.

17. **(D)** As the author states that the principle of tolerance must be accepted by both parties, his attitude toward civil disobedience is not one of hostility or contempt. Answers (C) and (E), then, are wrong. Choice (A) is also incorrect, as is choice (B), since the author does not totally admire civil disobedience. (D) is the best answer.

18. **(E)** The use of the word apartheid, which refers to the principles of racial separation practiced in South Africa, is not particularly relevant to answering the question. The focus of the passage is that civil disobedience is only proper when the laws broken are themselves the main focus of dissent. The incidental breaking of laws is not proper since there should be actions that spill over from the dissent into other areas of improper action. While the situation posed in the question stem does not specifically relate to the breaking of a law, the procedural concerns of the author are the ones that must be carried forward into the new situation. Therefore (E), which projects that the author would disapprove of the harm to innocent bystanders, is quite in accord with the focus in the passage on making sure that the actions of dissent are sharply focused on their object.

(A) and (D) are certainly not correct since the author has not indicated anything which would indicate to us his views about the issue at hand. Indeed, the issue being protested is not relevant to the author. It is true that he believes that only affronts to fundamental human values are the proper subject of civil disobedience, but we are not being asked to make such judgments, only to judge the procedural issues raised in the passage. Thus, (A) and (D) fail.

(B) is wrong since there is no basis on which to say that the author has or would have any opinion about the location of any business. On the contrary, the businesses are portrayed as the innocent bystanders (if the question says they are innocent bystanders, then they are innocent bystanders).

(C) is the converse of (E) and fails for all the reasons that (E) succeeds. The only merit of (C) is that it uses the word tolerant, which is certainly dear to the heart of the author. But the mere appearance of a word is not enough to make an answer correct.

19. **(D)** On structural grounds, (D) should be the answer choice to which you give first attention, quite apart from any matter of content. All four of the other answer choices are very strong statements with cannot or necessary. (D), on the other hand, only says "sometimes," which is much weaker.

(A) fails on grounds of meaning, since all civil disobedience is, by definition, illegal, and yet it is sometimes acceptable when it is done for the proper purposes and in the proper way.

(C) fails on careful reading since it is stating that the dissenters cannot use civil disobedience in a particular way, and the fact of the matter is that they can use it in any way they wish, but the author disapproves of their using it in this way.

(B) and (E) are the sort of statements that are hard to quarrel with, but they are not particularly relevant to this passage. The only requirement that the author imposes on the just society is that it be tolerant. This may not mean that it does or can accept immoral actions, whatever accept might amount to, but it certainly does not mean that the just society cannot accept these actions. (E) has problems with the idea of many authorities, since this is unclear from the passage, and, even more importantly, has the word free. There is absolutely nothing of any kind in the passage about a free society, but only about a just one. There may be a connection between the two ideas, but it is not made in the passage and thus we should not make it unless it is inescapable, which it isn't.

20. **(E)** (D) is of no interest to the author. (A), (B), and (C) are topics mentioned in the passage, but only as serving the general analysis of the Planning Commission's proposal. Thus, (E) is more descriptive of the actual passage.

21. **(D)** The author's argument essentially states that the commission may be right as far as it goes, but it is not that simple. This implies that the commission has been shortsighted. It is true that because of the shortsightedness, the author views the plan as foolish, and perhaps somewhat ignorant, but these derive from the shortsightedness, and the tone is respectful rather than condemnatory. (A) and (B) have no basis.

22. **(D)** (A) is attractive, but the word complete kills it. The author is clearly unsure of the number of beds that should be closed and sees that as a future issue. (B) and (C) fail for the same reason. (E) sounds good, but is not really mentioned.

23. **(C)** All of the statements are agreeable to the author, but (C) is specifically stated by the passage not to be properly addressed in the context of the commission's proposal. Because of (A) and (E), large hospitals may not be more efficient. (B) and (D) are both reasons why small hospitals should not be closed.

24. **(A)** (A) is only half agreeable. The author states the larger centers provide more complex care, and if the larger hospitals do not provide the most efficient care—as the author claims they don't—then it is certainly probable that they do not definitely provide the better care than smaller hospitals of the sort that can be received at both kinds of facilities.

    (B) is inferable from the statement that only overall costs are used to set rates. (C) is inferable from the author's support of the existence of institutions that can only provide that sort of care, while also supporting quality. (D) is stated to be a possible problem. (E) is inferable from the concern shown for greater or lesser access in the third and fifth paragraphs.

25. **(B)** The author knows that he cannot simply say to the commission that they shouldn't close the smaller hospitals. He must present evidence that it is not the best approach to the agreed-upon goal of saving money and closing unneeded beds—hence, (B). (A) is false since closing beds is agreed to by the author. (C) is true, but not as precise as (B); also the word another is troublesome since it is actually an alternative which is proposed. (D) is not currently at issue. (E) is appealing, but the inefficiencies of larger hospitals are not stated to be in the use of space.

26. **(A)** Prisons are, in a manner of speaking, service organizations (like hospitals), and thus very large ones may not be more efficient, according to the author; thus, (A). (B) is probably just what the author wants, since he is unsure of the number of beds that should be closed anyway. (C) is stated to be agreeable to the author in the last paragraph. (D) and (E) are indeterminable. There is no basis for agreement or disagreement given in the passage.

27. **(E)** The concern about possible *over*-centralization of ambulatory services is raised in the context of the proposal to close portions of the larger hospitals rather than the entirety of smaller hospitals. This juxtaposition of the two means that the author believes that closing parts of the larger hospitals might have the poor result of turning over so much space in those locations to ambulatory care that a disproportionate part of the ambulatory care system would reside at the larger hospitals. His use of the prefix over- indicates disapproval.

    The only references to the costs of ambulatory care are to its chaos and to some needs to keep it down. This implies a concern by the author that ambulatory care costs might increase, not that they might be decreased. Hence, (A) fails.

    (B) and (C) refer to connections that are not in the passage. The author refers to increasing the facilities for ambulatory services, but not to increasing the demand, which he seems to think is

there already. If you answered (C), you are answering from current events and not from the passage.

    (D) has the appeal of being something that the author would probably like to have happen, but it is not implicit in the passage that the Planning Commission has the power to bring it about, and he certainly does not ask it. Rather, the force of the argument about the use of the space left by the closed portions of larger medical centers is that this space would certainly not go to waste.

28. **(E)** Fetid means having a bad or offensive odor; thus, (E) is a very good opposite. Embryonic means not yet born or fully developed.

29. **(B)** Illusory means based on an illusion, thus not realistic. Nimble means agile and physically well coordinated.

30. **(A)** Dour means gloomy or sullen, and gay is an excellent opposite. Sweet plays on the idea of sour, which does have some real merit since a dour disposition can also be referred to as sour. However, since we are speaking of personalities, gay is a better opposite to dour/sour than is sweet, since a sweet disposition is not so much cheerful as amiable or gracious. They are fairly close, however.

31. **(C)** Mendacious means lying and untruthful, so (C) is a perfect opposite. Broken plays on the mend part of the word, as does destructive. Efficacious means efficient and effective.

32. **(B)** Enervate means to weaken significantly. Fortify means to strengthen. Debilitate means to weaken and is essentially a synonym, rare on the GRE as an answer choice.

33. **(B)** Discrete means separate, as in three discrete parts. One thing that you know about the word is that it is NOT discreet, which means tactful and quiet, thus (A) and (C) are incorrect. Combined is a good opposite, if not perfect.

34. **(D)** Primitive means basic, undeveloped, but not necessarily strong; thus, (C) is incorrect. Similarly, (A) is not connected. The other three answer choices are all referring to various levels of development of different ideas. The contrast between the answer choices shows that naive is a low level of development of understanding of the way things work, and is thus more of a synonym than an opposite. Sophisticated has to do with a highly developed understanding of something, while knowledgeable has to do with having a great deal of knowledge about something. Thus, sophisticated has the connotation of great development, which corresponds to the sense of primitive as having very little development.

35. **(B)** Partition means to divide into parts. Both (A) and (B) have some meaning of joining together, which is opposite to partition. In distinguishing solidify from unify, you might ask what the opposite of solid is. Since the opposite of solid is liquid, and partition refers to dividing into parts rather than liquefying, solidify is not correct. Parse means to separate into parts grammatically and is thus either the same as the stem word, or unrelated. Maintain is also unrelated. Enjoin is a word that has a superficial appeal since joining is what is wanted in an answer. However, enjoin means to legally forbid something from happening.

36. **(B)** Clandestine means secret, private, or concealed, usually on purpose. (A), (B), and (C) all have some merit. Outside, by itself, is not the opposite of hidden. Aboveground and public are therefore the two best answers, and both have a real oppositeness to clandestine. In choosing between them, the key factor is the very specific way in which aboveground works versus the more general meaning of public. The perfect opposite to aboveground is underground, which certainly means hidden, but public specifically means that it is revealed. Underground/aboveground refers more to the legitimacy of the activity—can it stand the light of day?—than to whether it is hidden or not. While it is true that clandestine activities by certain groups have, in recent years, been characterized as illicit, that is not part of the original meaning of the word clandestine. The shady flavor comes from the idea that a clandestine activity may be kept hidden by deception.

37. **(D)** Phlegmatic means cooly self-possessed and undemonstrative. Effusive means to make a great demonstration of feeling. Hoarse connects to the idea of phlegm in the throat, which might make one hoarse, but that is not helpful here.

38. **(E)** Manumit means to free a slave; hence enslave is a perfect opposite.

SECTION III

1. **(B)** In treating radicals (square roots), it is important to keep in mind that the numbers under the radicals may be combined only when the two radicals are being multipled, not when the radicals are being added. Thus $\sqrt{5}\sqrt{4}$ is the standard notation for $\sqrt{5} \times \sqrt{4}$; the symbol for multiplication is omitted just as it is in algebraic notation (e.g., a times b is written ab). In this problem, the indicated operation is addition, not multiplication. While $\sqrt{5}\sqrt{4} = \sqrt{20}$, $\sqrt{5} + \sqrt{4} \neq \sqrt{9}$. Having established that, the problem is now easily solved. We know that $\sqrt{9} = 3$. (Note: $\sqrt{9} = 3$ not $\sqrt{9} = +$ or $-$ 3.) The printed radical is by convention a *non-negative* number. Only when we have $x^2 = 9$,

do we have $x = \pm 3$, and that is because we are taking the square root of both sides of the equation:

$$x^2 = 9$$
$$x = \pm\sqrt{9}$$
$$x = \pm 3$$

Notice that the $\pm$ symbol was inserted in front of the radical *before* taking the square root of 9.

As for Column B, $\sqrt{4} = 2$. And we also know that $\sqrt{5} > \sqrt{4}$, so $\sqrt{5} > 2$. This means that Column B is 2 plus something greater than 2, and thus totals something greater than 4, so B must be greater than A.

2. **(A)** Knowing the common fraction-percent equivalents would make this problem a cinch: $\frac{1}{6} = 16\frac{2}{3}\%$. But even if one does not remember that, the problem is easily solved by dividing 6 into 1: $6)\overline{1.00} = .16\frac{2}{3}$. So, Column A is greater than Column B.

3. **(D)** Here we can use the information about positive and negative roots discussed in question 1 above. The direct attack here is to solve for x:

$$x^2 - 4 = 0$$
$$x^2 = 4$$
$$x = \pm\sqrt{4}$$
$$x = \pm 2$$

This shows that x might be either + or −2. To be sure, if $x = +2$, Column A is equal to Column B; but if $x = -2$, Column B is greater. This shows that our answer must be (D).

4. **(D)** Without knowing how much fruit costs per pound, we have no way of determining which costs more, three pounds of grapes or four pounds of bananas. We cannot assume that B is greater just because the bananas weigh more.

5. **(B)** You can solve this problem by performing the addition in Column A, but we have seen some problems in previous exercises in which the arithmetic would be too time-consuming. This problem borders on being one of those. If your first reaction was to add, and you then added the three numbers in less than 20 seconds, your're on firm ground. However, if you took 30 to 45 seconds to complete the addition, you should look for a shortcut. In this case, it is easy to see that the second and third terms are roughly 6 and 5. That will add up to 11. It remains only to ask whether the additional decimals in all three terms will total 1 (11 + 1 = 12). A quick glance shows that they do not add up to as much as 1, so Column B must be greater than Column A.

6. **(A)** Q and S are approximately equal, while P is much larger than R, thus making Column A larger. Since this is a chart, it is likely that the scale is true. Even if you calculated S as 20%, you

would then be left with the comparison $\frac{45\%}{20\%}$ to $\frac{15\%}{20\%}$, which need not be computed since the fractions can be compared on the basis of the denominators (bottoms) being equal and the numerators (tops) being different. The computation would show Column A as $\frac{9}{4}$ and Column B as $\frac{3}{4}$.

7. **(C)** We get started by filling in missing details. We are looking to connect our x's with a known shape.

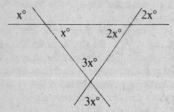

We complete the interior of the triangle using the principle that opposite angles are equal. Then, we know that the sum of the interior angles of a triangle is 180°, so:

$$x + 2x + 3x = 180°$$
$$6x = 180°$$
$$x = 30°$$

This shows that Column A and Column B are equal.

8. **(A)** Since the left expression is not factorable, the best way to begin is to multiply the right-hand expression and then strip everything from the comparison which will not make a difference: $(x + y)^2 = (x + y)(x + y) = x^2 + 2xy + y^2$. Now we see that we have an x^2 and a y^2 term on both sides of the comparison, so we strip them away (by subtracting x^2 and y^2 from both sides). This leaves 0 in Column A and $+2xy$ in Column B. But the centered information states that x is positive and y is negative. So $2xy$ must be *negative*, which makes it less than 0. Column B is less than Column A so the answer is (A).

9. **(A)** This is one of those cases where the algebraic statement is probably easier to grasp than the English equivalent: "x is 150% of y" means $x = 1.5y$. We can see from this that since $y > 0$, $1.5y$ must be larger than y.

10. **(A)** A complete revolution of the minute hand will cover 360° (there are 360° around the center of a circle). So if the minute hand covers 480°, it will make one full turn coming back to the 3, then it will continue for another 120°, which is a third of the circle. Since there are 12 numbers on the face of the clock, one-third of that is four numbers, so we add four numbers to the 3, arriving at 7. As for Column B, 720° is just two full turns, so the minute hand will go around twice, coming to rest again on the 3. So Column A is 7 while Column B is only 3.

11. **(C)** There are a couple of ways of approaching this problem. One is to do the indicated multiplication. The result in each case will be $a^2 - 2ab + b^2$, which shows that no matter what the values for a and b are, the expressions must be equal. Another approach is to notice that $a - b$ and $b - a$ both measure the distance from a to b. One of them does so by moving from positive to negative, the other does so by moving from negative to positive, but the absolute value is the same in both cases (the numerical value) though the signs are different. But when these values are squared, they both come out positive and therefore equal.

12. **(A)** 2 raised to the 6th power is 64, so m must be 6. 3 raised to the 4th power is 81, so n must be 4. 6 is greater than 4, so Column A is greater than Column B.

13. **(C)** We are looking to compare the perimeters, or the length of the walls, of the rooms. First we note that we are given information that all the angles are right angles. This is one point of similarity. Another point of similarity is that the two rooms are both 12 ft. by 8 ft. with a notch taken out. Since all the walls are at right angles, we know that the length of the right to left walls in each room must total 8 feet, plus the other two, which total 8 feet also, even though we do not know what x or y are. The two cross segments in room P, for instance, are x and $8 - x$ feet respectively. For Room Q they are y and $8 - y$ feet.

Similarly, the walls in the 12-foot direction must be 12 feet on each side of the room, even though broken up. Thus the total perimeter will be the same for both rooms. It is exactly 40 feet in both instances, though you do not need to compute it. For P it would be $12 + y + (12 - y) + x + (8 - x) + 8 = 40$, and similarly for Q. Note that you cannot make a comparison of the areas.

14. **(B)** Since x is an angle of an equilateral triangle $(6 = 6 = 6)$, we know that $x° = 60°$. Substituting 60° for x in the left-hand figure, we see that $60° + y° + 2y° = 180°$. So $3y = 120°$, and $y = 40°$. Now we know that $x = 60°$ and that $2y = 80°$, so Column B is greater than Column A.

15. **(C)** To compute the weight of the left-hand column, we must multiply x cartons by y pounds/cartons and get xy pounds. To compute the weight of the right-hand column we multiply y cartons by x pound/carton and get yx pounds. But since $xy = yx$, the columns must be equal.

16. **(D)** By multiplying out the given expression, we learn $w(x + y + z) = wx + wy + wz$, which shows

that (A) is an equivalent expression. Second, given that it does not matter in multiplication in which order the elements are listed (i.e., $2 \times 3 = 3 \times 3$), we can see that (B) is also an equivalent expression. From $wx + wy + wz$, we can factor the w's out of the first two terms: $w(x + y) + wz$, which shows that (E) is an equivalent expression. Finally, we could also factor the w's from the last two terms: $wx + w(y + z)$, which shows that (C) is an equivalent expression. (D) is not, however, equivalent: $w + w + w + x + y + z$. The 3 would make you suspicious of (D).

17. **(C)** The answers tell you that the issue is the decimal point. The percent sign signifies that the number has been multipled by 100. To convert a percentage to a decimal, we divide by 100 and drop the percent sign, and this is equivalent to moving the decimal point two places to the left and dropping the percent sign. Thus, $.1\% = .001$. Then when we multiply by ten, we move the decimal point one place to the right: $.001 \times 10 = .01$. So our answer is (C).

18. **(B)** The most direct solution to this problem is to substitute the value $+4$ for x: $(+4 - 7)(+4 + 2) = (-3)(6) = -18$. Substitute before multiplying.

19. **(B)** Here we need to solve the simultaneous equations. Though there are different methods, one way to find the values of x and y is first to redefine y in terms of x. Since $x + y = 2$, $x = 2 + y$. We can now use $2 + y$ as the equivalent of x and substitute $2 + y$ for x in the other equation:

$$2(2 + y) + y = 7$$
$$4 + 2y + y = 7$$
$$3y = 3$$
$$y = 1$$

Once we have a value of y, we substitute that value into either of the equations. Since the second is a bit simpler, we may prefer to use it: $x - 1 = 2$, so $x = 3$. Now we can determine that $x + y$ is $3 + 1$, or 4.

Another approach would be to add the two equations together so that the y term will cancel itself out:

$$2x + y = 7$$
$$+ (\ x - y = 2)$$
$$\overline{3x \qquad = 9}, \text{ thus } x = 3.$$

20. **(A)** Average speed requires total distance divided by total time. Therefore it is incorrect to average the two speeds together for, after all, the girl moved at the slower rate for three times as long as she moved at the faster rate, so they cannot be weighted equally. The correct way to solve the problem is to reason that the girl covered the 15 miles by bicycle in 1 hour. She covered the 15 miles by walking in 3 hours. Therefore, she travelled a total of 30 miles in a total of 4 hours. 30 miles/4 hours = 7.5 miles per hour.

21. **(D)** While we know by inspection that the shaded area is larger—the diagonal of a rectangle divides the rectangle in half—the answer choices tell us more is needed though (C) is eliminated. We begin by noting that the area which is left unshaded is a triangle with a 90° angle. This means that we have an altitude and a base at our disposal. Then we note that the shaded area is the area of the square minus the area of the triangle. So we are in a position to compute the area of the square, the triangle, and the shaded part of the figure. In the first place, the base of the triangle—which is the unshaded area of the figure—is equal to the side of the square, 4. The altitude of that triangle is four units long less the unknown distance x, or $4 - x$. So the area of the triangle, $\frac{1}{2}ab$, is $\frac{1}{2}(4 - x)(4)$. The area of the square is 4×4, or 16, so the shaded area is 16 minus the triangle, which we have just determined is $\frac{1}{2}(4 - x)(4)$. Let us first pursue the area of the triangle:

$$\tfrac{1}{2}(4 - x)(4) = (4 - x)(2) = 8 - 2x$$

Substituting in the shaded portion:

$$16 - (8 - 2x) = 8 + 2x$$

Now we complete the ratio. $8 + 2x$ goes on the top, since that is the shaded area, and $8 - 2x$ goes on the bottom, since that is the unshaded area: $\dfrac{8 + 2x}{8 - 2x}$. And we reduce by 2 to yield $\dfrac{4 + x}{4 - x}$.

22. **(D)** Since Linda is the youngest and the other ages are derived from hers, let us assign the value x for Linda's age. In that case Mike will be $2x$ years old, since he is twice as old as Linda. Finally, Ned will be $2x + 2$ since he is two years older than Mike. Our three ages are: Linda, x; Mike, $2x$; and Ned, $2x + 2$. We know that these three ages total 27. Hence, $x + 2x + 2x + 2 = 27$. And now we solve for x:

$$5x + 2 = 27$$
$$5x = 25$$
$$x = 5$$

So Linda is 5 years old. Then, if Linda is 5, Mike must be 10 years old.

23. **(D)** Since our rates are by fifths of a mile, let us begin the solution by figuring out how many fifths of a mile (or parts thereof) there are in this trip. In $2\frac{2}{5}$ miles there are 12 fifths. Then we add another fifth for the additional bit of distance between $2\frac{2}{5}$ and $2\frac{1}{2}$ miles. So the whole trip can be broken down into 13 segments of one-fifth (or part of one-fifth). For the first, the charge is $1.00. That leaves 12 more segments, the charge for each of which is 20¢, giving a total charge for those 12 segments of $2.40. Now, the total charge for the trip is $1.00 for the first one-fifth of a mile and $2.40 for the remaining segments, or $3.40.

24. **(E)** We know that the formula for the area of a square is $s^2 = $ area. So $s^2 = 36x^2$, and, taking the

square root of both sides we learn s = 6x. (Note: there is no question here of a negative solution since geometrical distances are always positive.)

25. **(A)** Since we do not know how much money Ed has, we must assign that amount the value of x. We now establish that Tom has x + $2 since he has $2 more than Ed; and we know that Susan has (x + $2) + $5, which is x + $7, since she has $5 more than Tom. We want to divide this money equally. The natural thing to do, then, is to add up all the money and divide it by 3. The total held by all three individuals is: x + x + 2 + x + 2 + 5 = 3x + 9. Dividing that by 3, we want everyone to have x + 3. Ed has x so he needs to receive 3. Tom has x + 2 so he needs to receive 1. Susan has x + 7 so she needs to rid herself of 4. Susan gets rid of this 4 by giving 1 to Tom and 3 to Ed, giving us answer choice (A).

    Some shortcutting is possible by considering that Susan has the most money, and then Tom and then Ed. Therefore, any answer which has Ed give up money cannot result in equal shares, eliminating (C) and (E). Furthermore, since Susan has the most, she must give up the most. In (D) Tom gives more than Susan, so this is eliminated. In (B), Susan gives out more than Tom, but she also receives from Tom, so her net giving out is only $1, compared to Tom's $4, so this is also wrong, which leaves (A).

26. **(C)** Proposition 1 is true. It is the geometry theorem that two lines parallel to a third must be parallel to each other. Proposition II is also necessarily true. Just as with lines, if two planes are parallel to a third plane, they must likewise be parallel to each other. Proposition III, however, is not necessarily true. Two lines might be drawn in a plane parallel to another plane and yet intersect with one another:

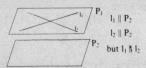

27. **(C)** We all know the simple formula that price minus discount equals discounted price—that much is just common-sense arithmetic. What we sometimes overlook, however, is the fact that the discounted price can be expressed either in monetary terms, e.g., $5.00 or 37¢, or in percentage terms, e.g., 50% of the original price. In this case, the discount is given as a percentage of the original price. So we have, original price − 90¢ = 90% of original price; or, using x for the original price: x − $.90 = .9x. This is an equation with only one variable, so we proceed to solve for x: .1x = $.90, so x = $9.00.

28. **(D)** We begin by computing the length of the side of the square ABCD. Since the x and y axes meet on the perpendicular, we have a right triangle formed by the origin (the point of intersection of x and y) and points A and B. Since point A has the coordinates (2,0), we know that OA is two units long—the x coordinate is 2. Similarly, point B is two units removed from O, so OB is also two units long. Thus, the two legs of our right triangle are 2 and 2. Using the Pythagorean Theorem:

$$2^2 + 2^2 = s^2, \text{ so } s = \sqrt{8} = 2\sqrt{2}$$

Now that we have the length of the side, we compute the area of ABCD by side × side: $(2\sqrt{2})(2\sqrt{2}) = 8$.

29. **(A)** This problem is particularly elusive since there is no really clear starting point. One way of getting a handle on it is to manipulate the expression $\frac{x}{y} + \frac{n}{m}$. If we add the two terms together using the common denominator of my, we have $\frac{mx + ny}{my}$. We can see that this bears a striking similarity to the first equation given in the problem: mx + ny = 12 my. If we manipulate that equation by dividing both sides by my, we have $\frac{mx + ny}{my} = 12$. But since $\frac{x}{y} + \frac{n}{m}$ is equivalent to $\frac{mx + ny}{my}$, we are entitled to conclude that $\frac{x}{y} + \frac{n}{m}$ is also equal to 12.

30. **(D)** This problem, too, is fairly difficult. The difficulty stems from the fact that its solution requires several different formulas. For example, we can conclude that (A) is necessarily true. MN is not a diameter. We know this since a diameter passes through the center of the circle. So whatever the length of MN, it is less than that of the diameter (the diameter is the longest chord which can be drawn in a circle). Since 2MO would be equal to a diameter (twice the radius is the diameter), and since MN is less than a diameter, we can conclude that MN is less than 2MO. We also know that z = y. Since MO and NO are both radii of circle O, they must be equal. So we know that in triangle MNO, MO = NO; and since angles opposite equal sides are equal, we conclude that z = y. (B) requires still another line of reasoning. Since MN is greater than NO, the angle opposite MN, which is x, must be greater than the angle opposite NO, which is y. So x is greater than y. Finally, (E) requires yet another line of reasoning. If MN were equal to NO, it would also be equal to MO, since MO and NO are both radii. In that case, we would have an equilateral triangle and all angles would be 60°. Since MN is greater than MO and NO, the angle opposite MN, which is x, must be greater than 60°. So (D) must be the correct answer. A moment's reflection will show that it is not necessarily true that x = y + z. This would be true only in the event that MNO is a right triangle, but there is no information given in the problem from which we are entitled to conclude that x° = 90°.

SECTION IV

1. **(B)** One sure approach to this problem is to perform the addition indicated in the right-hand column: $\frac{1}{0.1} + \frac{0.1}{10} = \frac{100 + 1}{10} = \frac{101}{10} = 10.1$. This shows that Column B is larger. A quicker way of finding the correct answer is to divide .1 into 1, which yields 10. Then, no matter what the second term of Column B turns out to be, when it is added to the first term, the sum must be greater than 10.

2. **(C)** Since l_1 and l_2 are parallel, the third line creates a whole set of angle relationships, e.g., alternate interior angles are equal, and so on. For this problem, all we really need to see is that x and y must be equal since the transverse cuts the parallel lines on the perpendicular (all angles created must be equal to 90°). Because x and y are both 90°, our answer must be (C).

3. **(C)** The first line of attack on a problem like this is to cancel, thereby simplifying the comparison:

$$\frac{3}{1} \times \frac{1}{2} \times \frac{6}{1} \times \frac{1}{6} = 1$$
$$\frac{4}{1} \times \frac{1}{4} \times \frac{7}{1} \times \frac{1}{7} = 1$$

It is clear that 1 is equal to 1, so our answer must be (C).

4. **(A)** Since we are asked about x, the first line of attack here must be to solve for x in the centered equation:

$$3x + 2 = 11$$
$$3x \quad\;\; = 9$$
$$x = 3$$

Since x is 3, and 3 is greater than 2, our answer must be (A). Merely substituting 2 for x would only eliminate (C).

5. **(D)** One approach is to recognize that no comparison of 5% of an unspecified number and 5% of a different unspecified number is possible. For those who had any difficulty with this insight, however, a good attack on the problem would be to divide both sides of the comparison by 5%. This effectively removes the 5%, reducing the comparison to x versus y. Now it is even easier to see that the answer must be (D) since no information is provided about x and y except the fact that each is greater than zero.

6. **(A)** This is a relatively difficult problem. To solve it, the student needs to recognize that if the triangle had dimensions of 3, 4, and 5 it would be a right triangle: $3^2 + 4^2 = 5^2$. That is to say, all triangles which have dimensions that satisfy the Pythagorean Theorem must have a 90° angle. If we knew that x was 90°, we would know that the remaining two angles would have to total to 90° because there are 180° in a triangle. But this is not a case of a 3–4–5 triangle, and 3, 4, and 5.1 will not satisfy the Pythagorean Theorem, so this is *not* a right triangle. Given that it is not a right triangle, then, we need to ask in what way does it differ from a right triangle. The answer is that the side 5.1 is slightly larger than 5, which would have given us a right triangle. So, too, angle x must be slightly larger than 90°. Now if x is slightly larger than 90°, the sum of the remaining two angles must be slightly less than 90° because, again, there are only 180° in a triangle. So x° must be greater than y° + z°.

7. **(A)** We begin our attack on this problem by solving for x and y in the equations given:

$$\frac{x}{3} - 16 = 32 \qquad \frac{y}{4} + 12 = 24$$
$$\frac{x}{3} = 48 \qquad\quad \frac{y}{4} = 12$$
$$x = 144 \qquad\quad y = 48$$

Since x is larger than y, our answer must be (A).

Another method would be to see that $\frac{x}{3}$ with 16 subtracted is larger than $\frac{y}{4}$ with 12 added. Thus $\frac{x}{3}$ is much larger, relatively speaking, than $\frac{y}{4}$ and, even though the 4 versus 3 in the denominator is a reason for $\frac{y}{4}$ to be smaller than $\frac{x}{3}$, it might seem clear that x must be larger. There is no problem with negative numbers since both $\frac{x}{3}$ and $\frac{y}{4}$ are positive, which means that both x and y are positive.

8. **(B)** Performing the indicated operations:

Column A	Column B
x(x + 3) + 2(x + 3)	$(x + 3)^2$
$x^2 + 3x + 2x + 6$	(x + 3)(x + 3)
$x^2 + 5x + 6$	$x^2 + 6x + 9$

Subtracting x^2, 5x, and 6 from both columns:

0	x + 3

Since x > 0, Column B is greater than 3, and therefore larger than Column A.

9. **(C)** Let us first draw the picture:

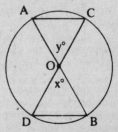

Now, most students will intuitively see that AB must be equal to CD no matter what the magnitudes of x and y are. (Note: We mean by 'intuitively' not measurement or reliance on eye-estimation, but merely the sort of thing where one says, "I can't prove it, but I know it must be correct.") A simple proof can also be given. Since x and y are equal (vertical angles are equal), they intercept equal arcs (cut off equal parts of the circle). The chords (AB and CD) subtend (join) equal arcs of the same circle and so must be equal.

Another way of proving that AC = BC is to point out that AO and CO are radii and are equal to CO and BO, which are also radii. Then we know that x and y are equal, so AOC and COB are congruent triangles. Consequently, the third sides must also be equal.

10. **(D)** At first glance, it might appear that x and y must be equal. After all, any number raised to the zero power is equal to 1. And this reasoning would be sound if the base were anything except 1. For 1 raised to any power is equal to 1:

$$1^{7-1} = 1^6 = 1$$
$$1^{7-5} = 1^2 = 1$$

So the values of x and y are not important: 1 raised to any power is still just 1.

11. **(A)** We begin by filling in more details:

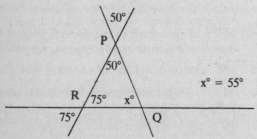

$$x° = 55°$$

This is because vertical angles are equal. Then we can compute the remaining angle as 55° (50° + 75° + x = 180°, x = 55°). Now, in any given triangle, the larger the angle the longer the side. Since PQ is opposite a 75° angle while RP is opposite a 55° angle, PQ must be larger than RP.

12. **(C)** It is possible to solve this comparison using simultaneous equations or substitution: Let x be the number of adult tickets, and let y be the number of children's tickets. Then x − y = 29, and 5x + 2.5y = 302.50. But there is an easier way. Let us assume, for the purposes of analysis, that the number of adult tickets sold was exactly 50. On that assumption, the receipts derived from adult tickets was $250. We know further, on that assumption, that 21 tickets were sold for $2.50, and total receipts from children's tickets would be $52.50. Combining our two totals, we come up with gross sales of $302.50. And since that is the total receipts specified in the centered information, we have proved that the number of adult tickets is 50.

If the resulting total dollars had not equalled what the problem told us it should, then (C) would be eliminated as a possible answer choice. If the total based on the assumption of the columns being equal was high, then fewer tickets were sold than assumed.

13. **(A)** This problem is solved by merely counting on one's fingers. The first multiple of 4 greater than 281 is 284 (284 divided by 4 = 71), the second is 288, the third is 292, the fourth is 296, and the fifth is 300. So there are five multiples of 4 between 281 and 301. The first multiple of 5 greater than 2401 is 2405, the second is 2410, the third is 2415 and that is the last one that is less than 2419. So there are only three multiples of 5 between 2401 and 2419. Since 5 is greater than 3, our answer choice must be (A).

Another method would be to notice that there are more numbers from 281 to 301 than from 2401 to 2419 and that you cover more ground with a multiple of 5 than a multiple of 4, so Column A would be a longer distance on the number line in smaller pieces, while Column B would be a smaller distance and larger pieces. The specification of multiples might work against that since we are not addressing the length, but the number of multiples, but Column A starts with a multiple of 4 while Column B starts just after a multiple of 5.

14. **(C)** This is a fairly difficult problem. The first thing to realize is that x = 60° and y = 30°. We learn this by a calculation. Since x is twice as large as y, we know that x = 26. Then we also know that x + y = 90. By substitution, we have y + 2y = 90, so y = 30 and x = 60. We can now see that we have the special case of the right, or 30:60:90, triangle. In such a triangle, the side opposite the 30° angle is equal to one-half the hypotenuse, and the side opposite the 60° angle is equal to one-half the hypotenuse times the square root of three:

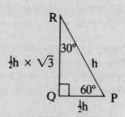

Since PR is the hypotenuse, PQ is the side opposite the 30° angle, and PQ = ½PR. So we can substitute ½PR for PQ in the right column: $\frac{\frac{1}{2}PR}{PR} = \frac{1}{2}$; so our two columns are equal.

15. **(C)** It is possible to go through an entire computation here. By the Pythagorean Theorem, DC and CB must be:

$$s^2 + s^2 = 1^2$$
$$2s^2 = 1$$
$$s = \sqrt{\tfrac{1}{2}}$$
$$s = \frac{1}{\sqrt{2}} = \frac{\sqrt{2}}{2}$$

Then DC and CB can function as altitude and base of DCB, and we use the formula for the area of a triangle: $\frac{1}{2}ab = \frac{1}{2}(\sqrt{2}/2)(\sqrt{2}/2) = \frac{1}{4}$. The area of the square is easily gotten as $1 \times 1 = 1$. So the area of the entire figure is $1 + \frac{1}{4}$ or 1.25. But there is an easier way to solve the problem:

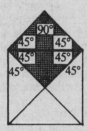

We can see intuitively that DCB is $\frac{1}{4}$ the area of the square. Since the area of the square is 1, the area of DCB must be $\frac{1}{4}$, and the combined areas are 1.25, the area of the entire polygon ABCDE.

16. **(D)** This is a relatively easy problem. It can be solved by doing the subtraction: $\frac{4}{5} - \frac{3}{4} = \frac{16 - 15}{20} = \frac{1}{20}$. In this case, a substitution of percentages for fractions might be useful if you are knowledgeable about the equivalencies: $\frac{4}{5} = 80\%$ and $\frac{3}{4} = 75\%$. $80\% - 75\% = 5\% = \frac{1}{20}$.

17. **(C)** First we must convert one and one-half yards into inches. There are 36 inches in a yard, so one and one-half yards must contain $36 + 18$ or 54 inches. Now, to determine how many two-inch segments there are in 54 inches, we just divide 54 by 2, which equals 27. So there must be 27 two-inch segments in a segment which is one and one-half yards long.

18. **(B)** It is important to remember that the positive x values are to the right of the origin (the intersection between the x and y axes), and that the negative values on the x axis are to the left of the origin. Also, the positive y values are above the origin, while the negative y values are below the x axis.

```
                 y
       (-,+)   |   (+,+)
               |
         II    |    I
               |
  ─────────────┼───────────── x
               |
        III    |    IV
               |
       (-,-)   |   (+,-)
               |
```

When reading an ordered pair such as (x,y) (called ordered because the first place is always the x-coordinate and the second place is always the y-coordinate), we know the first element is the movement on the horizontal or x axis, while the second element of the pair gives us the vertical distance. In this case, we are five units to the left of the origin, so that gives us an x value of negative 5. We are 2 units above the horizontal axis, so that gives us the second value (y) of +2. Thus our ordered pair is (−5,2), answer (B).

19. **(B)** The formula for computing the circumference of a circle is $2\pi r$. In this case our radius is 4, so the circumference of the circle is 8π. Now, P and Q will be as far apart as they can possibly be when they are directly opposite one another:

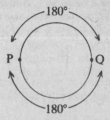

Or a half circle away from each other. So the maximum distance by which P and Q could be separated—measured by the circumference of the circle and not as the crow flies—is one-half the circumference, or 4π.

20. **(E)** Remember that a prime number is an integer which has only itself and 1 as integral factors. Thus, 13, 17, 41, and 79 are all prime numbers because their only factors are 13 and 1, 17 and 1, 41 and 1, and 79 and 1, respectively. 91, however, is not a prime number since it can be factored by 7 and 13 as well as by 1 and 91.

21. **(C)** The natural starting point here would be to draw the picture:

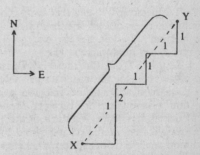

Since directions are perpendicular, we can perform the needed calculation with the Pythagorean Theorem. To simplify things, we can show that the above picture is equivalent to this:

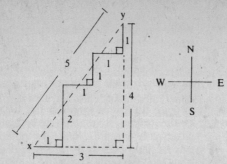

Now we can solve for the distance between X and Y with one use of the Pythagorean Theorem. Since the two legs of the right triangle are 3 and 4, we know that the hypotenuse must be 5. (Remember that 3, 4, and 5, or any multiples thereof such as 6, 8, and 10, always make a right triangle.)

22. **(C)** Let us begin by substituting x, y, and z for $\angle QPS$ and $\angle TPR$. Since $\angle QPS$ and $\angle TPR$ are equal, we know x + y = z + y, and since y = y, we know that x = z. As for (A) and (B), we do not know whether y is equal to x and z; it could be larger or smaller or equal:

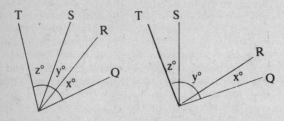

We can also eliminate (D) since we have no information that would lead us to conclude that all three are of equal measure.

23. **(D)** The footnote at the bottom of the chart tells us that the annual rate, that is shown in the table, is computed by taking the actual profits made in the quarter and multiplying by 4. An annual rate for a quarter shows how the store would do in a year if the quarter's activity were maintained for a whole year (over four quarters). So, to compute the actual profit for that quarter we need to divide by 4:

$$\frac{\$1.6 \text{ million}}{4} = \$.4 \text{ million}$$

24. **(D)** There are two interesting points to be made about this question. First, in dealing with a problem like this, you must start from the answer choices. In essence, the question asks "of the following five choices . . . ." It is often a waste of time to go first to the chart to find the quarter in which profits were actually the lowest for all quarters shown on the chart. That is, in fact, the first quarter of 1978, but that does not appear as

an answer choice. Second, although the number recorded by the graph is actually four times that of actual profits (see question 23 above), there is no need to divide each of these by four. Obviously, the greater the annual profit rate, the larger the actual profit made in the quarter. In this case, the smallest annual rate of the five listed in the problem occurred in the third quarter of 1978, about $0.75 million, so the actual profits must have been smallest in that quarter.

25. **(A)** This is a fairly simple problem. We need only consult the graph for that period to see that in six quarters, the annual profit rate exceeded $1.5 million: 2nd quarter of 1979 ($1.6 million), 3rd quarter of 1979 ($1.7 million), 4th quarter of 1979 ($1.9 million), 2nd quarter of 1980 ($1.8 million), 3rd quarter of 1980 ($2.1 million), and 4th quarter of 1980 ($2.3 million).

26. **(C)** Remember that the amount reported on the graph is four times the actual profits made in the quarter. So, if we take the annual profit rate for each quarter and divide it by four, we will have the actual profits for each quarter. We can then add those numbers up to get the annual profits (actual). It is a bit simpler, however, just to add the four annual rates and then divide the whole thing by 4:

1st	1.4 million
2nd	1.8 million
3rd	2.1 million
4th	2.3 million
Total	7.6 million

$7.6 million divided by four = $1.9 million. So the actual profit in that year was $1.9 million.

In practice, however, an estimate rather than a complete calculation will suffice since the answer choices are fairly far apart, though (C) and (D) are somewhat similar. The four quarters of 1980 go up, with the balance point or average somewhere around 1.8. Since that was the annualized figure, (C) would be good choice. (D) and (E) are impossible since each of the four quarters had rates above those choices, while (A) and (B) are figures beyond the highest reach of the chart.

27. **(C)** Again, we can simply use annual rates. There is no reason to divide everything by 4 for each quarter. The annual rates for 1977 are:

1st	1.3 million
2nd	1.1 million
3rd	0.9 million
4th	0.7 million
Total	4.0 million

We can retrieve the total for 1980 from question 26 above, and work the percentage change formula: $\frac{7.6 - 4.0}{4.0} = \frac{3.6}{4.0} = \frac{9}{10}$ which is 90%. Again, estimation can save work. The four quarters of

1977 are in orderly progression, with the midpoint being 0.9. As noted for problem 26, the 1980 profits can be estimated at 1.8 or slightly less (1st quarter is farther below 1.8 than other quarters are above 1.8). An increase from 0.9 to 1.8 would be a 100% increase, which is closest to (C).

28. **(A)** This problem is rather tedious, though it is not conceptually difficult. Let us start working in the interior:

$$4 - 3(2 + 1(3 - (2 + 3) + 2) + 2) + 4$$
$$4 - 3(2 + 1(3 - \quad 5 \quad + 2) + 2) + 4$$
$$4 - 3(2 + 1(\quad \quad 0 \quad \quad) + 2) + 4$$
$$4 - 3(2 + \quad \quad 0 \quad \quad + 2) + 4$$
$$4 - 3(\quad \quad \quad 4 \quad \quad \quad) + 4$$
$$4 \quad -12 \quad \quad \quad \quad + 4$$
$$- 4$$

29. **(C)** By this juncture the drill should be well known. We must begin by drawing a picture:

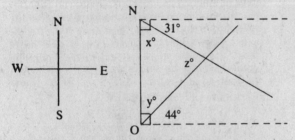

Now, since the angles at N and O are 90°, we can compute the magnitude of x and y: $x = 90° - 31° = 59°$, and $y = 90° - 44° = 46°$. Then, since x, y, and z are the interior angles of a triangle, we know $x + y + z = 180°$. Substituting for x and y, we have $59° + 46° + z = 180°$, and we solve for z: $z = 75°$. Since z is the angle of intersection between the two highways, our answer must be (C).

30. **(B)** Let us use x to represent the sum of money. Then we know that when x is divided equally by n, the result is $60; or, expressed in formal notation: $\frac{x}{n} = 60$. We then know that when x is divided by n + 1 (that is the original number plus another child), the result is $50, or $\frac{x}{n + 1} = 50$. Now, let us manipulate these equations so that we isolate n:

$$\frac{x}{n} = 60 \qquad \frac{x}{n + 1} = 50$$
$$\frac{x}{60} = n \qquad \frac{x}{50} = n + 1$$
$$\frac{x}{60} = n \qquad \left(\frac{x}{50}\right) - 1 = n$$

Since n = n, we know that $x/60 = x/50 - 1$, and we have an equation with only one variable: $x/60 - x/50 = -1$, so:

$$\frac{5x - 6x}{300} = -1$$
AND: $\quad -x = -300$
SO: $\quad x = 300$

The sum of money is $300 and our answer is (B). (Note that you could also solve for n; in this case n = 5, and $5 \times $60 = 300.)

SECTION V

Questions 1–4

Arranging the Information

This problem has two aspects, the order in which items have to be done and the times during the week when the various offices and individuals are available. Note that although the first statement in the information set does seem to give some feeling that thesis approval by the professors must come after the filling out of the application, this would be reading too much into the problem. In fact, the additional statements about the required order of events indicate, by silence about the timing of thesis approval, that the approval can come after the visit to the dean. Question 4 supports this by putting the approval process ahead of the other items. The filing at the Financial Aid Office must be last.

Since the information is given to us in terms of mornings and afternoons, that is the way to arrange it. There are no immediate interactions between the items of information (such as might have been the case if Professor Fansler's office hours were always three days after Professor Cross's, or if the Dean's hours were described in terms of those of the Financial Aid Office). Therefore, a straight listing of the information on hours is all that is required.

	MON.	TUES.	WED.	THUR.	FRI.
AM	Fin. Aid	Fin. Aid		Dean	Dean
	Fansler	Fansler			Fin. Aid
		Cross			Cross
PM	Dean	Dean			
			Fin. Aid		

DEAN MUST PRECEDE FIN. AID; FIN. AID LAST; PROF'S PRE/POST DEAN.

Answering the Questions

1. **(D)** Since the thesis must be approved by Fansler only and not by Cross, only Monday and Tuesday mornings are possibilities, which eliminates (C) and (E). The student also has to go to the Financial Aid Office after seeing the professor.

Since the Financial Aid Office is open on both Monday and Tuesday mornings, both of those times are good; hence, (D) rather than (A) or (B).

2. **(E)** This problem is, of course, separate from the preceding one, so we must consider that the student is starting out fresh and needs to see the Dean, a professor, and the Financial Aid Office. They are asking for what must be false, so we seek elimination by seeing possibilities.

I is not necessarily false, because it is possible to have thesis approval from Professor Cross and complete the job in one day. On Friday morning all three of the required parties are open for business and, ignoring waiting time (which you do because if they didn't bring it up, you shouldn't), there would be no problem. This eliminates answer choices (A) and (D).

II is false because Professor Fansler's approval can only be obtained on Monday or Tuesday morning. While it is true that both the Financial Aid Office and the Dean are open on Mondays and Tuesdays, the order is wrong. By the time the Dean is open for business the Financial Aid Office is closed, so the application cannot be filed that day. This eliminates answer (C).

III is also false because neither of the professors is available in the afternoon. Hence, (B) is out and (E) is correct.

3. **(D)** This problem does not require that the process be completed in any particular time, but only that all the action take place on Tuesdays and Thursdays. Since both professors have office hours on Tuesdays, statements I and II are not necessarily true. As it happens, this is enough to give you the answer since all of the answer choices except (D) allege that either I or II or both are true.

III is false because on Thursdays only the Dean is open, and because on Tuesdays the Financial Aid Office closes before the Dean opens, as was previously discussed.

IV requires you to interpret what a school week might be. If a mere seven-day period was intended (start on Thursday and complete on the following Tuesday), that would not be called a "school" week. A school week is Monday through Friday, and the application cannot be done on a consecutive Tuesday and Thursday. Thus, all four of the statements are false.

4. **(C)** On Wednesday and Thursday only one of the proper offices is open, so they are not possible one-visit days, but this only eliminates (D). Friday morning is a possible one-visit time, which eliminates answer choice (A). Monday and Tuesday mornings, while blessed with open offices for the professors and the Financial Aid Office, do not have the Dean, so (E) is eliminated (as is (D) for the second time).

Monday and Tuesday have the problem of order of office openings previously referred to, and thus are not one-visit days—which eliminates (B), leaving (C) as the answer.

5. **(C)** Notice that the student responds to the professor's comment by saying, "That can't be true," and then uses the Duchess of Warburton as a counter-example. The Duchess would only be a counter-example to the professor's statement had the professor said that women cannot inherit the estates of their families. Thus, (C) must capture the student's misinterpretation of the professor's statement. What has misled the student is that he has attributed too much to the professor. The professor has cited the general rule of primogeniture—the eldest male child inherits—but he has not discussed the special problems which arise when no male child is born. In those cases, presumably a non-male child will have to inherit. (E) incorrectly refers to inheriting from a mother, but the student is discussing a case in which the woman inherited her father's estate. (D) is wrong for the student specifically mentions the conditions which make a child legitimate: born to the wife of her father. (A) was inserted as a bit of levity: Of course, only men can *father* children of either sex. Finally, first-born or not, a daughter cannot inherit as long as there is any male child to inherit, so (B) must be incorrect.

6. **(D)** The key phrase in this paragraph is "beef costs more per pound than fish." A careful reading would show that (A) is in direct contradiction to the explicit wording of the passage. (B) cannot be inferred since the dietician merely says, "I pay." Perhaps he intends to keep the price of a meal stable by cutting back in other areas. In any event, this is an example of not going beyond a mere factual analysis to generate policy recommendations, unless the question stem specifically invites such an extension, e.g., which of the following courses of action would the author recommend? (C) makes an unwarranted inference. From the fact that beef is more costly one would not want to conclude that it is more profitable. (E) is wrong for this reason also. (D) is correct because it focuses upon the per measure cost of protein, which explains why a fish meal will cost the dietician more than a beef meal, even though fish is less expensive per pound.

Questions 7–9

Arranging the Information

The question stems and the original information indicate that the items of interest will be what projections can be made on the basis of the given information. This means that there will be less time spent on arranging and more spent on working out the problems.

The starting information boils down to the conclusion that the subject got off at the third, fourth, fifth, or seventh floor. Since there were only three people on the elevator, this should immediately raise in your mind the possibility of subterfuge.

Answering the Questions

7. **(B)** The question stem adds a condition that builds on the fact that someone obviously pressed buttons for more than one floor, since the elevator carrying only three people, stopped four times and no one got on the elevator. There is no reason to assume on the test that either of the other two riders pushed two buttons, though in real life it is certainly a possibility. Rather, the limitation is that the subject, who is the likeliest to have pressed two buttons, would not have pressed two buttons so long as there were others in the elevator. Therefore, the second button pressed by the subject must have been after the other two riders got off the elevator. The earliest stop at which both could have gotten off the elevator is the third floor.

   If we assume, as we must for the problem, that at most three buttons were pressed when the elevator started (one for each rider), then the subject could have pressed the extra button either after the third floor (if both other riders got off there) or after the fourth floor (if one rider got off at each of the third and fourth floors). Therefore, the subject did not get off at the third floor but may have gotten off at any one of the other floors. Thus, answer choice (E) is eliminated for saying that the subject may have gotten off at the third floor. Each of the other answers is possible, but we are looking for the safest conclusion, which is the one which has the least chance of being wrong. (B) is the safest conclusion because it is definitely correct within the parameters of the question. (A) omits the possibility that the subject got off at the fourth floor, (C) the fourth and seventh, and (D) the seventh.

8. **(B)** The preceding discussion in 7 indicates that there are only three possible floors on the way up the building. However, that deduction is based on the detective's assumption as stated in the question stem. This assumption does NOT carry over into the problem. If we do not have the limitation on the actions of the subject posited in 7, then the first upward ride of the elevator yields four possible floors on which the subject may have left the elevator. The downward empty return from seven limits nothing.

   The second up-and-down trip described in this question stem mentions two additional floors, two and six, but only six is a possible location of the subject. The elevator stopped at two on the way up, and therefore could not have brought the

subject to two. The stairs are closed. If the subject got off on seven the first trip, then he may have gone down to six on the second trip, thus three, four, five, six, and seven are all possibilities, hence, answer (B).

9. **(E)** This seems a peculiar result, but we must be certain that we do not assume more than the problem gives us. The problem does not tell us that the subject was on the elevator when it reached the fourth floor. He may have exited on the third floor. Also, he may have exited on the fourth floor since we only know what is explicitly stated. The detective might have learned this piece of information indirectly, rather than from the people getting on and off the elevator. In any case, he knows only what they say.

   The original reason for putting the subject on the top two floors was the fact that there were more stops than people, but this proves to be false for this problem. Thus, the person getting on at four may have been going to the fifth or seventh floor, leaving the other as well as three and four as possible exits for the subject. Thus, (E).

10. **(A)** Statements I and II combine to give us (A). If all wheeled conveyances which travel on the highway are polluters, and a bicycle does not travel on the highway, then a bicycle cannot be a polluter. If (A) is correct, (B) must be incorrect because bicycles do not travel on the highways at all. (C) and (D) make the same mistake. III must be read to say "if I am driving, it is raining," not "if it is raining, I am driving." (E) is clearly false since my car is driven on the highway. Don't make the problem harder than it is.

11. **(E)** Picking up on our discussion of (C) and (D) in the previous question, III must read "if I am driving, then it is raining." Let that be: "If P, then Q." If we then had not-Q, we could deduce not-P. (E) gives us not-Q by changing IV to "it is not raining." Changing I or II or even both is not going to do the trick, for they don't touch the relationship between my driving my car and rain— they deal only with pollution and we need the car to be connected. Similarly, if we change III to make it deal with pollution, we have not adjusted the connection between my driving and rain, so (C) must be wrong. (D) is the worst of all the answers. Whether rainwater is polluted or not has nothing to do with the connection between my driving and rain. Granted, there is the unstated assumption that my car only pollutes when I drive it, but this is O.K.

Questions 12–16

Arranging the Information

If we indicate the idea of "some" by putting the number of the proposition with a question mark over the two areas of a Venn diagram, we will get the following for propositions I, II, and III:

Diagram 1:

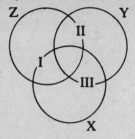

Adding the information from proposition IV, we get:

Diagram 2:

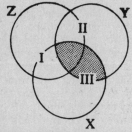

Answering the Questions

12. **(E)** Refer to Diagram 1. The three statements we are dealing with here are simply indications as to where some things are and say nothing about where things aren't. Thus, (A) cannot be known to be true from I, II, and III, and is eliminated.

The same general argument eliminates answer choices (B), (C), and (D). Since the "some" statements covered areas divided into two parts in the diagram, we cannot know which of the two areas is the actual inhabited location, or perhaps both are. The areas pointed to in the three answer choices are indicated here:

Diagram 3:

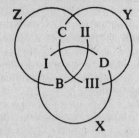

13. **(A)** Referring to Diagram 2, we see that one of the areas at first thought to be possibly inhabited in accordance with statement III is rendered impossible by statement IV's obliteration of the overlap between X and Y. This, in turn, means that only the area of X has something in it. Hence, (A) is impossible and the answer sought.

(B) and (C) refer to the two areas governed by statement I, and we do not know whether one or both of these has members. Similar reasoning applies to answer choice (D).

14. **(D)** I is already known since statement IV of the original information forbids X to be also Y. II is known for the same reasons that (A) in 13 is false. III is uncertain since II of the original information says only that there is either some member of Y + Z, or both, Hence, (D).

15. **(C)** (A) is possibly true since the Z-things which are not also Y-things might not have characteristic X. (B) is possibly true since the pure Y region is left open (logically possible). For the same reason (D) is possible: the open pure Y region does not assert there are pure Y-things—only that they are possible. (E) is incorrect since (A), (B), and (D) are possibly true. (C), however, is equivalent to "All X are Z" and that is inconsistent with the diagram.

16. **(D)** Coding in the additional information gives us this diagram:

Diagram 4:

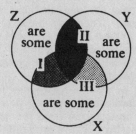

From this diagram we see that there are some individual items which are only X, others only Y, and others only Z. No overlap of any sort is permitted. (D) falsely states that Z must be X. (E) states that you cannot find a Z except for those Z that are not Y, which is correct.

Questions 17–22

Arranging the Information

Previewing the question stems for this set of questions shows that there is only one conditional question and it is based on a new individual. This leads you to suppose that you should be able to completely describe this situation. In addition, a preview of the general information at the start of the problem set indicates that there are only two ways in which the pandas are to be related to each other and that the two ways—wet/dry and fat/slim—are both separate.

Let us first arrange the information into a usable format, starting with the fat/slim idea. Each piece of information must fit in with some previously arranged piece of information in order to create a complete and valid arrangement. Since each panda's name begins with a different letter, we can use single letters to indicate each panda.

←FATTER————SLIMMER→

B fatter
than G

B   G

C slimmer than F—
can't do now

D fatter than B	D	B	G		
E slimmer than G	D	B	G	E	
F slimmer than E	D	B	G	E	F

C slimmer than F—
can do now

	D	B	G	E	F	C

G fatter than F—
redundant

Now we can do the dry/wet idea.

←DRIER————WETTER→

| B drier than E | B E | |

C wetter than G—
can't do now

D wetter than G—
can't do now

| E drier than C | B E C |

C wetter than G—
can do now

B E C

← G

D wetter than G—
can do now

B E C

————G D→

| F drier than B | F B E C |

————G D→

| G wetter than B | F B E C |

————G D→

Answering the Questions

17. **(C)** Only B is on the fatter (left) side of E and also on the drier (left) side of G.

18. **(D)** Only C is both slimmer (right) and wetter (right) than E.

19. **(B)** Only D is both fatter (left) and wetter (right) than G. Even though the exact wetness position of D is not known, it is wetter than G.

20. **(D)** F is the driest (left-most) in the final diagram.

21. **(B)** I is not false for sure because the exact wetness relationship between D and C is not known. D might be wetter or drier than C. II is definitely false since F is drier than D. III is not knowable from the given information since the exact amounts by which the various pandas are fatter or slimmer is not stated. D is fatter than G, but not necessarily by three inches. However, the statement is not false because it might be true. Thus, only II is definitely false.

22. **(E)** The exact rank cannot be determined because the new panda Y's being slimmer than B and fatter than F leaves unclear the relationship between Y and pandas G and F.

23. **(B)** We have seen examples of the form of argument Holmes has in mind before: "P or Q; not-P; therefore, Q." Here, however, the first premise of Holmes' argument is more complex: "P or Q or R . . . S," with as many possibilities as he can conceive. He eliminates them one by one until no single possibility is left. The logic of the argument is perfect, but the weakness in the form is that it is impossible to guarantee that all contingencies have been taken into account. Maybe one was overlooked. Thus, (B) is the correct answer. (A), (C), and (E) are wrong for the same reason. Holmes' method is designed to answer a particular question—in this case, "Where did the body come from?" Perhaps the next step is to apply the method to the question of the identity of the murderer as (E) suggests, but at this juncture he is concerned with the preliminary matter of how the murder was committed. In any event, it would be wrong to assail the logic of Holmes' deduction by complaining that it does not prove enough. Since (A) and (C) are even more removed from the particular question raised, they, too, must be wrong. Finally, (D) is nothing more than a reiteration of Watson's original comment, and Holmes has already responded to it.

24. **(A)** Although we do not want to argue theology, perhaps a point taken from that discipline will make this question more accessible: "If God is only good, from where does evil come?" Rousseau, at least as far as his argument is characterized here, faces a similar problem. If man is by his very nature sympathetic, what is the source of his non-sympathetic social institutions? (A) poses this critical question. The remaining choices each commit the same fundamental error. Rousseau *describes* a situation. The paragraph never suggests that he proposed a *solution*. Perhaps Rousseau considered the problem of modern society irremediable.

25. **(E)** Here we are looking for the unstated or hidden assumptions of the author. (A) is one because the author dates the building by measuring the wear and tear on the threshold, but if that were a replacement threshold installed, say, 50 years after the building was first built, the author's calculations would be thrown off completely. So, to reach the conclusion he does, he must have assumed that he was dealing with the original threshold. (C) is very similar. The calculations work—based as they are on the estimated capacity of the monastery—only if the author is right about the number of people walking across the door sill. So it also follows that (D) is something he assumes. After all, if marble tended

to wear out spontaneously instead of under use—if sometimes it just evaporates—then the whole process of calculating time as a function of wear would be ill-founded. (E) is correct. The author uses the wars he cites to help him date *this particular group* of buildings. He never suggests that this has occurred often.

SECTION VI

Questions 1–3:

Arranging the Information

Previewing the questions indicates that the complex issue is the fighting. Thus, the diagram must keep track of combinations.

$$F \leftarrow \text{not with any} \rightarrow \quad \text{G with H} \quad \text{J}$$

not
with
↓
K

Answering the Questions

1. **(C)** I is not inferable since there is no reason to prefer F to K as an addition to G and H. We are not given any reason to prefer eating to non-fighting and thus cannot judge the relative problems with F and K. II is not inferable since there is nothing that tells us that G and H will fight with each other, only with K. III is inferable since the only combinations available have to include fighters. If F is included, there is likely to be fighting. If F is not included, then G, H, and K will fight.

2. **(C)** If G and J go home, then only H, K, and F are left. All of these cats will fight with each other for reasons similar to those outlined for question 1. Therefore, two new cats are needed to combine with either H or K.

3. **(C)** Since the purposes of a cat cast are established in the situation description, we know that an available cast means one that will have a good chance of succeeding. With F calmed down, the only remaining problem is the fighting between G, H, and K. However, G and H should be together since we are told that they eat well together, and that is the goal of the commercial filming. Thus, we have G and H, who can be with J or with F, and we have F with K and J. Although we do not know how well K and J eat, they will at least not

fight and that is sufficient for them to qualify as available. Thus, there are three possible casts available.

4. **(B)** The proposition that you cannot argue with taste says that taste is relative. Since we are looking for an answer choice inconsistent with that proposition, we seek an answer choice that argues that taste, or aesthetic value, is absolute, or at least not relative—that there are standards of taste. (B) is precisely that.

    (C) and (D) are just distractions, playing on the notion of taste in the physical sense and the further idea of the distasteful; but these superficial connections are not strong enough.

    (A), (B), and (E) are all activities in which there is some element of aesthetic judgment or appreciation. In (A), the holding of an exhibition, while implying some selection principle and, thus, some idea of a standard of taste, does not purport to truly judge aesthetics in the way that (B), precisely a beauty *contest,* does. The exhibition may be of historical or biographical interest, for example. (E) also stresses more of the exhibition aspect than the judging aspect. You should not infer that all movie festivals are contests, since the word festival does not require this interpretation and, in fact, there are festivals at which the judging aspect is minimal or non-existent. The Cannes Film Festival, while perhaps the best-known, is not the only type of movie festival there is. The questions are not tests of your knowledge of the movie industry.

5. **(C)** Take careful note of the exact position the author ascribes to the analysts: They *always* attribute a sudden drop to a crisis. The author then attacks this simple causal explanation by explaining that, though a crisis is followed by a market drop, the reason is not that the crisis causes the drop but that both are the effects of some common cause, the changing of the moon. Of course, the argument seems implausible, but our task is not to grade the argument, only to describe its structure. (A) is not a proper characterization of that structure since the author never provides a specific example. (B), too, is inapplicable since no statistics are produced. (D) can be rejected since the author is attacking generally accepted beliefs rather than appealing to them to support his position. Finally, though the author concedes the reliability of the reports, (E), in question, he wants to draw a different conclusion from the data.

6. **(A)** Given the implausibility of the author's alternative explanation, he is probably speaking tongue-in-cheek, that is, he is ridiculing the analysts for *always* attributing a drop in the market to a political crisis. But whether you took the argument in this way or as a serious attempt to explain the fluctuations of the stock market, **(A)**

will be the correct answer. (E) surely goes beyond the mere factual description at which the author is aiming, as does (D) as well. The author is concerned with the *causes* of fluctuations; nothing suggests that he or anyone else is in a position to exploit those fluctuations. (C) finds no support in the paragraph, for nothing suggests that he wishes to attack the credibility of the source rather than the argument itself. Finally, (B) is inappropriate to the main point of the passage. Whether the market ultimately evens itself out has nothing to do with the causes of the fluctuations.

Questions 7–11

Arranging the Information

This problem set describes a layout or map situation. One clue is its being a set of regular shapes and the other is the use of compass directions. You have to distinguish between conditions which lead to definite squares being definite crops and ones which simply describe relationships between crops.

If two sides of the field run east-west, the other sides run north-south, and the field is aligned with the compass.

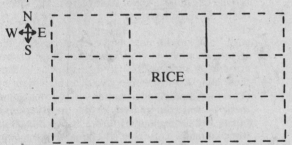

The information about wheat and barley cannot be coded into the diagram now, nor can the information about the soybeans, but peanuts can.

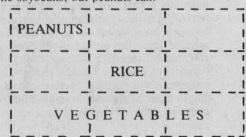

Answering the Questions

Questions 7, 8, and 9 refer to five squares. Let us locate them on the map:

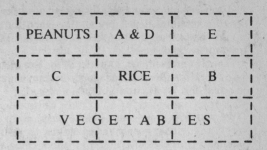

If the four unallocated fields are to be planted with one field of wheat, one of barley, and two of soybeans, the wheat and barley have to be two of the upper right-hand fields in order to be next to each other.

7. **(E)** If field (E) is planted with soybeans, then the wheat and barley cannot be next to each other.

8. **(C)** If (C) is planted with wheat, the barley cannot be next to it.

9. **(E)** Although there are two fields next to the peanuts, we have already eliminated (C) from consideration as a wheat field. Thus, the wheat must be in the field just north of the rice (A)/(D), and the barley must be in field (E) to be next to the wheat.

10. **(D)** The rice is in the middle, so the tomatoes cannot be next to the soybeans, eliminating II— AND answer choices (B) and (E). Either of the fields to the east or west of the rice field could be planted with the soybeans, as previously discussed; thus, I and III are possible, and (D) is correct.

    Note that the squash actually must be next to the soybeans, but that also means it is possible.

11. **(B)** It is a fair assumption that the other crops mentioned are to be planted and only the ones specifically omitted are not planted (to do otherwise would be mere nitpicking). This means that there will be one field of rice and barley, and two of soybeans—leaving five for vegetables.

Questions 12–15

Arranging the Information

This is a problem in which the main issue is the overlapping of different sets of groups, which means that Venn diagrams are a good method of arranging the information. This type of problem usually requires that the majority of your time be spent in arranging the information and somewhat less in answering the questions. However, a preview of the questions indicates that some of the statements might contradict some of the other statements. Question 13 indicates that statements I, II, and III are to be taken as true, and question

12, which asks about contradiction, only asks about possible contradiction after I, II, and III. Thus, it would seem that I, II, and III could be arranged without any problems.

The most efficient arrangement of the information of I and II is in a three-circle (Venn) diagram with circles standing for L, M, and Z. Remember that a Venn diagram is only good for up to three categories.

We will now draw a three-circle diagram for L, M, and Z. Statement I only indicates that there is some possibility of there being each of the four categories. It does not mean, for instance, that there will be an L by itself that is not any of the others, etc. This does not affect the diagram.

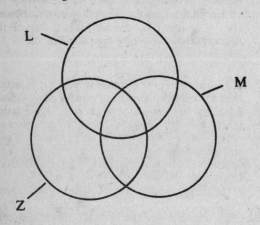

Statement II is coded into the diagram by marking out the parts of the diagram where M is not L.

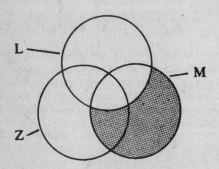

Statement III is coded into the diagram by eliminating the parts of the diagram where L is not Z, leaving us with this:

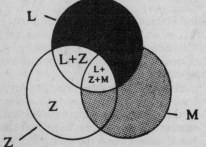

Thus, what remains possible is L with Z, L with M and Z, and Z by itself.

Answering the Questions

12. **(B)** Statement III was successfully integrated with the previous statements without encountering any problem, so answer choice (A) is eliminated. Statement IV, however, does present a problem. If no M are Z, this means that there can be no M found inside the Z circle. However, the only place where M can be found, after coding the first three statements, is inside the Z circle. The elimination of the possibility of having L, M, and Z together will eliminate the possibility of having M altogether, which is forbidden by statement I. Thus, answer choice (B) is correct. Note that one must proceed in order in this particular problem because the question asks about contradictions with all previous statements, which means that the first one with a contradiction must be the answer sought. Both statements V and VI are fully compatible with the following diagrams:

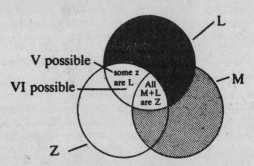

13. **(C)** In the previous question we saw that statement IV was contradictory to the previous statements, which excludes it from being deducible from statements II and III, eliminating answer choices (A) and (D). Statement V is not deducible from the others because it states that there are actually some Z. The existence of any Z is definitely not known since statements II and III only discuss the relationships that pertain to the groups if there happen to be any members of the groups. This eliminates answer choices (B) and (D) (again), and (E).

Answer choice (C) is deducible because the only place that L and M overlap is in the location where L and M and also Z apply. Thus, anything, such as P, which is going to be both L and M must also be Z.

14. **(D)** From the diagram we can see that there are two possible locations within the L area. One location is the LMZ area and the other is the LZ area. Thus, all L are Z, as statement III has said. The only reason that you would use the diagram instead of just relying on the original statement is

to make sure that there was no further limitation that had snuck in, as happened with M, all of which are also Z (ignoring the contradiction problem). You cannot make any statement about the overlap between P and X because statement VI only states where P will not be found and makes no promises that there are P's that actually are M and L, etc.

15. **(D)** The diagram shows that there is a definite possible area of Z which does not overlap any part of the L or M areas; therefore, it is still possible for Z to be by itself. It would be wrong to say that there definitely was some Z by itself, but it is also wrong to say that there cannot be any Z by itself.

(A) is not false since statement I states that L is possible. (B) is not known to be true or false. The statement that some Z are L does not make it false or true to say some Z are not L. As discussed in the previous problem, the actual occurrence of P's other than under M and L is still an open question, and (C) is, thus, not false. (E) is eliminated with the discovery that (D) is false.

Questions 16–22

Arranging the Information

Previewing the questions shows that most of them are conditional questions, and the setup of the situation is of that nature, too. This means that most of the work will be in answering the questions rather than in determining the arrangement of the information.

At least 2 of D E F

Either 1 or 2 from L M N P

Total of 4

N not=P

E not=L

D not=N, thus, if N, neither P or D

Answering the Questions

16. **(C)** If Nancy is chosen, then both David and Paul are out. Since at least two out of the trio of David, Erica, and Francis must be chosen, the elimination of David results in the forced selection of Erica and Francis, which eliminates answer choices (A) and (E). Since Nancy will not work with Paul, he cannot be a member of the crew, and answer choice (D) is eliminated. Since Erica is selected, as previously noted, and Erica will not work with Larry, answer choice (B) is eliminated, and we find that the crew will be David, Erica, Mary, and Nancy.

17. **(E)** If Paul is chosen, the only direct restriction is that Nancy is eliminated from the crew. This leaves only the restriction of the grinders versus the sail trimmers. If you wanted to select answer choice (A) because you thought there could only be two grinders, you missed the fact that the only restriction on the numbers of grinders versus sail trimmers was that AT LEAST two of the crew additions had to be grinders, which leaves open the possibility of all three of the grinder candidates being accepted. Thus, answer choice (A) is possible.

Answer choice (E), however, is not possible because Erica will not work with Larry as the answer choice requires. The other answer choices, (B), (C), and (D), do not violate any of the restrictions laid down by the problem.

18. **(C)** I must be true because if David is rejected, then the only two remaining grinder candidates—Erica and Francis—must be chosen. The selection of Erica means the elimination of Larry, leaving Mary, Nancy, and Paul. However, since Nancy will not work with Paul, only one of those two may be chosen, which gives Mary a definite berth on the boat.

II follows from the first sentence of the discussion of I.

III does not have to be true. The selection of David permits the selection of a crew such as David, Francis, Mary, and Paul or the selection of a crew without Paul—such as David, Francis, Mary, and Larry.

Thus, the answer is that I and II must be true and III is a maybe.

19. **(E)** As hinted at by the structure of the three Roman-numeral propositions, the acceptance of Larry as a crew member eliminates Erica from consideration, and thus requires the selection of David and Francis. The selection of David means that Nancy cannot be chosen, which leaves either Mary or Paul as acceptable candidates to fill the last sail trimmer slot with Larry. I and III are, thus, possible and II is not.

20. **(C)** I must be true since the choice of Larry eliminates Erica and requires the choice of David and Francis, as noted in question 19.

II is not necessarily true since the choice of Mary imposes no further restrictions on the choice of crew, so Mary and Nancy may or may not crew together.

III is also necessarily true. If Larry is chosen, Erica cannot be chosen; and this means David and Francis must be picked to meet the minimum number of two grinders. With David on the crew, Nancy cannot be on the crew.

21. **(B)** The choice of Paul eliminates Nancy, and, thus, answer choices (C) and (D). The omission of David forces the choice of Erica and Francis, which in turn eliminates Larry, and, thus, answer choices (A) and (E), leaving only Mary to fill out the crew, as stated in answer choice (B).

22. **(A)** If Erica makes the crew and Francis does not, this leaves David to fill in the second grinder slot. Erica's presence eliminates Larry, and David's eliminates Nancy, leaving a crew of David, Erica, Mary, and Paul. Thus, both I and II must be true.

23. **(D)** It is important not to attribute more to an author than he actually says or implies. Here the author states only that Ronnie's range is narrow so he will not be an outstanding vocalist. Vocalizing is only one kind of music career, so I, which speaks of professional musicians, takes us far beyond the claim the author actually makes. II also goes beyond what the author says. He never specifies what range an outstanding vocalist needs, much less what range is required to vocalize without being outstanding. Finally, III is an assumption since the author moves from a physical characteristic to a conclusion regarding ability.

24. **(C)** Ann's response would be appropriate only if Mary had said, "All of the students at State College come from Midland High." That is why (C) is correct. (D) is wrong because they are talking about the background of the students, not the reputations of the schools. (E) is wrong, for the question is from where the students at State College come. (B) is superficially relevant to the exchange, but it, too, is incorrect. Ann would not reply to this statement, had Mary made it, in the way she did reply. Rather, she would have said, "No, there are some Midland students at State College." Finally, Ann would correctly have said (A) only if Mary had said, "None of the students from North Hills attends State College," or, "Most of the students from North Hills do not attend State College." But Ann makes neither of these responses, so we know that (A) cannot have been what she thought she heard Mary say.

25. **(A)** Perhaps a small diagram is the easiest way to show this problem.

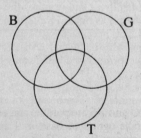

We will show that "all B are T" by eliminating that portion of the diagram where some area of B is not also inside T:

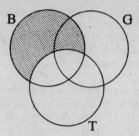

Now, let us put an x to show the existence of those B's which are G's:

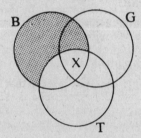

The diagram shows us that I is true. Since the only areas left for B's are within the T circle, the G condition is unimportant. II is not inferable. Although there is some overlap of the G and T circles, there is also some non-overlap. This shows that it may be possible to be a T without also being a G. III is not inferable since our diagrams are restricted to the three categories B, G, and T and say nothing about things outside of those categories.

SECTION VII

1. **(B)** $40\% = \frac{2}{5}$
   $\frac{2}{5} \times \frac{10}{7} = \frac{4}{7}$

2. **(D)** 27 and 51 are each divisible by 3. 17 and 59 are prime numbers. Hence, I and IV only.

3. **(A)** Angle DOC = 6 + x
   Angle AOC = (6 + x) + x = 180 − 20
   6 + 2x = 160
   2x = 154
   x = 77

4. **(D)** Let C = the capacity in gallons. Then $\frac{1}{3}$C + 3 = $\frac{1}{2}$C. Multiplying through by 6, we obtain 2C + 18 = 3C, or C = 18.

5. **(E)** $\dfrac{91 + 88 + 86 + 78 + x}{5} = 85$
   343 + x = 425
   x = 82

6. **(C)** $12 \times .39 = 4.68$ inches; that is, between $4\frac{1}{2}$ and 5.

7. **(D)**

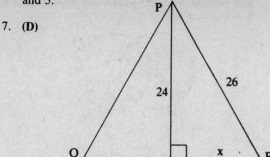

In the figure above, $PS \perp QR$. Then, in right triangle PSR:

$$x^2 + 24^2 = 26^2$$
$$x^2 = 26^2 - 24^2$$
$$x = \sqrt{100} = 10$$

So $QR = 20$.

You might also have noticed that 24 and 26 are twice 12 and 13, respectively. 5, 12, and 13 are Pythagorean numbers (like 3, 4, and 5), so the missing length, x, must be twice 5, or 10.

8. **(C)** All terms involving x are 0. Hence, the equation reduces to:

$$0 - 7y + 15 = 0$$
$$\text{or } 7y = 15$$
$$y = 2\frac{1}{7}$$

9. **(E)** Let s = number of shirts t = number of ties, where s and t are integers:

$$\text{Then } 7s + 3t = 81$$
$$7s = 81 - 3t$$
$$s = \frac{81 - 3t}{7}$$

Since s is an integer, t must have an integral value such that $81 - 3t$ is divisible by 7. Trial shows that $t = 6$ is the smallest such number, making $s = \frac{81 - 18}{7} = \frac{63}{7} = 9$. Hence, $s:t = 9:6 = 3:2$

10. **(C)** Rate $= \frac{\text{distance}}{\text{time}} = \frac{\frac{2}{5}\text{ mile}}{\frac{5}{60}\text{ hour}} = \frac{\frac{2}{5}}{\frac{1}{12}}$ rate $= \frac{2}{5} \cdot \frac{12}{1}$

$= \frac{24}{5} = 4\frac{4}{5}$ miles per hour.

11. **(D)** Draw the altitudes indicated. A rectangle and two right triangles are produced. From the figure, the base of each triangle is 20 feet. By the Pythagorean Theorem, the altitude is 15 feet. Hence, the area:

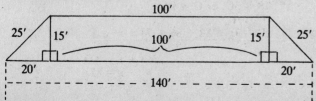

Area = Triangle + Rectangle + Triangle
= $(\frac{1}{2} \cdot 15 \cdot 20)$ + $(100 \cdot 15)$ + $(\frac{1}{2} \cdot 15 \cdot 20)$
= 150 + 1500 + 150
= 1800 square feet

12. **(E)** If $1 + \frac{1}{t} = \frac{t+1}{t}$, then the right-hand fraction can also be reduced to $1 + \frac{1}{t}$, and we have an identity, which is true for all values of t except 0.

13. **(E)** All points 6 inches from A are on a circle of radius 6 with center at A. All points 1 inch from b are on 2 straight lines parallel to b and 1 inch from it on each side. These two parallel lines intersect the circle in 4 points.

14. **(E)** Let $R = 5P$ and $S = 5Q$ where P and Q are integers. Then $R - S = 5P - 5Q = 5(P - Q)$ is divisible by 5. $RS = 5P \cdot 5Q = 25PG$ is divisible by 25. $R + S = 5P + 5Q = 5(P + Q)$ is divisible by 5. $R^2 + S^2 = 25P^2 + 25Q^2 = 25(P^2 + Q^2)$ is divisible by 5. $R + S = 5P + 5Q = 5(P + Q)$, which is not necessarily divisible by 10.

15. **(D)** $\frac{1}{2} \cdot 7 \cdot h = \pi \cdot 7^2$. Dividing both sides by 7, we get $\frac{1}{2}h = 7\pi$, or $h = 14\pi$.

16. **(E)**

$$\frac{9}{13} = \begin{array}{r} .69 \\ \overline{)9.00} \\ 78 \\ \hline 120 \\ 117 \end{array} \qquad \frac{13}{9} = \begin{array}{r} 1.44 \\ \overline{)13.00} \\ 9 \\ \hline 40 \\ 36 \\ \hline 40 \\ 36 \end{array} \qquad \begin{array}{l} 70\% = .7 \\[6pt] \frac{1}{.70} = \frac{1}{7} \\ \quad\quad 10 \end{array}$$

$$= \begin{array}{r} 1.42 \\ \overline{7)10.00} \\ 7 \\ \hline 30 \\ 28 \\ \hline 20 \end{array}$$

Correct order is $\frac{9}{13}$, 70%, $\frac{1}{.70}$, $\frac{13}{9}$; or I, III, IV, II.

17. **(D)**

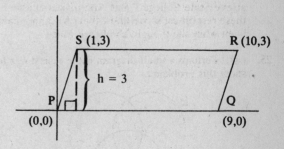

Since PQ and RS are parallel and equal, the figure is a parallelogram of base = 9 and height = 3. Hence, area $= 9 \cdot 3 = 27$.

18. **(A)**

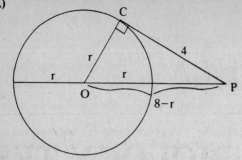

From the figure, in right △PCO:

$$PO^2 = r^2 + 4^2$$
$$(8 - r)^2 = r^2 + 16$$
$$64 - 16r + r^2 = r^2 + 16$$
$$48 = 16r$$
$$r = 3$$

Hence, diameter = 6.

19. **(B)** Area of wall = $4 \cdot \frac{60}{3} = 4 \cdot 20 = 80$ sq. yd.
Cost = $80 \times \$10.50 = \$840.00$.

20. **(D)** Using the distance formula, derived from the Pythagorean Theorem, that the distance from (a,b) to (c,d) is $\sqrt{(a-c)^2 + (b-d)^2}$:
Distance of $(4,4)$ from origin = $\sqrt{16 + 16} = \sqrt{32} < 7$
Distance of $(5,5)$ from origin = $\sqrt{25 + 25} = \sqrt{50} > 7$
Distance of $(4,5)$ from origin = $\sqrt{16 + 25} = \sqrt{41} < 7$
Distance of $(4,6)$ from origin = $\sqrt{16 + 36} = \sqrt{52} > 7$
Hence, only II and IV are outside circle.

21. **(A)** Let x = the cost.

Then $x + \frac{1}{4}x = 80$
Multiplying by 4: $4x + x = 320$
Adding like terms: $5x = 320$
Dividing by 5: $= \$64$ (cost)

$$\frac{\text{Cost}}{\text{S.P.}} = \frac{64}{80}$$
$$= \frac{4}{5}$$

22. **(C)**

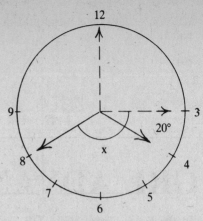

At 3:00, large hand is at 12 and small hand is at 3. During the next 40 minutes, large hand moves to 8 and small hand moves $\frac{40}{60} = \frac{2}{3}$ of the distance between 3 and 4; $\frac{2}{3} \times 30° = 20°$. Since there is a 30° arc between two numbers on a clock $\angle x = 5(30°) - 20° = 150° - 20° = 130°$.

23. **(B)** Area of sector = $\frac{120}{360} \cdot \pi \cdot 15^2$
$= \frac{1}{3} \cdot \pi \cdot 15 \cdot 15$
$= 75\pi$

24. **(D)** $\frac{17}{10}y = 0.51$
Multiplying both sides by 10, we get $17y = 5.1$, or $y = .3$.

25. **(D)** $40\% = \frac{2}{5} \times 50 = 20$ girls attended
$50\% = \frac{1}{2} \times 70 = 35$ boys attended

$$\frac{55}{50 + 70} = \frac{55}{120} = \frac{11}{24}$$

$$\begin{array}{r} .458 = 45.8\% \\ 24\overline{)11.000} \\ \underline{96} \\ 140 \\ \underline{120} \\ 200 \\ \underline{192} \end{array}$$

Approx. 46%

Part Five

GRE ADVANCED BIOLOGY TEST

GRE ADVANCED BIOLOGY TEST

The GRE Advanced Biology Test is designed to measure an applicant's ability to understand basic biological concepts and scientific processes and to evaluate and interpret data using scientific techniques. The test also measures an individual's knowledge of the subject matter typically presented in undergraduate biological science programs.

The GRE Advanced Biology Test is composed of approximately 210 multiple-choice questions, each of which has five possible answer choices. You will be given two hours and 50 minutes to complete the test.

Three primary areas of biology are tested: Cellular and Subcellular, Organismal, and Population Biology. Approximately 70 questions pertain to each of these subject areas. The test is not divided into separate sections; questions from each area are intermingled throughout the test.

You will receive a total score and three subscores (Cellular and Subcellular, Organismal, Population) when you take the test. Your raw scores are computed as follows: one point is given for each correct answer and one-fourth point is deducted for each wrong answer. Points are not given or deducted for questions left unanswered. The raw scores are then converted to scaled scores.

There is a penalty for wrong answers, so you should guess the answer to a question only when you can narrow down the number of possible answers by eliminating one or more answer choices as incorrect. If you have no idea of the correct answer to a question, it is probably better to leave the question unanswered.

ANSWER SHEET FOR THE GRE ADVANCED BIOLOGY PRACTICE EXAMINATION

1 Ⓐ Ⓑ Ⓒ Ⓓ Ⓔ   26 Ⓐ Ⓑ Ⓒ Ⓓ Ⓔ   51 Ⓐ Ⓑ Ⓒ Ⓓ Ⓔ   76 Ⓐ Ⓑ Ⓒ Ⓓ Ⓔ   101 Ⓐ Ⓑ Ⓒ Ⓓ Ⓔ

2 Ⓐ Ⓑ Ⓒ Ⓓ Ⓔ   27 Ⓐ Ⓑ Ⓒ Ⓓ Ⓔ   52 Ⓐ Ⓑ Ⓒ Ⓓ Ⓔ   77 Ⓐ Ⓑ Ⓒ Ⓓ Ⓔ   102 Ⓐ Ⓑ Ⓒ Ⓓ Ⓔ

3 Ⓐ Ⓑ Ⓒ Ⓓ Ⓔ   28 Ⓐ Ⓑ Ⓒ Ⓓ Ⓔ   53 Ⓐ Ⓑ Ⓒ Ⓓ Ⓔ   78 Ⓐ Ⓑ Ⓒ Ⓓ Ⓔ   103 Ⓐ Ⓑ Ⓒ Ⓓ Ⓔ

4 Ⓐ Ⓑ Ⓒ Ⓓ Ⓔ   29 Ⓐ Ⓑ Ⓒ Ⓓ Ⓔ   54 Ⓐ Ⓑ Ⓒ Ⓓ Ⓔ   79 Ⓐ Ⓑ Ⓒ Ⓓ Ⓔ   104 Ⓐ Ⓑ Ⓒ Ⓓ Ⓔ

5 Ⓐ Ⓑ Ⓒ Ⓓ Ⓔ   30 Ⓐ Ⓑ Ⓒ Ⓓ Ⓔ   55 Ⓐ Ⓑ Ⓒ Ⓓ Ⓔ   80 Ⓐ Ⓑ Ⓒ Ⓓ Ⓔ   105 Ⓐ Ⓑ Ⓒ Ⓓ Ⓔ

6 Ⓐ Ⓑ Ⓒ Ⓓ Ⓔ   31 Ⓐ Ⓑ Ⓒ Ⓓ Ⓔ   56 Ⓐ Ⓑ Ⓒ Ⓓ Ⓔ   81 Ⓐ Ⓑ Ⓒ Ⓓ Ⓔ   106 Ⓐ Ⓑ Ⓒ Ⓓ Ⓔ

7 Ⓐ Ⓑ Ⓒ Ⓓ Ⓔ   32 Ⓐ Ⓑ Ⓒ Ⓓ Ⓔ   57 Ⓐ Ⓑ Ⓒ Ⓓ Ⓔ   82 Ⓐ Ⓑ Ⓒ Ⓓ Ⓔ   107 Ⓐ Ⓑ Ⓒ Ⓓ Ⓔ

8 Ⓐ Ⓑ Ⓒ Ⓓ Ⓔ   33 Ⓐ Ⓑ Ⓒ Ⓓ Ⓔ   58 Ⓐ Ⓑ Ⓒ Ⓓ Ⓔ   83 Ⓐ Ⓑ Ⓒ Ⓓ Ⓔ   108 Ⓐ Ⓑ Ⓒ Ⓓ Ⓔ

9 Ⓐ Ⓑ Ⓒ Ⓓ Ⓔ   34 Ⓐ Ⓑ Ⓒ Ⓓ Ⓔ   59 Ⓐ Ⓑ Ⓒ Ⓓ Ⓔ   84 Ⓐ Ⓑ Ⓒ Ⓓ Ⓔ   109 Ⓐ Ⓑ Ⓒ Ⓓ Ⓔ

10 Ⓐ Ⓑ Ⓒ Ⓓ Ⓔ   35 Ⓐ Ⓑ Ⓒ Ⓓ Ⓔ   60 Ⓐ Ⓑ Ⓒ Ⓓ Ⓔ   85 Ⓐ Ⓑ Ⓒ Ⓓ Ⓔ   110 Ⓐ Ⓑ Ⓒ Ⓓ Ⓔ

11 Ⓐ Ⓑ Ⓒ Ⓓ Ⓔ   36 Ⓐ Ⓑ Ⓒ Ⓓ Ⓔ   61 Ⓐ Ⓑ Ⓒ Ⓓ Ⓔ   86 Ⓐ Ⓑ Ⓒ Ⓓ Ⓔ   111 Ⓐ Ⓑ Ⓒ Ⓓ Ⓔ

12 Ⓐ Ⓑ Ⓒ Ⓓ Ⓔ   37 Ⓐ Ⓑ Ⓒ Ⓓ Ⓔ   62 Ⓐ Ⓑ Ⓒ Ⓓ Ⓔ   87 Ⓐ Ⓑ Ⓒ Ⓓ Ⓔ   112 Ⓐ Ⓑ Ⓒ Ⓓ Ⓔ

13 Ⓐ Ⓑ Ⓒ Ⓓ Ⓔ   38 Ⓐ Ⓑ Ⓒ Ⓓ Ⓔ   63 Ⓐ Ⓑ Ⓒ Ⓓ Ⓔ   88 Ⓐ Ⓑ Ⓒ Ⓓ Ⓔ   113 Ⓐ Ⓑ Ⓒ Ⓓ Ⓔ

14 Ⓐ Ⓑ Ⓒ Ⓓ Ⓔ   39 Ⓐ Ⓑ Ⓒ Ⓓ Ⓔ   64 Ⓐ Ⓑ Ⓒ Ⓓ Ⓔ   89 Ⓐ Ⓑ Ⓒ Ⓓ Ⓔ   114 Ⓐ Ⓑ Ⓒ Ⓓ Ⓔ

15 Ⓐ Ⓑ Ⓒ Ⓓ Ⓔ   40 Ⓐ Ⓑ Ⓒ Ⓓ Ⓔ   65 Ⓐ Ⓑ Ⓒ Ⓓ Ⓔ   90 Ⓐ Ⓑ Ⓒ Ⓓ Ⓔ   115 Ⓐ Ⓑ Ⓒ Ⓓ Ⓔ

16 Ⓐ Ⓑ Ⓒ Ⓓ Ⓔ   41 Ⓐ Ⓑ Ⓒ Ⓓ Ⓔ   66 Ⓐ Ⓑ Ⓒ Ⓓ Ⓔ   91 Ⓐ Ⓑ Ⓒ Ⓓ Ⓔ   116 Ⓐ Ⓑ Ⓒ Ⓓ Ⓔ

17 Ⓐ Ⓑ Ⓒ Ⓓ Ⓔ   42 Ⓐ Ⓑ Ⓒ Ⓓ Ⓔ   67 Ⓐ Ⓑ Ⓒ Ⓓ Ⓔ   92 Ⓐ Ⓑ Ⓒ Ⓓ Ⓔ   117 Ⓐ Ⓑ Ⓒ Ⓓ Ⓔ

18 Ⓐ Ⓑ Ⓒ Ⓓ Ⓔ   43 Ⓐ Ⓑ Ⓒ Ⓓ Ⓔ   68 Ⓐ Ⓑ Ⓒ Ⓓ Ⓔ   93 Ⓐ Ⓑ Ⓒ Ⓓ Ⓔ   118 Ⓐ Ⓑ Ⓒ Ⓓ Ⓔ

19 Ⓐ Ⓑ Ⓒ Ⓓ Ⓔ   44 Ⓐ Ⓑ Ⓒ Ⓓ Ⓔ   69 Ⓐ Ⓑ Ⓒ Ⓓ Ⓔ   94 Ⓐ Ⓑ Ⓒ Ⓓ Ⓔ   119 Ⓐ Ⓑ Ⓒ Ⓓ Ⓔ

20 Ⓐ Ⓑ Ⓒ Ⓓ Ⓔ   45 Ⓐ Ⓑ Ⓒ Ⓓ Ⓔ   70 Ⓐ Ⓑ Ⓒ Ⓓ Ⓔ   95 Ⓐ Ⓑ Ⓒ Ⓓ Ⓔ   120 Ⓐ Ⓑ Ⓒ Ⓓ Ⓔ

21 Ⓐ Ⓑ Ⓒ Ⓓ Ⓔ   46 Ⓐ Ⓑ Ⓒ Ⓓ Ⓔ   71 Ⓐ Ⓑ Ⓒ Ⓓ Ⓔ   96 Ⓐ Ⓑ Ⓒ Ⓓ Ⓔ   121 Ⓐ Ⓑ Ⓒ Ⓓ Ⓔ

22 Ⓐ Ⓑ Ⓒ Ⓓ Ⓔ   47 Ⓐ Ⓑ Ⓒ Ⓓ Ⓔ   72 Ⓐ Ⓑ Ⓒ Ⓓ Ⓔ   97 Ⓐ Ⓑ Ⓒ Ⓓ Ⓔ   122 Ⓐ Ⓑ Ⓒ Ⓓ Ⓔ

23 Ⓐ Ⓑ Ⓒ Ⓓ Ⓔ   48 Ⓐ Ⓑ Ⓒ Ⓓ Ⓔ   73 Ⓐ Ⓑ Ⓒ Ⓓ Ⓔ   98 Ⓐ Ⓑ Ⓒ Ⓓ Ⓔ   123 Ⓐ Ⓑ Ⓒ Ⓓ Ⓔ

24 Ⓐ Ⓑ Ⓒ Ⓓ Ⓔ   49 Ⓐ Ⓑ Ⓒ Ⓓ Ⓔ   74 Ⓐ Ⓑ Ⓒ Ⓓ Ⓔ   99 Ⓐ Ⓑ Ⓒ Ⓓ Ⓔ   124 Ⓐ Ⓑ Ⓒ Ⓓ Ⓔ

25 Ⓐ Ⓑ Ⓒ Ⓓ Ⓔ   50 Ⓐ Ⓑ Ⓒ Ⓓ Ⓔ   75 Ⓐ Ⓑ Ⓒ Ⓓ Ⓔ   100 Ⓐ Ⓑ Ⓒ Ⓓ Ⓔ   125 Ⓐ Ⓑ Ⓒ Ⓓ Ⓔ

126 Ⓐ Ⓑ Ⓒ Ⓓ Ⓔ	143 Ⓐ Ⓑ Ⓒ Ⓓ Ⓔ	160 Ⓐ Ⓑ Ⓒ Ⓓ Ⓔ	177 Ⓐ Ⓑ Ⓒ Ⓓ Ⓔ	194 Ⓐ Ⓑ Ⓒ Ⓓ Ⓔ
127 Ⓐ Ⓑ Ⓒ Ⓓ Ⓔ	144 Ⓐ Ⓑ Ⓒ Ⓓ Ⓔ	161 Ⓐ Ⓑ Ⓒ Ⓓ Ⓔ	178 Ⓐ Ⓑ Ⓒ Ⓓ Ⓔ	195 Ⓐ Ⓑ Ⓒ Ⓓ Ⓔ
128 Ⓐ Ⓑ Ⓒ Ⓓ Ⓔ	145 Ⓐ Ⓑ Ⓒ Ⓓ Ⓔ	162 Ⓐ Ⓑ Ⓒ Ⓓ Ⓔ	179 Ⓐ Ⓑ Ⓒ Ⓓ Ⓔ	196 Ⓐ Ⓑ Ⓒ Ⓓ Ⓔ
129 Ⓐ Ⓑ Ⓒ Ⓓ Ⓔ	146 Ⓐ Ⓑ Ⓒ Ⓓ Ⓔ	163 Ⓐ Ⓑ Ⓒ Ⓓ Ⓔ	180 Ⓐ Ⓑ Ⓒ Ⓓ Ⓔ	197 Ⓐ Ⓑ Ⓒ Ⓓ Ⓔ
130 Ⓐ Ⓑ Ⓒ Ⓓ Ⓔ	147 Ⓐ Ⓑ Ⓒ Ⓓ Ⓔ	164 Ⓐ Ⓑ Ⓒ Ⓓ Ⓔ	181 Ⓐ Ⓑ Ⓒ Ⓓ Ⓔ	198 Ⓐ Ⓑ Ⓒ Ⓓ Ⓔ
131 Ⓐ Ⓑ Ⓒ Ⓓ Ⓔ	148 Ⓐ Ⓑ Ⓒ Ⓓ Ⓔ	165 Ⓐ Ⓑ Ⓒ Ⓓ Ⓔ	182 Ⓐ Ⓑ Ⓒ Ⓓ Ⓔ	199 Ⓐ Ⓑ Ⓒ Ⓓ Ⓔ
132 Ⓐ Ⓑ Ⓒ Ⓓ Ⓔ	149 Ⓐ Ⓑ Ⓒ Ⓓ Ⓔ	166 Ⓐ Ⓑ Ⓒ Ⓓ Ⓔ	183 Ⓐ Ⓑ Ⓒ Ⓓ Ⓔ	200 Ⓐ Ⓑ Ⓒ Ⓓ Ⓔ
133 Ⓐ Ⓑ Ⓒ Ⓓ Ⓔ	150 Ⓐ Ⓑ Ⓒ Ⓓ Ⓔ	167 Ⓐ Ⓑ Ⓒ Ⓓ Ⓔ	184 Ⓐ Ⓑ Ⓒ Ⓓ Ⓔ	201 Ⓐ Ⓑ Ⓒ Ⓓ Ⓔ
134 Ⓐ Ⓑ Ⓒ Ⓓ Ⓔ	151 Ⓐ Ⓑ Ⓒ Ⓓ Ⓔ	168 Ⓐ Ⓑ Ⓒ Ⓓ Ⓔ	185 Ⓐ Ⓑ Ⓒ Ⓓ Ⓔ	202 Ⓐ Ⓑ Ⓒ Ⓓ Ⓔ
135 Ⓐ Ⓑ Ⓒ Ⓓ Ⓔ	152 Ⓐ Ⓑ Ⓒ Ⓓ Ⓔ	169 Ⓐ Ⓑ Ⓒ Ⓓ Ⓔ	186 Ⓐ Ⓑ Ⓒ Ⓓ Ⓔ	203 Ⓐ Ⓑ Ⓒ Ⓓ Ⓔ
136 Ⓐ Ⓑ Ⓒ Ⓓ Ⓔ	153 Ⓐ Ⓑ Ⓒ Ⓓ Ⓔ	170 Ⓐ Ⓑ Ⓒ Ⓓ Ⓔ	187 Ⓐ Ⓑ Ⓒ Ⓓ Ⓔ	204 Ⓐ Ⓑ Ⓒ Ⓓ Ⓔ
137 Ⓐ Ⓑ Ⓒ Ⓓ Ⓔ	154 Ⓐ Ⓑ Ⓒ Ⓓ Ⓔ	171 Ⓐ Ⓑ Ⓒ Ⓓ Ⓔ	188 Ⓐ Ⓑ Ⓒ Ⓓ Ⓔ	205 Ⓐ Ⓑ Ⓒ Ⓓ Ⓔ
138 Ⓐ Ⓑ Ⓒ Ⓓ Ⓔ	155 Ⓐ Ⓑ Ⓒ Ⓓ Ⓔ	172 Ⓐ Ⓑ Ⓒ Ⓓ Ⓔ	189 Ⓐ Ⓑ Ⓒ Ⓓ Ⓔ	206 Ⓐ Ⓑ Ⓒ Ⓓ Ⓔ
139 Ⓐ Ⓑ Ⓒ Ⓓ Ⓔ	156 Ⓐ Ⓑ Ⓒ Ⓓ Ⓔ	173 Ⓐ Ⓑ Ⓒ Ⓓ Ⓔ	190 Ⓐ Ⓑ Ⓒ Ⓓ Ⓔ	207 Ⓐ Ⓑ Ⓒ Ⓓ Ⓔ
140 Ⓐ Ⓑ Ⓒ Ⓓ Ⓔ	157 Ⓐ Ⓑ Ⓒ Ⓓ Ⓔ	174 Ⓐ Ⓑ Ⓒ Ⓓ Ⓔ	191 Ⓐ Ⓑ Ⓒ Ⓓ Ⓔ	208 Ⓐ Ⓑ Ⓒ Ⓓ Ⓔ
141 Ⓐ Ⓑ Ⓒ Ⓓ Ⓔ	158 Ⓐ Ⓑ Ⓒ Ⓓ Ⓔ	175 Ⓐ Ⓑ Ⓒ Ⓓ Ⓔ	192 Ⓐ Ⓑ Ⓒ Ⓓ Ⓔ	209 Ⓐ Ⓑ Ⓒ Ⓓ Ⓔ
142 Ⓐ Ⓑ Ⓒ Ⓓ Ⓔ	159 Ⓐ Ⓑ Ⓒ Ⓓ Ⓔ	176 Ⓐ Ⓑ Ⓒ Ⓓ Ⓔ	193 Ⓐ Ⓑ Ⓒ Ⓓ Ⓔ	210 Ⓐ Ⓑ Ⓒ Ⓓ Ⓔ

GRE ADVANCED BIOLOGY PRACTICE EXAMINATION

Time: 2 hours 50 minutes

Directions: Each question in this section is followed by five choices, one of which is correct. Choose the best answer among the choices.

1. All of the following statements concerning vitamins are correct *except* that

   (A) vitamin C regulates the manufacture of a cementing substance that binds cells together
   (B) intestinal bacteria synthesize many of the B vitamins
   (C) folic acid plays a role in the metabolism of nucleotides
   (D) thiamine prevents the deficiency disease called pellagra
   (E) none of these

2. Of the following, the one which is an example of a buffer system in blood is

   (A) hemoglobin and oxyhemoglobin
   (B) oxygen and carbon dioxide
   (C) albumin and globulin
   (D) sodium bicarbonate and carbonic acid
   (E) oxygen and carbon monoxide

3. A *Drosophila* fly having two X chromosomes and three sets of autosomes is called

   (A) female   (C) supermale
   (B) intersex   (D) superfemale
                (E) male

4. The type of kidney found in fully matured reptiles, birds, and mammals is the

   (A) mesonephros
   (B) ananephros
   (C) metanephros
   (D) pronephros
   (E) none of these

5. Of the following, the vitamin that forms part of two coenzymes, $NADP^+$ and NADPH, is

   (A) ascorbic acid
   (B) biotin
   (C) riboflavin
   (D) nicotinic acid
   (E) ergosterol

6. Scientists discovered the source of the oxygen liberated by algae primarily through the use of

   (A) the electron microscope
   (B) microdissection instruments
   (C) the phase microscope
   (D) the ultracentrifuge
   (E) isotopes

7. External fertilization is most likely to be

carried on by organisms that live in

(A) deserts
(B) meadows
(C) forests
(D) tundra
(E) ponds

8. Hormones extracted from some plants that can induce earlier blooming in other plants are known as

(A) chromogens
(B) aerogens
(C) anthogens
(D) zymogens
(E) androgens

9. The sea anemone and the hermit crab live in a relationship which is

(A) parasitic
(B) mutually helpful
(C) helpful to the anemone but destructive to the crab
(D) helpful to the crab but destructive to the anemone
(E) commensalistic

10. Nitrogen tetroxide has been discovered in the atmosphere of the planet Venus. This discovery is related to the

(A) lack of free oxygen in the atmosphere of Venus
(B) lack of plant life on Venus
(C) pattern of radio waves received from Venus
(D) soil of Venus
(E) lack of animal life on Venus

11. A bacteriophage and a yeast cell are alike in that both

(A) carry on intracellular digestion
(B) can carry on aerobic respiration
(C) contain nucleic acids
(D) have a cell wall
(E) must have living cells to grow on

12. Oxygen enters the cells of *Hydra* by

(A) cyclosis
(B) hydrolysis
(C) osmosis

(D) plasmolysis
(E) diffusion

13. Hereditary variations in plants have been produced by which one of the following?

(A) auxins
(B) DDT
(C) 2,4D
(D) gibberellins
(E) colchicine

14. In vascular plants, the stele is surrounded by

(A) collenchyma
(B) meristem
(C) endodermis
(D) phellogen
(E) epidermis

15. The scientist who first synthesized DNA was

(A) Kornberg
(B) Ochoa
(C) Sanger
(D) du Vigneaud
(E) Barnard

16. Dinosaurs were abundant during the geologic period called the

(A) Devonian
(B) Eocene
(C) Mississippian
(D) Pennsylvanian
(E) Jurassic

17. For which one of the following processes is an appropriate photo-period necessary?

(A) the onset of pollination
(B) the onset of flowering
(C) onset of vernalization
(D) osmosis
(E) diffusion of materials into and out of cells

18. If an organism uses carbon dioxide as a hydrogen acceptor, it is most likely

(A) a yeast
(B) an alga
(C) a protozoan

(D) a virus
(E) a rickettsian

19. The transport of which one of the following is a function of human blood but not a function of grasshopper blood?

(A) nutrients
(B) antibodies
(C) hormones
(D) wastes
(E) oxygen

20. An albino corn plant lacks chlorophyll and therefore cannot carry on photosynthesis. Continuation of this genetic trait in corn plants occurs because

(A) albino plants become green in the sunlight
(B) self-pollination occurs in albino plants
(C) green plants may carry the albino gene
(D) the gene for albinism is sex-linked
(E) none of these

21. Book lungs may be found in dissections of which one of the following?

(A) aphids
(B) spiders
(C) silverfish
(D) finches
(E) clams

22. Two insects that belong to different orders are

(A) cricket and grasshopper
(B) bee and ant
(C) cicada and dragonfly
(D) butterfly and moth
(E) termite and cockroach

23. Which one of the following is an intermediate product of metabolism that cells can convert to protein, fat, or carbohydrate?

(A) vitamin K
(B) pyruvic acid
(C) carbonic acid
(D) glucose-6-phosphate
(E) vitamin E

24. Thomas Hunt Morgan and his co-workers were the first to offer experimental proof that

(A) during formation of gametes there is separation of maternal and paternal factors
(B) genes are located in chromosomes in a linear arrangement
(C) a single phenotype may be the result of more than one gene
(D) non-allelomorphic factors segregate independently
(E) a single phenotype may be the result of only one gene

25. With a genotype, AaBb, the fraction of gametes that will be ab is

(A) $1/16$
(B) $1/4$
(C) $1/2$
(D) $3/4$
(E) $1/8$

26. Of the following, the one which is an example of an inactive form of an enzyme is

(A) pepsinogen
(B) coenzyme A
(C) gastrin
(D) secretin
(E) insulin

27. An anthropologist believes that the first men from outer space to be seen by earth men will be bimanous, quadrupedal hexapods. Such outer space men will

(A) have four limbs
(B) have six feet
(C) have two hands
(D) not be bilaterally symmetrical
(E) not be able to interpret sense reception

28. The glacier that covered New York State during the Ice Age originated in

(A) Greenland
(B) Siberia
(C) Alaska
(D) Labrador
(E) Antarctic

29. A cloaca is *not* found in which one of the following?

    (A) turtles
    (B) salamanders
    (C) rays
    (D) sparrows
    (E) sunfish

30. Unicellular organisms ingest large molecules into their cytoplasm from the external environment without previously digesting them. This process is called

    (A) diffusion
    (B) peristalsis
    (C) plasmolysis
    (D) osmosis
    (E) phagocytosis

31. *Negative practice* in learning a skill does *not* refer to

    (A) breaking undesirable habits
    (B) learning what not to do
    (C) practicing unrelated incorrect skills
    (D) unlearning interfering habits
    (E) learning interfering habits

32. Organelles which serve as sensory receptors in unicellular organisms are which one of the following?

    (A) myonemes
    (B) chromatophores
    (C) flagella
    (D) neurofibrils
    (E) cilia

33. Balanced lethals are used in *Drosophila* crosses to

    (A) determine on which chromosome a recessive mutant gene is located
    (B) show the effect of hypostatic alleles
    (C) prove that a fly is heterozygous for a selected trait
    (D) test for sex-linkage
    (E) test for linkage

34. Studies made by Tatum and Beadle have increased our knowledge in the field of

    (A) animal parasitology
    (B) biochemical genetics
    (C) comparative histology
    (D) plant ecology
    (E) animal and plant evolution

35. The hormone that speeds the conversion of glucose to glycogen is

    (A) insulin
    (B) heparin
    (C) acetylcholine
    (D) oxytocin
    (E) somatotrophin

36. Which sugar is obtained from the hydrolysis of RNA?

    (A) glucose
    (B) sucrose
    (C) ribose
    (D) dextrose
    (E) uracil

37. The coccyx in man is a vestigial

    (A) turbinate bone
    (B) caudal appendage
    (C) colonic caecum
    (D) accessory mammary
    (E) frontal appendage

38. The DNA code is directly dependent upon the

    (A) number of carbons in the sugars
    (B) number of deoxyribose molecules
    (C) arrangement of purine-pyrimidine pairs
    (D) position of the phosphate groups
    (E) number of phosphate groups

39. The effects of alcohol upon a person who drinks may last several hours with all the following effects *except*

    (A) slower reaction of eyes, hands, and feet to signals
    (B) wandering attention
    (C) recklessness due to impaired judgment
    (D) increased resistance to contagious diseases
    (E) decreased sensitivity to surroundings

40. Of the following senses, the one most seriously affected by weightlessness dur-

ing space flight would be the

(A) auditory
(B) visual
(C) tactile
(D) vestibular
(E) kinesthetic

41. In experiments to determine how honeybees react to simple sounds, it was found that sound at a frequency of 600 cycles per second at about 120 decibels "stops honeybees in their tracks." They remain frozen as long as the sound continues, but return to full activity as soon as the sound is stopped. The sound described is

(A) audible only to insects
(B) lethal to bees if continued for as much as 120 seconds
(C) not audible to human beings
(D) audible only to human beings
(E) so loud that some form of ear protection is needed for beekeepers hearing it

42. The history of early man dates back to which one of these periods?

(A) Jurassic
(B) Pleistocene
(C) Paleocene
(D) Permian
(E) Devonian

43. Of the following, the most significant weakness in Darwin's theory of evolution was his belief in

(A) germplasm
(B) mutation
(C) natural selection
(D) pangenes
(E) somatoplasm

44. Which one of the following is not found in the skull?

(A) turbinals
(B) hyoid
(C) mastoid
(D) parietal
(E) frontal

45. Examination of soils in some areas has shown that what is now maple and basswood forestland was once occupied by lakes. The lake first choked up with water plants, and swamp vegetation appeared. Then spruce and pine grew. Finally basswood and maple became the dominant forms. The above process is best known as

(A) ecological succession
(B) geological evidence
(C) natural selection
(D) survival of the fittest
(E) variation

46. Autocatalysis in cytology refers to

(A) protein digestion
(B) hormonal activity
(C) bacterial disintegration
(D) gene duplication
(E) assimilation

47. Pyrenoids are associated with which one of the following?

(A) mitochondria
(B) nuclei
(C) chloroplasts
(D) ribosomes
(E) Golgi bodies

48. It is generally agreed by scientists that the number of years which have elapsed since the retreat of the last continental ice sheet which covered the northern United States is closest to which one of the following?

(A) 5,000
(B) 10,000
(C) 15,000
(D) 20,000
(E) 50,000

49. Cattle may develop the condition known as blind staggers after ingesting feed containing

(A) xenon
(B) cobalt
(C) manganese
(D) thorium
(E) selenium

50. On the average, Americans will be adding only five years to their life spans during the years 1959 to 1999, in contrast to the gain of 22 years in the period 1900 to 1958. It appears at present that these future gains will depend mostly on

    (A) widespread immunization procedures against infectious diseases
    (B) further reduction of infant mortality
    (C) more widespread use of polio vaccines
    (D) shorter working hours
    (E) controlling such diseases as cancer and cardiovascular-renal diseases

51. Charles Darwin, in his *Origin of Species,* formulated the theory of

    (A) mutations producing new species
    (B) natural selection producing new species
    (C) radiation producing mutations
    (D) use and disuse in forming new species
    (E) allopatric speciation

52. The 1961 Nobel Prize in Medicine for discoveries concerning the physical mechanisms of stimulation within the cochlea was awarded to

    (A) Lederberg
    (B) Von Békésy
    (C) Tatum
    (D) Calvin
    (E) Banting and Best

53. The most obvious change of climate during the past century has been a tendency toward

    (A) increased rainfall
    (B) decreased rainfall
    (C) warmer winters
    (D) colder winters
    (E) none of these

54. *Zinjanthropus boisei* has been estimated to have lived 1,750,000 years ago. By what dating method was this estimate made?

    (A) carbon-14
    (B) neon-sodium
    (C) nitrogen-krypton

    (D) uranium-lead
    (E) potassium-argon

55. Which instrument has played a major role in permitting scientists to discover the chemical makeup of a mitochondrion?

    (A) electron microscope
    (B) phase microscope
    (C) microdissection apparatus
    (D) microtome
    (E) ultracentrifuge

56. The frequency of crossing-over of genes tends to vary

    (A) inversely with the distance between genes in allelic chromosomes
    (B) inversely with the number of genes near the centromere
    (C) directly with the character of the gene
    (D) inversely with the increasing complexity of the organism
    (E) none of these

57. Which of the following instruments can measure the activities of the cerebral cortex?

    (A) pneumonometer
    (B) sphygmomanometer
    (C) pneumograph
    (D) electrocardiograph
    (E) electroencephalograph

58. A plant that carries on very little transpiration in its natural environment would most likely have a

    (A) thick leaf cuticle, few stomata, and hairy leaves
    (B) thick leaf cuticle, many stomata, and smooth leaves
    (C) thin leaf cuticle, few stomata, and smooth leaves
    (D) thin leaf cuticle, many stomata, and smooth leaves
    (E) thin leaf cuticle, few stomata, and hairy leaves

59. The incidence of type A blood increases with increase of latitude in North America. Which of the following statements is in best agreement with our understanding of this problem?

(A) The incidence of persons of North European descent increases with latitude in North America.

(B) The incidence of type A blood is influenced by temperature during pregnancy.

(C) The incidence is related to the percentage of Indian blood in the population.

(D) The incidence of type A blood is influenced by atmospheric pressure during late pregnancy.

(E) At present there is no explanation for the observation.

60. Among normal members of *Homo sapiens,* the size of the brain

(A) is directly related to body type
(B) is unrelated to intelligence
(C) varies consistently from one race to another
(D) varies directly with intelligence
(E) is directly related to intelligence and body type

61. Which has the *longest* wavelength?

(A) blue light
(B) cosmic rays
(C) orange light
(D) X-rays
(E) ultraviolet light

62. The parasympathetic system

(A) speeds up the heartbeat
(B) is composed of chains of ganglia parallel to the spinal cord
(C) produces cholinesterase to stimulate muscle contraction
(D) opposes the action of the sympathetic system
(E) none of these

63. Which of the following wavelengths of light, if withheld from a geranium plant would most limit the rate of photosynthesis?

(A) red
(B) green
(C) orange
(D) ultraviolet

(E) blue

64. Which one of the following compounds stores energy that is immediately available for active muscle cells?

(A) creatine phosphate
(B) glycogen
(C) glucose
(D) glycine
(E) glycerol

65. Genes will *not* be found in gene pairs in the

(A) sperm cells of a frog
(B) guard cells of a leaf
(C) muscle cells of a worm
(D) air sacs of a grasshopper
(E) uterine cells of a dog

66. Viruses and chloroplasts behave alike in that they

(A) replicate in living cells only
(B) are essentially made up of DNA
(C) are saprophytic
(D) reproduce in a cell-free medium
(E) are parasitic

67. Adult birds normally possess only one functional

(A) ureter
(B) ovary
(C) kidney
(D) testis
(E) lung

68. The tubercle bacillus is best stained with

(A) hematoxylin
(B) acid-fast stain
(C) chromic acid
(D) glacial acetic acid
(E) Gram's stain

69. Variations in the colors of wheat kernels is best ascribed to the effects of

(A) xenia
(B) maternal inheritance
(C) multiple alleles
(D) photoperiodism
(E) solar radiation

70. The color of certain *Hydrangea* flowers may be changed to blue by the addition to the soil of

    (A) SO_2
    (B) Al
    (C) CO
    (D) CaO
    (E) $Al(OH)_3$

71. The coeliac ganglion of the autonomic nervous system helps to control activities of the

    (A) bronchioles
    (B) heart
    (C) liver
    (D) urinary bladder
    (E) trachea

72. The direction in which the Ice Sheet travelled over New York State may be most directly determined by an examination of

    (A) kames
    (B) kettle holes
    (C) drumlins
    (D) pot holes
    (E) none of these

73. Of the following, the one that is closely associated with the contraction of the muscle fibers is

    (A) actinomycin
    (B) actin
    (C) nigrosin
    (D) interferon
    (E) norepinephrine

74. Which of the following is most likely to excrete most of its nitrogenous waste as ammonia?

    (A) bean plant
    (B) grasshopper
    (C) tree ferns
    (D) man
    (E) paramecium

75. The ciliary muscle is used for the process of

    (A) locomotion
    (B) food transportation
    (C) blinking
    (D) dust removal

    (E) accommodation

76. To which of the following choices can many plant movements best be attributed?

    (A) gibberellins
    (B) kinetins
    (C) contractile substances
    (D) a combination of turgor and growth differentials
    (E) auxins, kinetins, and contractile substances

77. $R-\underset{\underset{H}{|}}{\overset{\overset{NH_2}{|}}{C}}-COOH$ represents the general formula for

    (A) glucose
    (B) a fat
    (C) glycogen
    (D) a carbohydrate
    (E) an amino acid

78. An organism that reproduces asexually normally produces offspring that are

    (A) genetically alike
    (B) an improvement over the parent
    (C) better adapted to their environment
    (D) better equipped for survival
    (E) examples of hybrid vigor

79. Peripheral resistance is controlled by the

    (A) aorta
    (B) arterioles
    (C) capillaries
    (D) carotid artery
    (E) veins

80. A result of the widespread use of DDT is

    (A) the control of mosquitoes
    (B) the development of insects immune to DDT
    (C) the development of fishes immune to DDT
    (D) the destruction of harmful birds
    (E) none of these

81. Which adaptation has made possible the separation of oxygenated blood from deoxygenated blood?

(A) development of lungs in air-breathing vertebrates

(B) appearance of aortic arches in the annelids

(C) single ventricle in the frog's three-chambered heart

(D) four-chambered double heart in mammals

(E) single auricle in the tadpole's two-chambered heart

82. *Homo neanderthalensis* lived

(A) less than 4,000 years ago

(B) between 5,000 and 10,000 years ago

(C) between 20,000 and 30,000 years ago

(D) not less than 200,000 years ago

(E) between 40,000 and 80,000 years ago

83. Some fish migrate thousands of miles each year to lay their eggs and then return to the same area from which they had migrated. Reasons for this behavior are

(A) related to undersea pressures

(B) related to availability of polarized light

(C) related to ocean currents

(D) related to ocean temperatures

(E) not known

84. An example of a plant that has its seeds dispersed chiefly by animals is which one of the following?

(A) ash

(B) burdock

(C) maple

(D) thistle

(E) corn

85. Hybrid cotton has been produced by a method called

(A) carcinogenation

(B) detasseling

(C) selective gametocide

(D) self-pollination

(E) cross-pollination

86. Tissue culture has been extensively used as a research method in all of the following fields of biological investigation *except*

(A) photosynthesis

(B) virology

(C) development of nerve cells

(D) experimental embryology

(E) none of these

87. Of the following, the one that is a cellular enzyme that is involved in the production of pigment is

(A) acetyl coenzyme A

(B) acetyl cholinesterase

(C) tyrosinase

(D) ribonuclease

(E) none of these

88. Cranial capacity is a measurement of

(A) intelligence

(B) cephalic index

(C) internal volume of the brain case

(D) the size of the cerebellum

(E) memory

89. Of the following, the one which is an example of a useful American animal that has become extinct because of bad conservation practices is the

(A) bison

(B) dodo

(C) condor

(D) southeastern opossum

(E) passenger pigeon

90. A sound wave at a frequency of 30,000 vibrations per second would

(A) have an extremely long wavelength

(B) sound very loud to the normal person

(C) have a velocity greater that onc at 10,000 vibrations per second

(D) be inaudible to the normal person

(E) none of these

91. Of the following, the pair most closely related is:

(A) bluejay and grackle

(B) flicker and sandpiper

(C) hermit thrush and veery

(D) crow and ovenbird

(E) raven and owl

92. Which one of the following minerals is commonly found in granite rocks?

    (A) calcium
    (B) gold
    (C) silver
    (D) iron
    (E) mica

93. A level of 160 decibels, a very loud noise, has been found lethal for some animals. This occurs through

    (A) causing malfunction of the liver
    (B) impairment of hearing
    (C) raising body temperature
    (D) reduction in sleep
    (E) causing malfunction of the heart

94. The structure in a mammal that carries sperm cells from the testes to the urethra is the organ called the

    (A) seminiferous tubule
    (B) urachis
    (C) ureter
    (D) vas deferens
    (E) none of these

95. A blood vessel that is functional during development of mammals but normally becomes closed at birth is the

    (A) duct of Cuvier
    (B) ductus arteriosis
    (C) foramen ovale
    (D) thoracic duct
    (E) none of these

96. The first living organisms probably were able to obtain energy directly from

    (A) enzymes in the environment
    (B) oxygen in the atmosphere
    (C) carbon dioxide and water
    (D) organic molecules in the water
    (E) inorganic molecules in the water

97. A tree which has leaf venation similar to that of the maple is the

    (A) chestnut
    (B) gingko
    (C) oak
    (D) elm
    (E) sycamore

98. The chromosome number of unicellular organisms that reproduce sexually is maintained by the process of

    (A) mitosis and cytoplasmic division
    (B) mitosis and fertilization
    (C) meiosis and mitosis
    (D) meiosis and fertilization
    (E) meiosis and cytoplasmic division

99. Which statement concerning an allelic pair of genes controlling a single characteristic in man is true?

    (A) Both genes come from the father.
    (B) Both genes come from the mother.
    (C) One gene comes from the father and one gene comes from the mother.
    (D) The genes come randomly in pairs from either the father or the mother.
    (E) Both genes are the direct result of mutations occurring simultaneously to both the mother and father.

100. When a strong beam of light is passed through smoke, the beam is partly scattered and becomes visible. This phenomenon is known as the

    (A) Compton effect
    (B) Bothe effect
    (C) Zernicke effect
    (D) Zummer effect
    (E) Tyndall effect

101. The code of messenger RNA is directly dependent upon the

    (A) number of ribose sugars in RNA
    (B) purine and pyrimidine pairs in RNA
    (C) amino acid content of the cytoplasm
    (D) sequence of nucleotides in the associated DNA
    (E) glucose content and configuration in the cytoplasm

102. Of the following, the one which is an organ of equilibrium found in some invertebrates is the

    (A) labyrinth
    (B) cochlea
    (C) semicircular canal
    (D) statocyst
    (E) larynx

103. If the organism converts pyruvic acid to ethyl alcohol and carbon dioxide, it is most likely

    (A) a rickettsian
    (B) an alga
    (C) a protozoan
    (D) a virus
    (E) a yeast

104. An eosinophil is identified as a

    (A) type of cell in the gastric mucosa
    (B) red blood corpuscle
    (C) white blood corpuscle
    (D) type of neutrophil
    (E) type of cell in the trachea

105. Of the following, the plants that grow best in shady environments are

    (A) bur-reeds
    (B) cattails
    (C) ferns
    (D) goldenrods
    (E) rushes

106. An American tree which disease has rendered almost extinct in the United States is the

    (A) tulip tree
    (B) chestnut
    (C) elm
    (D) horse chestnut
    (E) horse tulip

107. The witch hazel is an unusual shrub because it

    (A) grows in an unusual habitat
    (B) is saprophytic
    (C) blooms in the fall
    (D) shows marked thigmotropic responses
    (E) is autotrophic

108. The discovery that the human chromosome number was 46 came as the result of using which one of the following pairs of cytological techniques?

    (A) chromatography and electron microscopy
    (B) x-ray diffraction studies and ultraviolet microscopy

(C) Feulgen stains
(D) fluorescein dyes and human tissue cultures
(E) action of colchicine and treatment with hypotonic saline solution

109. Of the following, which one probably gives the correct succession of early man?

    (A) Neanderthal—Piltdown—Sinanthropus
    (B) Sinanthropus—Pithecanthropus
    (C) Cro-Magnon—Neanderthal
    (D) Pithecanthropus—Neanderthal—Cro-Magnon
    (E) Cro-Magnon—Piltdown

110. Which one of the following would *not* likely be captured from a pond by means of a net?

    (A) larvae of dragonflies
    (B) flatworms
    (C) *Fucus*
    (D) *Elodea*
    (E) water spiders

111. With respect to the endocrine gland involved, the one term that does *not* belong with the others listed is

    (A) exopthalmia
    (B) cretinism
    (C) myxedema
    (D) Addison's disease
    (E) simple goiter

112. Stimulation of the vagus nerve will cause

    (A) secretion of gastric juice
    (B) dilation of the bronchial tubes
    (C) inhibition of peristalsis
    (D) an increase in the heart rate
    (E) none of these

113. Of the following, the crop that would be most likely to deplete the soil of its nitrates is

    (A) alfalfa
    (B) soybeans
    (C) clover
    (D) corn
    (E) legumes

114. The concept of the "constancy of the internal environment" is attributed to

    (A) Claude Bernard
    (B) Louis Pasteur
    (C) Arthur Sherrington
    (D) Linus Pauling
    (E) Charles Darwin

115. Of the following crosses, the one that is most likely to produce the largest number of recessive offspring is

    (A) AA × Aa
    (B) Aa × Aa
    (C) Aa × aa
    (D) AA × aa
    (E) AA × AA

116. Many plants store proteins in the form of which one of the following structures?

    (A) elaioplasts
    (B) starch grains
    (C) chromoplasts
    (D) aleurone grains
    (E) mitochondria

117. Of the following, the one which is an enzyme that catalyzes the reaction
    $$2H_2O_2 \rightarrow 2H_2O + O_2 \text{ is}$$

    (A) lipase
    (B) catalase
    (C) phosphorylase
    (D) invertase
    (E) maltase

118. A dog learns to salivate at the sound of a bell. This type of behavior is most closely associated with the research of

    (A) Lysenko
    (B) Watson
    (C) Pavlov
    (D) Dewey
    (E) Lamarck

119. A luciferin-luciferase system refers to which one of the following?

    (A) visual pigments in fish
    (B) photosynthesizing pigments of bacteria
    (C) transformation in bacteria
    (D) bioluminescence
    (E) transduction

120. When a patch of white hair is shaved from a Himalayan rabbit, the hair grows back black in color if the rabbit is maintained at a low temperature during this period of new growth of hair. This is due to the fact that the

    (A) expression of a gene is a result of heredity and environment
    (B) gene for white is recessive
    (C) genes have mutated
    (D) white is the phenotype, not the genotype
    (E) gene for white is dominant

121. Among the following, the first plants to reappear in a badly burned forest area will most probably be

    (A) mosses
    (B) ferns
    (C) liverworts
    (D) dandelions
    (E) grasses

122. The role of receptor organs in the body is to

    (A) transmit impulses to the spinal cord
    (B) transform stimuli into nerve impulses
    (C) mediate nervous reactions
    (D) act as reflex centers
    (E) receive stimuli from motor neurons

123. Companion cells are most closely associated with which one of the following groups?

    (A) tracheids
    (B) vessels
    (C) gametes
    (D) gonads
    (E) sieve-tubes

124. The concept that the DNA content of an egg holds the information needed to control its development agrees most closely with the doctrine of

    (A) vitalism
    (B) teleology
    (C) preformation

(D) epigenesis
(E) scienticism

125. When two organisms, each hybrid for a given trait, are crossed, a large progeny will show which one of the following percentage of hybrids?

(A) 100 percent
(B) 75 percent
(C) 50 percent
(D) 25 percent
(E) 80 percent

Directions: Each set of five choices precedes a set of questions. Choose the answer to each question from the choices directly above. An answer may be correct once, more than once, or not at all.

(A) *Plasmodium*
(B) *Ascaris*
(C) *Schistosoma*
(D) *Trypanosoma*
(E) *Entamoeba*

126. Cause of African sleeping sickness

127. Its most virulent species is *falciparum*

128. Has a snail as intermediate host

129. Its sole vector is the mosquito

130. Causes dysentery but generally no other symptoms

(A) glyoxysomes
(B) microbodies
(C) lysosomes
(D) cisternae
(E) cristae

131. Folds of the mitochondria's inner lining

132. Vesicles containing hydrolytic enzymes important in assimilation

133. Eukaryotic sites of amino acid oxidases

134. Inner compartments formed by foldings in the endoplasmic reticulum

135. Another name for this is *peroxisomes*

(A) Coelenterata
(B) Arthropoda
(C) Mesozoa
(D) Echinodermata
(E) Chordata

136. Simplest multicellular organisms

137. Possesses bilateral symmetry as larva and radial symmetry as adult

138. Radially symmetrical as adult and as larva

139. Bilaterally symmetrical organisms whose anus derives from the embryonic blastopore

140. Organism in which the blastopore becomes only the adult's mouth

(A) endoderm
(B) ectoderm
(C) mesoderm
(D) gastrula
(E) blastula

141. The first embryonic stage containing an inner cavity

142. Germ layer that forms the brain

143. Last germ layer formed during development

144. Stage during which the blastopore is formed

145. Germ layer that forms the digestive and respiratory organs

(A) metanephros
(B) Malpighian tubule
(C) flame cell
(D) contractile vacuole
(E) nephridium

146. The major excretory organ of the earthworm

147. Part of a mammal's excretory system

148. Removes wastes from a turbellarian

149. Concentrates wastes in insects

150. Removes water from protozoans

(A) monocot
(B) monoecious
(C) dicot
(D) dioecious
(E) monotreme

151. No self-pollination

152. A primitive thermoregulator

153. Vascular tubes in the young arranged in a circle or fused to form a tubular cylinder

154. For example, grass, corn, and wheat

155. Unless it is specialized for outbreeding, a single individual organism of this type can found a community

    (A) sympatry
    (B) allopatry
    (C) protandry
    (D) polyandry
    (E) polygyny

156. The phalarope provides one of the few cases of this

157. The most common mode of speciation requires this as a precondition

158. A male fish changes into a female upon reaching a certain size

159. *Rana pipiens* and *Rana buffo* have overlapping ranges

160. The Australian aborigine's social system involves this

    (A) chiasma
    (B) chi-square
    (C) synapsis
    (D) tetrad
    (E) translocation

161. Region of apparent contact between non-sister chromatids in a bivalent

162. Condition existing at the end of telophase II

163. A step in protein synthesis

164. Precise alignment between homologous sister chromatid pairs

165. Attachment of a chromosome fragment to a nonhomologous chromosome

    (A) vitamin
    (B) nucleic acid
    (C) carbohydrate
    (D) protein
    (E) lipid

166. Chemically, a substance consisting of a long hydrocarbon chain and an esterified carboxylic acid group

167. A trace organic element needed as a coenzyme

168. The type of molecule in which over half of all organic carbon is found

169. A macromolecule usually containing tyrosine and tryptophan

170. Of the above, the most versatile type of biological substance

Directions: This section contains experimental data. Each experiment is described and is followed by two or more questions. Choose the answers to the questions based upon the results presented and upon your knowledge of biology.

Questions 171-174

The diagram shows the daily insolation in cal/cm²/day received at the earth's surface in the absence of an atmosphere.

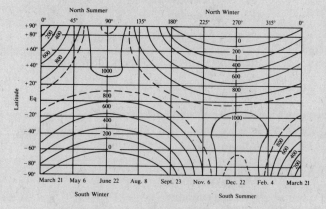

171. During the northern summer the North Pole receives the maximum daily insolation. This might be accounted for by the

    (A) delineation of the sun's axis toward the earth
    (B) ice and snow of that region reflecting more of the sun's rays
    (C) length of the Arctic summer day
    (D) soil of that area absorbing heat more rapidly
    (E) pressure exerted by gravity

172. The total radiation received by the southern hemisphere during the southern summer is greater than the amount received by the northern hemisphere during its summer. This is probably best accounted for by the fact that

(A) during the southern summer the earth is nearer the sun than during the northern summer

(B) fewer observations of insolation are taken in the southern hemisphere than in the northern hemisphere

(C) the northern summer is shorter than the southern summer

(D) the southern hemisphere contains less land and more water than the northern

(E) none of these

173. Assuming a 40 percent loss in insolation due to atmospheric conditions at the equator on June 22, how many calories of insolation would reach an area of one square foot in that one day (1 cm = .3937 inches)?

(A) $\dfrac{144\,(800)\,(.60)}{(.3937)^2}$

(B) $\dfrac{(12)^2\,(.3937)^2\,(800)}{.40}$

(C) $\dfrac{(.3937)^2\,(.60)}{(144)\,(800)}$

(D) $(800)\,(.40)\,(.3937)\,(12)$

(E) none of these

174. Assuming atmospheric absorption to be constant, which of the following locations (time and latitude) is likely to be the warmest?

(A) January 1, $+40°$
(B) July 1, $-40°$
(C) March 1, $+60°$
(D) February 1, $+20°$
(E) May 1, $-40°$

Questions 175–180

Following is a human pedigree tracing the occurrence of a trait through several generations.

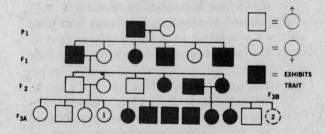

175. How may the trait best be described?

(A) autosomal dominant
(B) autosomal recessive
(C) autosomal, incompletely dominant
(D) sex-linked dominant
(E) sex-linked recessive

176. What is the chance that individual 1 exhibits the trait?

(A) 0
(B) $\frac{1}{4}$
(C) $\frac{1}{3}$
(D) $\frac{1}{2}$
(E) $\frac{3}{4}$

177. What is the chance that individual 2 exhibits the trait?

(A) $\frac{1}{4}$
(B) $\frac{1}{2}$
(C) $\frac{3}{4}$
(D) $\frac{6}{7}$
(E) 1

   I. Heterosis
  II. Linkage
 III. Inbreeding

178. Which of the above is (are) demonstrated in the pedigree?

(A) I, II, III
(B) I and II, only
(C) II and III, only
(D) I only
(E) III only

179. What human trait could be represented by the above pedigree?

(A) hemophilia
(B) albinism
(C) Tay-Sachs disease
(D) sickle-cell anemia
(E) brachydactyly

180. In which group of offspring does the phenotypic ratio differ significantly from expectation? (Omit individuals 1 and 2.)

(A) F_1
(B) F_2
(C) F_{3A}
(D) F_{3B}
(E) in no group

Questions 181-183

The table shows some radioactive isotopes, the kind of radiation emitted and their half-life. (Half-life is the time required for the disintegration of half of the atoms in a sample of some specific radioactive substance.)

ISOTOPE	RADIATION EMITTED	HALF-LIFE
Nitrogen-16	beta and gamma	7.4 seconds
Sulfur-37	beta and gamma	5 minutes
Sodium-24	beta and gamma	15 hours
Gold-108	beta and gamma	2.7 days
Iodine-131	beta and gamma	8 days
Iron-59	beta and gamma	45 days
Cobalt-60	beta and gamma	5.2 years
Strontium-90	beta	28 years
Radium-226	alpha and gamma	1,620 years
Carbon-14	beta	5,600 years
Chlorine-36	beta	310,005 years
Uranium-235	alpha, beta, gamma and neutrons	710 million years

181. Which one of the following statements is most nearly correct?

(A) The greater the number of kinds of radiation emitted, the longer the half-life of the isotope.
(B) Filtering out the beta radiation and leaving the gamma rays will decrease the half-life of sulfur-37.
(C) Carbon-14 cannot be used for dating archeological artifacts more than 5,600 years old.
(D) There appears to be some relationship between kind of radiation emitted and length of half-life.
(E) none of these

182. Which one of the isotopes listed below has a half-life nearest the time required for iodine-131 to have expended $63/64$ of its radiation?

(A) sodium-24
(B) gold-108
(C) iron-59
(D) cobalt-60

(E) strontium-90

183. How long does it take a radioactive isotope to lose at least 99 percent of its radioactivity?

(A) two half-lives
(B) four half-lives
(C) seven half-lives
(D) fifteen half-lives
(E) twenty half-lives

Questions 184-188

Ten judges were asked to judge the relative sweetness of five compounds (A, B, C, D, and E) by the method of paired comparisons. In judging each of the possible pairs they were required to unequivocally state which of the two compounds was the sweeter—a judgment of equality or no difference was not permitted.

The results of their judgments are summarized in the table below. In studying the table, note that each cell entry shows the number of comparisons in which the *row* compound was judged to be sweeter than the *column* compound.

	A	B	C	D	E
A		5	8	10	2
B	5		3	9	6
C	2	7		7	8
D	0	1	3		4
E	8	4	2	6	

184. How many comparisons did each judge make?

(A) 5
(B) 10
(C) 15
(D) 20
(E) 25

185. Which compound was judged to be sweetest?

(A) A
(B) B
(C) C
(D) D
(E) E

186. Which compound was judged to be *least* sweet?

(A) A
(B) B
(C) C
(D) D
(E) E

187. Which one of the following statements is most nearly correct?

(A) There was almost perfect agreement among the ten judges.
(B) The clearest discrimination was between B and C.
(C) The judges were not expert in discriminating sweetnesses.
(D) Compound D was most clearly discriminated from the other four compounds.
(E) none of these

188. Between which two compounds was the discrimination least consistent?

(A) A and D
(B) C and D
(C) C and E
(D) D and E
(E) B and A

Questions 189-191

Color Class, and Frequency Expected in F_2
(1 "Capital Letter Gene" = 1 Unit of Color)

Genotype	4	3	2	1	0
AABB	1/16				
AABb		2/16			
AAbb			1/16		
AaBB		2/16			
AaBb			4/16		
Aabb				2/16	
aaBB			1/16		
aaBb				2/16	
aabb					1/16
TOTALS, as fraction of F_2 population	1/16	4/16	6/16	4/16	1/16

Among the problems that did not yield readily to a Mendelian analysis in the early days of genetics were those involving quantitative variation, as seen in such characteristics as weight, length, intelligence, and color. Nevertheless, inheritance in such quantitative traits may be brought within the conceptual scheme of genetics, as was first shown by the Swedish geneticist H. Nilsson-Ehle in 1909.

Nilsson-Ehle had two strains of wheat, one with dark-red kernels, the other with white kernels. When these two were crossed they gave an F_1 that was very uniform and of an intermediate shade. The F_2 kernels could be sorted out into five color classes, ranging from the dark red of one parental strain to the white of the other. About $1/16$ of the F_2 were white, and $1/16$ were dark red.

Such results can be easily explained on the assumption that two pairs of alleles are involved, say A and a, and B and b; each capital letter allele gives one unit of color to the wheat kernels, and A and B are indistinguishable phenotypically. The genotypes AAbb, aaBB, and AaBb all look alike. On such a hypothesis we may work out the expected F_2, as shown in the table. The frequencies expected in each color class (see bottom row) were verified by Nilsson-Ehle.

189. Assuming that the color of human skin follows the same laws as above and that AABB represents a black and aabb a white, an individual represented by AaBb would appear to be

(A) a mulatto
(B) a black
(C) a white
(D) an Indian
(E) something other than any of the four choices above

190. The best definition for *alleles* is

(A) chromosomes containing color genes
(B) genes causing contrasting characteristics
(C) genes from pure-breeding plants or animals
(D) wheat color genes
(E) none of these

191. Why is the denominator of each fraction given in the table 16 and not 9?

(A) According to Mendel the denominator *would* be 9, but Nilsson-Ehle modified this law.

(B) Sufficient information is not given.

(C) The table shows characteristics of F_2; F_1 accounts for the remaining possibilities.

(D) There are 10 genotypes in the F_2 generation.

(E) There are 16 genotypes in the F_2 generation.

Questions 192-196

Fourth-day parasite counts were accumulated on 449 White Rock chicks inoculated at 6-8 days of age with 16×10^6 parasitized red cells. Analysis by sex showed that for 222 females the counts averaged 62.3 percent (S.E. = 1.2), whereas for 227 males the counts averaged 53.8 percent (S.E. = 1.2).

To determine whether the sex difference in parasite counts could be experimentally increased, male and female sex hormones of proven activity in chicks were administered. Ninety infected chicks were divided into 3 equal groups. Each chick in group A was injected intramuscularly with 0.1 mg. of testosterone propionate in 0.1 cc. of corn oil daily for 6 days, beginning on the day before the inoculation. Chicks in group B were similarly injected with 0.1 mg. of α-estradiol benzoate, and each of the controls in group C received 0.1 cc. of corn oil alone daily for the same period. The difference in parasite counts in the two sexes was not significantly increased by the administration of male or female sex hormones under the conditions of these experiments.

The incidence of exoerythrocytic schizonts in the capillary endothelium of the brain of chicks examined at various intervals after inoculation of sporozoites is presented in Table 1.

Parasite-count differences between the males and females were observed also in 418 blood-inoculated chicks treated with a suppressive level of quinine hydrochloride (Table 2).

TABLE 1

INCIDENCE OF EXOERYTHROCYTIC SCHIZONTS IN THE CAPILLARY ENDOTHELIUM OF THE BRAIN OF CHICKS EXAMINED 6-12 DAYS AFTER THE INTRAMUSCULAR INJECTION OF SPOROZOITES OF *P. GALLINACEUM*

	6th-10th day		11th day		12th day	
	No. examined	% positive	No. examined	% positive	No. examined	% positive
Females	61	65.6	41	90.2	40	92.5
Males	67	43.3	55	69.1	57	91.2
diff.* / S.E. diff.		2.59		2.71		not significant

* diff. / S.E. diff. represents the ratio of the observed difference to its Standard Error. Values greater than 2.00 are considered significant.

TABLE 2

FOURTH-DAY PARASITE COUNTS OF INFECTED CHICKS TREATED WITH QUININE.

	Number treated	Average count	Chicks showing count of 30% and above	
			Number	%
Females	212	7.28%	15	7.1
Males	206	4.60%	5	2.4
diff. / S.E. diff.		2.55%		2.3

192. Differences in infections of the chicks are attributable to the

   (A) age of the chicks
   (B) method of statistical analysis
   (C) sex of the host
   (D) type of inoculation
   (E) height and weight of the chicks

193. As compared with the males, the female chicks showed higher parasite counts

   (A) and earlier endothelial invasion

   (B) and later endothelial invasion
   (C) after the experimental period
   (D) prior to the experimental period
   (E) none of these

194. As compared with the females, the male chicks were

   (A) almost equally protected by quinine
   (B) less effectively protected by quinine
   (C) not examined
   (D) not protected by quinine
   (E) more effectively protected by quinine

195. Statistical significance is represented by

   (A) a comparison of percentages in terms of expected variation due to sampling
   (B) comparison of female and male chicks
   (C) percentage of parasite counts among infected chicks
   (D) percentage of positive reactions after intramuscular injections
   (E) comparison of height and weight of chicks

196. The null hypothesis, the use of which is implied by the fourth-day parasite counts of infected chicks treated with quinine, was

   (A) inadequate
   (B) not helpful
   (C) proved untenable
   (D) shown to be acceptable
   (E) not ascertained

Questions 197-201

In the course of a comprehensive investigation dealing with the influence of heredity on the carotene content of corn, crude carotene values were determined on the grain from all possible single cross combinations of 10 inbred lines of yellow dent corn, all of the same general maturity class and grown during the 1946 season. A 7×7 triple lattice design was used in the field experiment, thus providing for analysis three replicate samples of grain for each single cross. In the field experiment, the soil type and fertilizer treatment were the same on the three plots.

The corn was harvested at maturity, and the shelled corn was air-dried at room temperature for 10 days and stored in airtight containers at $0°C$. until it was analyzed. Carotene estimations were made by the official A.O.A.C. method, modified by the use of Hyflo Supercel and magnesium oxide, 3:1, as the chromatographic adsorbent.

Seed was not available for the Iowa $1205 \times$ Ohio 28 cross; hence, the carotene value for this combination is missing from the data. The range of yields of the other single cross combinations tested was from 71 to 123 bushels/acre.

The average difference between the highest and lowest of the three carotene values for the individual single crosses was of the order of 17 percent, the values given in Table 1 being the means for three duplicate estimations.

CAROTENE CONTENT OF CORN
(mg./lb — 15.5 percent moisture basis)

		Nebraska 6	Wisconsin 8	Illinois M14	Illinois A	Indiana WF9	Ohio 28	Wisconsin 32	Ohio 51A	Wisconsin 22	Iowa 1205
Nebraska	6			1.64	1.50	1.41	1.30	1.48	1.09	1.08	.67
Wisconsin	8	1.91	1.91	1.68	1.27	1.27	1.17	1.31	1.01	.88	1.07
Illinois	M14	1.64	1.68		1.26	1.23	1.03	.93	1.17	.84	.70
Illinois	A	1.50	1.27	1.26		.97	.95	.95	.93	.79	.66
Indiana	WF9	1.41	1.27	1.23	.97		.93	.98	.79	.74	.62
Ohio	28	1.30	1.17	1.03	.95	.93		.88	.66	.72	——
Wisconsin	32	1.48	1.31	.93	.95	.98	.88		.79	.73	.58
Ohio	51A	1.09	1.01	1.17	.93	.79	.66	.79		.60	.53
Wisconsin	22	1.08	.88	.84	.79	.74	.72	.73	.60		.69
Iowa	1205	.67	1.07	.70	.66	.62	——	.58	.53	.69	

Least significant difference between single crosses = .19 mg.

197. Which of the single cross combinations tested showed the highest per acre yield?

    (A) Ohio 28 and Nebraska 6
    (B) Ohio 28 and Iowa I205
    (C) Wisconsin 8 and Illinois M14
    (D) Wisconsin 8 and Nebraska 6
    (E) Insufficient data are given to answer the question.

198. On the average, the crosses involving which line produced corn of the highest carotene content?

    (A) Illinois A
    (B) Iowa I205
    (C) Nebraska 6
    (D) Ohio 51A
    (E) Ohio 28

199. The use of an experimental design which provided for repetition of the experiment would

    (A) be desirable only with reference to the inbred lines of corn
    (B) help to control soil type and fertilizer treatment
    (C) probably give identical results
    (D) provide more adequate experimental evidence
    (E) provide inadequate experimental evidence

200. The experiment reported here shows that

    (A) carotene is probably the most important nutritive factor in the development of new corn hybrids
    (B) different strains of yellow corn do not vary widely in carotene content
    (C) the carotene content of corn must be estimated on a percent moisture basis
    (D) the genetic constitution of corn may be largely responsible for its carotene content
    (E) none of these

201. The experiment reported indicates that the carotene content of the stored corn is

    (A) affected by temperature
    (B) associated with genetic factors
    (C) influenced by humidity

    (D) related to its weight
    (E) influenced by pressure

Questions 202-207

Certain investigators found that the effect of pH and salt concentration upon the solubility of β-lactoglobin, a globular protein, in water at 25° C. can be summarized by the following graph:

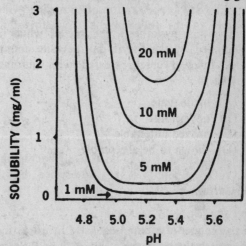

Figures refer to the concentration of NaCl.

The average interionic distance in NaCl solutions is known and includes the following experimental data:

Concentration (M)	Distance (A)
0.001	94
0.010	44
0.100	20
0.150	19
1.000	9.4

202. Of the following, β-lactoglobulin has the least solubility at a salt concentration of

    (A) 0.001 M
    (B) 0.005 M
    (C) 0.010 M
    (D) 0.100 M
    (E) 1.000 M

203. From the data, as interionic distance increases, solubility of β-lactoglobulin

    (A) increases continuously
    (B) decreases continuously
    (C) increases, then decreases
    (D) decreases, then increases
    (E) varies with pH

204. At a NaCl concentration of 1 mM, the average distance between Na^+ and Cl^- ions is, in microns (micrometers)

    (A) 9.4×10^{-5}
    (B) 9.4×10^{-4}
    (C) 9.4×10^{-3}
    (D) 9.4
    (E) 9.4×10^{-2}

205. At a salt concentration of 10 mM, at which pH of the following is β-lactoglobulin likely to be most soluble?

    (A) 4.7
    (B) 4.9
    (C) 5.1
    (D) 5.3
    (E) 5.5

206. The effect NaCl has on β-lactoglobulin's solubility is best described by the term

    (A) catalysis
    (B) precipitation
    (C) neutralism
    (D) salting-in
    (E) pH buffer

207. At zero salt concentration, β-lactoglobulin is least soluble at a pH best known as its

    (A) terminal pH
    (B) insoluble pH
    (C) pH of greatest acidity
    (D) isoelectric pH
    (E) pH of greatest basicity

Questions 208-210

Plant flowering is dependent upon light period in many species. Some species flower only when the photoperiod is short, others only when it is long. Cockleburs and soybeans, short-day plants, were used for experiments described below.

Two cocklebur plants were joined by a graft, but kept in separate light-tight compartments; one was exposed to a short-day, the other to a long-day photoperiod. Plates A-D describe the temporal sequence of the development of the plants. (The burs in the picture are the plant's flowers.)

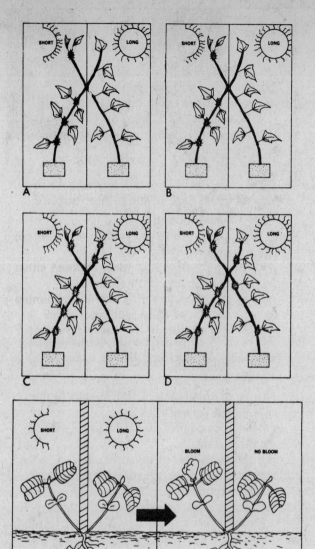

Two soybean plants were grafted together; each received separate amounts of light, as shown by the drawings. In Plate F, the leaves of the plant exposed to a long day have been removed. In Plate G, the plant on the right remains in total darkness.

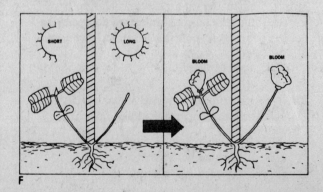

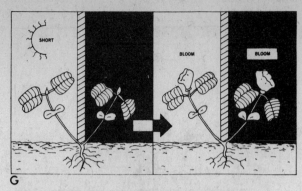

G

208. The leaves of the soybean evidently

    (A) inhibit flowering
    (B) inhibit flowering when exposed to long days only
    (C) inhibit flowering when exposed either to long days or total darkness
    (D) stimulate flowering when a minimum amount of daily light is provided
    (E) play no part in the plant's flowering

209. The cocklebur exposed to short days af-

fected the plant exposed to long days by, most probably,

    (A) destroying the inhibitor produced by the latter
    (B) sending nervous impulses stimulating flowering
    (C) transmitting a hormone to the latter
    (D) sending "primordial" flowering cells through the graft to the latter
    (E) supplying the latter with the pigment phytochrome

210. Critical day length is a (an) _____ value for short-day plants and a (an) _____ value for long-day plants.

    (A) minimum; minimum
    (B) minimum; maximum
    (C) maximum; minimum
    (D) unimportant; minimum
    (E) maximum; unimportant

ANSWER KEY FOR THE GRE ADVANCED BIOLOGY PRACTICE EXAMINATION

1.	D	39.	D	77.	E	115.	C
2.	D	40.	D	78.	A	116.	D
3.	B	41.	E	79.	B	117.	B
4.	C	42.	B	80.	B	118.	C
5.	D	43.	D	81.	D	119.	D
6.	E	44.	B	82.	E	120.	A
7.	E	45.	A	83.	B	121.	E
8.	C	46.	D	84.	E	122.	B
9.	B	47.	C	85.	C	123.	E
10.	A	48.	E	86.	A	124.	D
11.	C	49.	E	87.	C	125.	C
12.	E	50.	E	88.	C	126.	D
13.	E	51.	B	89.	E	127.	A
14.	C	52.	B	90.	D	128.	C
15.	A	53.	C	91.	C	129.	A
16.	E	54.	E	92.	E	130.	E
17.	B	55.	E	93.	C	131.	E
18.	B	56.	B	94.	D	132.	C
19.	E	57.	E	95.	B	133.	B
20.	C	58.	A	96.	D	134.	D
21.	B	59.	E	97.	E	135.	B
22.	C	60.	B	98.	D	136.	C
23.	B	61.	C	99.	C	137.	D
24.	B	62.	D	100.	E	138.	A
25.	B	63.	A	101.	D	139.	E
26.	A	64.	A	102.	D	140.	B
27.	C	65.	A	103.	E	141.	B
28.	D	66.	A	104.	C	142.	B
29.	E	67.	B	105.	C	143.	C
30.	E	68.	B	106.	B	144.	E
31.	C	69.	A	107	C	145.	A
32.	A	70.	D	108.	E	146.	E
33.	C	71.	C	109.	D	147.	A
34.	B	72.	C	110.	C	148.	C
35.	A	73.	B	111.	D	149.	B
36.	C	74.	E	112.	A	150.	D
37.	B	75.	E	113.	D	151.	D
38.	C	76.	D	114.	A	152.	E

153.	C	168.	C	183.	C	198.	C
154.	A	169.	D	184.	B	199.	C
155.	B	170.	D	185.	A	200.	D
156.	D	171.	C	186.	D	201.	B
157.	B	172.	A	187.	D	202.	A
158.	C	173.	A	188.	E	203.	B
159.	A	174.	E	189.	A	204.	C
160.	E	175.	A	190.	B	205.	A
161.	A	176.	A	191.	E	206.	D
162.	D	177.	C	192.	C	207.	D
163.	E	178.	E	193.	A	208.	B
164.	C	179.	E	194.	E	209.	C
165.	E	180.	E	195.	A	210.	C
166.	E	181.	D	196.	C		
167.	A	182.	C	197.	E		

EXPLANATORY ANSWERS FOR THE GRE ADVANCED BIOLOGY PRACTICE EXAMINATION

1. **(D)** Thiamine prevents the deficiency disease beri-beri. Pellagra, characterized by skin irritations and disorders of the digestive and nervous systems, is a deficiency disease attributed to lack of niacin.

2. **(D)** Buffers are substances which make it possible for the blood to take up large amounts of acid or base without a marked change in reaction or pH. The sodium combined with bicarbonate is available to neutralize any acid at once. Carbonic acid that is formed immediately dissociates into water and CO_2. The latter stimulates the respiratory center to remove the excess CO_2.

3. **(B)** Chromosomes which are the same in both sexes are termed autosomes. The configuration for an intersex fly in *Drosophila*, having two X chromosomes and three sets of autosomes is AAA-XX (karyotype). This fruit fly is predominately a female. This leads to the conclusion that there must be many minor sex-determining genes. Bridge's explanation is that the X chromosome alone is responsible for the production of femaleness, while one or more of the autosomes alone is responsible for the production of maleness.

4. **(C)** The metanephros is found in amniote vertebrates, acquiring a special duct, ureter, which grows into it from the original pronephric duct. It becomes the functional kidney of late embryo and adult.

5. **(D)** Nicotinic acid is a vitamin essential for the synthesis of $NADP^+$ and NADPH, which are essential in cellular metabolism as hydrogen acceptors. NADP is the abbreviation for nicotinamide adenine dinucleotide phosphate; the related electron-acceptor NAD is nicotinamide adenine dinucleotide.

6. **(E)** Radioactive isotopes of oxygen (O^{18}) are used to trace the pathway of this vital element through its developmental and sequential events within the algae cell. Radioactive carbon (C^{14}) is also employed in a similar manner to trace the role of carbon during photosynthesis.

7. **(E)** Invertebrates, fish, and amphibians inhabit pond waters. The eggs of the female are discharged into the water where the male discharges sperm over them, accomplishing fertilization. Since this process occurs outside the body of the female, external fertilization is said to take place.

8. **(C)** Anthogens are hormones which stimulate the production of anthocyanins, chemicals that are responsible for red, blue, and violet pigmentation in some flowers. An administration of anthogens will induce earlier blooming among these flowers and fruits.

9. **(B)** Mutualism is illustrated by this unusual symbiotic relationship. The hermit crab wanders into a shell that has a sea anemone attached. The anemone serves as protection for the crab, paralyzing attackers with its stinging tentacles. The hermit crab benefits the sea anemone by ripping and tearing food, which in turn floats upward, coming into contact with the aforesaid tentacles and ingested.

10. **(A)** The cloudy atmosphere of Venus is mostly carbon dioxide, containing perhaps a little water, but mostly devoid of free oxygen. Nitrogen tetroxide (N_2O_4) dissociates into nitric oxide and oxygen at very high temperatures. However, very little if any free oxygen is found in the atmosphere.

11. **(C)** Bacteriophage organisms are viruses that inject their DNA into host bacteria, eventually killing their victim. Yeast cells also contain nucleic acids, but are not parasitic in nature.

12. **(E)** *Hydra,* a coelenterate, does not possess any

complex organized respiratory system. Oxygen simply diffuses into the epidermal cells that come into contact with the watery medium in which the hydra is found.

13. **(E)** In 1937, it was discovered that colchicine acts as a mitotic poison, freezing the cell in metaphase. Polyploid plants are thus produced, exhibiting extremely large fruits and other mutant characteristics.

14. **(C)** The stele (vascular cylinder) is a collective term for the vascular and allied tissues in plants. The endodermis is a single layer of cells between the vascular cylinder and cortex. Its function is thought to be the prevention of water loss from stele to cortex region.

15. **(A)** In 1958, Arthur Kornberg perfected the enzymatic synthesis of DNA molecules in a test tube.

16. **(E)** The Jurassic period of the Mesozoic Era was characterized by conditions that were warmer and moister than conditions in the other periods of this era. During these ideal climatic circumstances, the dinosaurs reached the pinnacle of their success and became the dominant animal forms on the earth.

17. **(B)** The length of daylight hours seem to trigger the necessary plant hormones that directly control the flowering processes. Short- and long-day plants are thus classified according to their photoperiod requirements.

18. **(B)** Algae manufacture their own food by means of photosynthesis. During this complex process, carbon dioxide serves as a hydrogen acceptor for the split water molecule.

19. **(E)** Hemoglobin, in red blood corpuscles, combines with oxygen to transport oxyhemoglobin to the cells of humans. Grasshoppers obtain their oxygen by simply having the gas enter through openings in the body called spiracles. The gas then comes into contact with the cells directly, eliminating the need for a complex respiratory system in this respect.

20. **(C)** Albinism is a recessive trait and can manifest itself only when two such genes meet. However, "normal" photosynthetic plants can transmit this gene via their heterozygous genetic makeup. The plants possessing this hybrid condition are completely normal as far as ability to manufacture food is concerned, but they serve as carriers for this detrimental condition.

21. **(B)** The book lungs are peculiar to arachnids, serving to accomplish respiration. Each such structure consists of 15 to 20 horizontal plates containing blood vessels. Air entering the external slit on

the abdomen circulates between the plates, where the exchange of gases occurs.

22. **(C)** Cicadas belong to the order Homoptera, characterized by four membranous wings. Dragonflies are members of Odonata, possessing two pairs of transparent membranous wings with complex cross venation.

23. **(B)** Pyruvic acid is necessary for carbohydrate combustion (respiration) to occur. It is also a key ingredient in the combustion of many other types of fuels. Like carbohydrates, fats and proteins may also contribute to pyruvic acid formation. In each case a separate breakdown sequence exists, yielding greater or lesser net amounts of energy.

24. **(B)** Thomas Hunt Morgan (1926) formulated the "gene theory." It was concluded that the genes must be circumscribed corpuscles of some sort, each with a definite locus in the chromosome, arranged in linear order, each one different in substance from all of the others.

25. **(B)** There are only four out of sixteen ($^4/_{16} = ^1/_4$) possible gamete formations involving a dihybrid: AB, Ab, aB, ab.

26. **(A)** Pepsinogen is an enzyme precursor or zymogen in the digestive tract that is activated to prevent the exposure of cell proteins to possible destructive effects of the enzymes. Pepsinogen is hydrolyzed to yield pepsin and is catalyzed by a hydrogen ion. The suffix "-ogen" indicates an inactive enzyme form, as in pepsinogen—pepsin and fibrinogen—fibrin.

27. **(C)** Bimanous means "having two hands." Quadrupedal hexapods are conflicting terms meaning "four-footed" and "six-footed" respectively. Therefore, bimanous gives us choice (C).

28. **(D)** One of the three regions in North America in which the snow and ice was thickest, and from which the ice radiated in all directions, was the Labrador center, east of Hudson Bay. From this great ice accumulation came the ice sheet that covered eastern Canada and the northeastern United States.

29. **(E)** The cloaca is the terminal portion of the digestive, excretory, and reproductive passageways in various vertebrates, such as reptiles, amphibians, and birds. Some fish such as rays, sharks, and some bony fishes, possess this anatomical region. The sunfish does not contain a cloaca and is an exception.

30. **(E)** Large molecules adhere to the surface of the cell membrane, which then infolds or invaginates. Eventually, the sides of the pocket meet, trapping the large molecules within the cytoplasm. Special

digestive structures within the cytoplasm convert these large insoluble molecules into a soluble form.

31. **(C)** Certain birds' learning not to crouch is a negative process. Another example is that of pike learning *not* to hunt sticklebacks. Young pike will often try to snap up sticklebacks, only to find that the raised spines of the smaller fish prevent the pike from swallowing the smaller fish.

32. **(A)** Myonemes are contractile fibrils that occur in certain protozoans such as Vorticella and Stentor. These sensitive receptors extend and withdraw the cell as stimulated.

33. **(C)** Lethal genes kill homozygous individuals, but not heterozygous ones. If a fruit fly is crossed with a known heterozygous lethal gene carrier, its genotype can be ascertained from the number and type of progeny produced.

34. **(B)** Beadle and Tatum demonstrated that genes control the biosynthesis of essential amino acids and other nutritional compounds. The bread mold, *Neurospora crassa,* was utilized to form the "one gene-one enzyme" theory. Mutations were obtained and were shown to interfere with the vital biochemical sequences involved in the synthesis of indole.

35. **(A)** Insulin decreases the blood sugar level by suppressing the breakdown of liver glycogen to glucose, and encouraging building up of muscle glycogen from glucose.

36. **(C)** Ribonucleic acid is composed of a ribose sugar group which is set free during hydrolysis. This reaction involves the union of a salt and water to form an acid and a base.

37. **(B)** The coccyx bone in humans is the remnant of fused tail vertebrae, or a caudal appendage. This is an example of a vestigial structure which suggests common ancestry. This vestigial structure was, at one time, useful and functional, but through the ages lost its beneficial use.

38. **(C)** The stepwise (lengthwise) configuration of the single and double ring compounds arranged within the DNA molecule determines the genetic code, its meaning, and net effect.

39. **(D)** There is no evidence that alcohol is beneficial to the lining of the respiratory passages or to antibody production. Increased resistance to infectious diseases is attributed to vitamins A and C in particular.

40. **(D)** The vestibular apparatus affects balance; relies on gravity's pull on fluid in the inner ear; becomes nonfunctional in the absence of gravity.

41. **(E)** 120 decibels is on the threshold of pain level. Unless proper equipment is worn to muffle and baffle the sound intensity, severe damage will occur to the cochlea.

42. **(B)** The Age of Man (Quaternary Period) includes the final million and a half years of the earth's history. This period is composed of two epochs, the Pleistocene and the Recent. Primitive man first appeared during the Pleistocene epoch.

43. **(D)** Charles Darwin stated that each tissue or organ of the parent contributed "pangenes" which were incorporated into the egg or sperm and thus transmitted to the offspring, where they directed development, so as to produce in the offspring a duplicate of the tissue or organ from which they came. No evidence for such a belief has ever been obtained.

44. **(B)** The hyoid bone (lingual bone) is suspended from the tips of the styloid processes of the temporal bones by ligaments. It consists of five segments: a body, two greater cornua, and two lesser cornua.

45. **(A)** Succession is the gradual change in composition of plant life (population) from initial appearance to attainment of climax form.

46. **(D)** Autocatalysis refers to a gene catalyzing its own production. A single gene is capable of replicating itself exactly, catalyzing its own required molecules from component parts in the nucleoplasm.

47. **(C)** Pyrenoids are protein synthesis regions located along the spiral chloroplast of spirogyra and other algae. They are surrounded by a sheath composed of starch.

48. **(D)** It is believed that the last recession of the ice sheets took place perhaps 25,000 years ago, and many scientists speculate that we are now in a warm interglacial period which will be followed by the return of the ice sheets.

49. **(E)** Selenium in itself is non-poisonous, but many of its compounds are exceedingly toxic. One such compound, selenium hydride, is chemically related to arsenic and is a deadly poison. Cattle, upon ingesting feed containing selenium, produce this compound which will soon kill the animals.

50. **(E)** The leading causes of death at the present time are attributed to circulatory disease, cancer, and kidney disease. These diseases strike primarily the aged, as most infectious maladies have been controlled through vaccination, antibiotics, etc.

51. **(B)** In 1858 Charles Darwin published his theory of natural selection advanced to explain the evolution of living things. Its four fundamental concepts are overproduction, struggle for existence, variations, and survival of the fittest.

52. **(B)** Georg von Békésy demonstrated that the electrical potentials of the microphonic type generated by the inner ear of an experimental animal could be detected. When the vibrations of the eardrum are transmitted to the organ of Corti, the microphonic potentials of the vibrations can be picked up at the round window of the cochlea and displayed on the face of an oscilloscope.

53. **(C)** According to the theory of the seasons, the coldest portion of the year should be on or about December 21st. However, examination of temperature statistics indicates that there is a distinct lag in the seasons, the coldest period hovering around February 1st. This would markedly raise the average temperature range for winter, signifying a tendency toward warmer weather.

54. **(E)** *Zinjanthropus boisei,* a tool-using vegetarian australopithecine, was uncovered by the famous Leakeys. This specimen died in a stream of lava. Its age was determined by extracting radioactive potassium from the volcanic cover and bed that contained the fossil skull. By measuring potassium's slow decay into argon, the age was set at 1,750,000 years.

55. **(E)** By subjecting microscopic entities to extreme high-speed revolutions, different sedimentation layers are noted in accordance with the relative weights of the molecules contained therein. The chemical makeup of many cytoplasmic organelles has been determined by ultracentrifugation.

56. **(B)** Crossing-over of genes most often involves those units farthest away from the centromere. Experiments with *Drosophila* reveal that genes farthest away from the centromere exhibited this phenomenon 60:1 when compared with genes whose loci were very close to this point. Therefore, it can be stated that the frequency of crossing-over tends to vary inversely with the number of genes near the centromere.

57. **(E)** Brain wave patterns are measured electrically by the electroencephalograph. By comparing "normal" brain patterns with the subject under similar conditions, tumors, psychiatric conditions, blood disorders, etc., can be diagnosed.

58. **(A)** Transpiration is the evaporation of water from a leaf. Plants that live in areas void of plentiful rainfall (for example, a desert) possess numerous adaptations to retard water loss by means of transpiration. They exhibit few stomata, hairy leaves, and thick cuticles, all specifically serving to conserve water within the plant.

59. **(E)** No acceptable reason for this occurrence has been presented. The link, if any, between latitude and blood type cannot be explained according to any of our present genetic concepts.

60. **(B)** The size of the brain is no measure of intelligence—however, the number of convolutions per surface area is. Albert Einstein, for example, was rated a genius yet had a brain smaller in size than the average man.

61. **(C)** The wavelength of orange light is around 650 μ, exhibiting the longest wavelength of visible light next to red and far-red light.

62. **(D)** The autonomic nervous system is divided into the sympathetic and parasympathetic systems. These two subdivisions work in direct opposition to each other, maintaining their individual control and regulation.

63. **(D)** Red light is absorbed more than any other color by green plants for photosynthesis.

64. **(A)** Creatine phosphate participates in muscle metabolism by virtue of the freely reversible reaction with ATP:

$$\text{creatine} + \text{ATP} \rightleftharpoons \text{ADP} + \text{creatine phosphate}$$

The phosphoamide structure of this compound is highly reactive with respect to phosphate group transfer.

65. **(A)** Gametes possess the haploid number of chromosomes, thereby containing a single gene for a particular trait. It is not until fertilization occurs, restoring the diploid number to the species, that gene pairs exist.

66. **(A)** Viruses inject their DNA strands into a living host's cell which then manufacture more of the same virus organisms. Chloroplasts are organelles which can be formed only by living green plant cells, as dictated by their associated DNA pattern.

67. **(B)** The female reproductive system of a bird develops only on its left side. There is only one ovary located near the kidney and close to the open oviduct. In nonlaying birds the ovary is small, but during the egg-laying season it is much enlarged.

68. **(B)** The tubercle bacillus stains red against a blue background. Another name for the acid-fast stain is the Ziehl-Neelsen method, a routine staining procedure for the mycobacteria.

69. **(A)** Wheat endosperms will be colored with either genotype CCc or Ccc, while only those

with ccc will be white. Correns discovered that the sperm nucleus, when carrying a dominant gene, can determine this character even in the triploid endosperm. This phenomenon is referred to as xenia.

70. **(D)** *Hydrangea* flowers contain a litmus-like dye that changes from pink to blue in the presence of an alkali. Calcium oxide, when added to the soil, combines with water to form calcium hydroxide, a base, to effectuate this reaction.

71. **(C)** The hepatic plexus is the largest offset from the coeliac ganglia, receiving filaments from the left vagus and right phrenic nerves. Branches from this plexus accompany all the divisions of the hepatic artery.

72. **(C)** Drumlins are long, smooth, oval-shaped hills composed of till. They usually occur in groups in which all the hills point in the direction of glacier movement. They have the shapes of overturned canoes, with their steep ends facing the direction from which the glacier came.

73. **(B)** The first event to occur following the stimulation of a muscle is the initiation and propagation of an electrical response (muscle action potential). The calcium released by this reaction causes the protein actin to slide past the protein myosin, contracting the sarcomere.

74. **(E)** Protozoans lack the complex excretory systems necessary to convert proteins into nitrogenous wastes, such as urea and uric acid. One-celled animals simply produce ammonia, a gas that diffuses through the cell membrane into the surrounding watery medium.

75. **(E)** Accommodation is the automatic adjustment of the eye to focus light from a nearby object onto the retina. This is brought about by a contraction of the ciliary muscle, by which the choroid coat is pulled forward and the tension on the suspensory ligaments of the lens is lessened.

76. **(D)** A turgor movement is one which results from a change in turgor or water pressure. This can occur in many ways, such as guard cells' losing water from their large central vacuole. This will cause the cell to shrink, opening the stomata wider. Growth differentials are the results of unequal rates of growth in different parts of an organ. For example, plants move towards light (phototropism) when auxins in the leaves and stems accumulate in their dark regions, stimulating the growth of those cells with which they come into contact.

77. **(E)** The COOH group denotes an organic acid. The NH_2 group is an amine. Therefore, both together are part of an amino acid.

78. **(A)** Since only one parent is involved, and hence only one set of genes, the offspring are identical with the parent and with one another. There can be no variation because no additional corresponding conflicting genes can come into play.

79. **(B)** Peripheral resistance refers to the resistance offered by arterioles to the flow of blood. These tiny vessels maintain a high pressure behind them in the larger arteries and a lower pressure in front of them in the veins. They function as "nozzles" that gently spray blood into the capillaries. The amount of resistance to flow varies with the size of the lumens of the arterioles.

80. **(B)** With exposure, eventually a mutant resistant to DDT will be produced. This insect will be fitted for survival, and will pass on the beneficial gene to its descendants. It will not take long before an entire population of insects has these beneficial genes offering them immunity to DDT.

81. **(D)** The septum completely separates the deoxygenated blood in the right side of the heart from the oxygenated blood in the left side. The right auricle and ventricle receive deoxygenated blood and pump it to the lungs for aeration. The oxygenated blood then returns to the left auricle and ventricle for distribution throughout the body.

82. **(E)** The Neanderthal man actually existed between 35,000 and 110,000 years ago.

83. **(E)** There are many theories advanced to explain the reasons for fish migration. However, to date no one theory has definitely been accepted. Only by continued application of tagging experiments can we hope to solve this great mystery.

84. **(B)** Burdock seeds contain sharp, spiny projections radiating from a hard, dry seed coat. As fur-bearing animals brush against these seeds, the sharp spines catch onto and adhere to their bodies. It may be several miles before the animal realizes that one is attached and then proceeds to shake or scratch it free, thereby serving to disperse the new generation over a wide area.

85. **(C)** By artificially destroying those cotton plants with undesirable characteristics, the breeders prevent the unwanted genes from being passed onto the offspring plants. Eventually a hybrid cotton line will be attained, exhibiting only those desirable traits for which selection was originally made.

86. **(A)** Tissue culture technique is used for growing viruses and other cells outside of the body on cells immersed in a nutrient-complex solution. Photosynthesis experiments can easily be per-

formed with plants growing in soil, without the expensive and elaborate equipment needed for tissue culture experimentation.

87. **(C)** Tyrosinase catalyzes the formation of tyrosine. Tyrosine forms a compound called dihydroxyphenylalanine, which is the beginning chemical for a series of reactions ending in the production of melanin, the dark pigment. Albinos lack an enzyme necessary for the catalysis of one of these reactions.

88. **(C)** The measurement of one's cranial capacity indicates the internal size or volume of the skull (cranium).

89. **(E)** The passenger pigeon is now extinct because of the uncontrolled hunting and destruction by humans of breeding and feeding grounds. No law enforcement measures were employed to save these birds from the ravages of the sportsmen, who turned out to be, in reality, murderers.

90. **(D)** The upward limits of the human ear is approximately 20,000-25,000 cycles (vibrations). A sound wave of 30,000 cycles would, therefore, not be heard.

91. **(C)** The hermit thrush and the veery are both thrushes, belonging to the family Turdidae. These birds are characterized by brown backs and spotted breasts, song-producing, long legs, large eyes, and moderately slender beaks.

92. **(E)** Mica is found in thin, shiny, flat plates or flakes in granite, some sandstones and many other rocks.

93. **(C)** Fur-bearing animals, in particular, absorb sound waves and transform them into heat energy. If such an animal is placed in a controlled environment and subjected to very loud noises, the animal dies, not because of the sound's high intensity but rather from the increase in body temperature.

94. **(D)** The vas deferens is able to convey spermatozoa from the testes to the urethra by possessing a ciliated epithelium which functions to create a current by which the gametes are transported.

95. **(B)** In all amniotes, the ductus arteriosus (duct of Bothallus) functions until hatching or birth, transferring blood from the right ventricle into the aorta. However, when the branches of the pulmonary artery have developed sufficiently, the ductus arteriosus becomes attached to the left pulmonary artery. The evolutionary significance of this structure serves as a reminder of the emergence from an aquatic to a terrestrial mode of life among the vertebrates.

96. **(D)** The first organisms, having arisen in a sea

of organic molecules, and in contact with an atmosphere free of oxygen, presumably obtained energy by the fermentation of certain of these organic substances.

97. **(E)** Maple and sycamore trees exhibit netted venation and palmately lobed leaves. Dicot leaves show multibranching of veins (netted). Palmately lobed leaves contain several main veins which branch into the leaf blade at the tip of the petiole. Indentations extend toward the base of the leaf.

98. **(D)** The chromosome (diploid) number of chromosomes of any organism that reproduces sexually is maintained by the processes of meiosis (reduction division) and fertilization. Meiosis occurs during the formation of the gametes, reducing the chromosome number in half (haploid). During fertilization, the male and female gamete unite, each contributing a haploid set of genes and chromosomes, resulting in the restoration of the original diploid number.

99. **(C)** Alleles are two genes that occupy the same relative position (locus) on homologous chromosomes, and therefore, when in the same cell, undergo pairing during meiosis, but produce different effects on the same developmental processes. One gene is contributed by the female and the corresponding one by the male to complete the allelic pair.

100. **(E)** When a strong beam of light is passed through a region containing no fine particles, it is not visible from the side. If, however, the beam is intercepted by fine particles, such as smoke, dust, or other colloidal suspensions, the beam is partly scattered and becomes visible (Tyndall effect). The color and the intensity of the scattered light depend on the size of the particles.

101. **(D)** The messenger RNA is manufactured from DNA in the nucleus. The vital part of the DNA molecule is the linear arrangement of its nucleotide pairs (purine-pyrimidine configurations). Since DNA serves as the blueprint with which to manufacture a representative molecule of messenger RNA, the sequence of the said nucleotides are of prime importance.

102. **(D)** A statocyst is a small organ of equilibrium in which a particle rests among hair-like projections on sensory cells. Any change in position brings the particle (statolith) against one or another of the receptors, which transmits an impulse indicating the body position in respect to gravity. Statocysts are found in molluscs, jellyfishes, ctenophores, and crustaceans.

103. **(E)** Yeast converts pyruvic acid, in the absence of oxygen (anaerobically), to ethyl alcohol and

carbon dioxide during the process of fermentation.

104. **(C)** An eosinophil is a polymorphonuclear leukocyte containing granules staining in acid dyes such as eosin. In human beings, these white blood corpuscles comprise approximately 2 to 5 percent of all leukocytes, but increase in number during certain allergic and parasitic manifestations.

105. **(C)** Ferns grow prolifically in warm, tropical, wet areas. In the jungle, ferns never attain the tremendous height of angiosperms, being content to grow on the forest floor which is quite dark. The interlocking crowns of the large trees overhead block out most of the sunlight, yet ferns are able to survive because of the extremely wet conditions.

106. **(B)** *Endothia parasitica,* the infective agent and cause of chestnut blight, practically eradicated all of our chestnut trees. These ascomycetes attack the leaves of the tree, eventually destroying them and killing the organism.

107. **(C)** Members of the witch hazel family (Hamamelidaceae) produce flowers in spikes or heads consisting of approximately 4 to 5 separate petals. The plant blooms in the fall, making it different from most other plants that bloom in the spring.

108. **(E)** In tissue culture, colchicine is administered to stop mitosis at metaphase. The cells are then immersed in a hypotonic saline solution which causes them to swell. The chromosomes are then caused to disperse so that they can be photographed.

109. **(D)** The Java man *(Pithecanthropus erectus)* dates back to the Pleistocene period, and is considered to be one of the most primitive ape-men. The Neanderthal man *(Homo neanderthalensis)* dates back to approximately 150,000 years, and became extinct only about 25,000 years ago. The Cro-Magnon man *(Homo sapiens)* is modern man, whose first fossils date back 15,000 to 60,000 years.

110. **(C)** *Fucus* is a brown alga (seaweed) found only in marine water. No fresh water (pond) species exist, and therefore fucus cannot be obtained from this habitat by any means.

111. **(D)** Exopthalmia, cretinism, myxedema, and simple goiter are all abnormalities resulting from thyroxin imbalance, and hence the thyroid gland is responsible. Addison's disease is caused by lack of cortisone, a result of the malfunctioning of the adrenal glands.

112. **(A)** The vagus nerve sends branches to the bronchi, causing constriction of the passages; inhibitory fibers to the heart; constriction of various digestive passageways; and secretory fibers to the stomach and pancreas, stimulating the flow of gastric and pancreatic juices.

113. **(D)** Alfalfa, soybeans, and clover are all leguminous crops possessing nodules on their roots. Within these swellings live nitrogen-fixing bacteria, so vital in the nitrogen cycle, converting nitrogen into nitrates. Corn depletes the soil by using up these vital nitrates.

114. **(A)** Claude Bernard discovered the role of the liver in storing carbohydrates. He found out that the liver keeps the glucose concentration of the blood constant throughout the day.

115. **(C)** Whenever a hybrid is crossed with a recessive, the offspring are 50 percent hybrid and 50 percent recessive. None of the other crosses produce any recessive offspring, except the second, which produces 25 percent.

116. **(D)** Many proteins are stored as reserve foods in plant cells in the form of distinct bodies called aleurone grains. These are especially abundant in corn and wheat.

117. **(B)** Catalase is capable of bringing about the decomposition of 5 million molecules of hydrogen peroxide per minute. This substance is toxic, and is produced as a byproduct in a number of enzyme reactions. Catalase protects the cell by destroying the peroxide.

118. **(C)** Ivan Pavlov demonstrated conditioning using dogs. The dogs salivated at the sound of a bell, expecting to receive food. Substituting a secondary stimulus for the original stimulus is a definition of conditioned behavior.

119. **(D)** W. D. McElroy demonstrated that bioluminescence in fireflies involves luciferin (the substrate) and luciferase (the enzyme). ATP supplies the energy for the reaction, and, under certain conditions, the amount of light emitted is proportional to the amount of ATP present.

120. **(A)** Two colors are based upon a pair of allelic genes, with one being dominant over the other. Sometimes the wild type gene has mutated in more than one way, so that a series of three alleles has been formed (multiple alleles). Such a third gene causes the Himalayan rabbit to be white except for its extremities. The external temperature is the dominant factor in the expression of this characteristic. The rabbits of a certain genotype will be black if raised in a cold temperature and all white if raised in a hot, humid room. This gene determines a threshold temperature above which pigment cannot be formed.

121. **(E)** Of the choices given, only grasses and dandelions can exist in soil that does not have an excessive amount of moisture. Seeds of dandelions are wind blown and would be consumed by fire. Grass seeds become buried under the soil, and so would escape the ravages of a forest fire.

122. **(B)** Receptor organs contain many sensory neurons which receive stimuli and convert them to nervous impulses. Receptor organs are the eyes, ears, tongue, etc.

123. **(E)** Companion cells and sieve tubes are associated with the phloem transportation system of a plant. The cytoplasm in sieve tubes is continuous from cell to cell through the sieve pores of the end walls. Companion cells are elongated, and border upon the sieve tubes. These cells aid in conduction and/or store foods which are taken from the sieve tubes. They also possess very thin-walled, perforated areas which enhance the passage of materials from cell to cell.

124. **(D)** The epigenesis concept, formulated by Kaspar F. Wolff, stated that the structures of the embryo develop in succession. DNA composes genes, and directs epigenetic development.

125. **(C)** When a hybrid and recessive are crossed (Aa times aa), 50 percent of the offspring show the hybrid characteristic and 50 percent show the recessive trait.

126. **(D)**
127. **(A)**
128. **(C)**
129. **(A)**
130. **(E)**

Plasmodium sp., a member of class Sporozoa of the Phylum Protozoa, is an obligate intracellular parasite with two hosts in the life cycle, the *Anopheles* mosquito and man. The parasite reproduces sexually inside the mosquito and asexually inside of human red blood cells. In humans, the parasite causes malaria, of which the most virulent form, falciparum malaria, is caused by *Plasmodium falciparum*. The mosquito is called the vector for this disease because it is responsible for introducing it to man. The mosquito does this by biting his skin, depositing sporozoites into the bloodstream.

Ascaris lumbricoides is a nematode parasite of man that lives in the intestine and passes eggs out the feces, which can infect hosts when unwashed vegetables grown in dirty soil are ingested.

Schistosoma sp. is a blood fluke, a member of class Trematoda, phylum Platyhelminthes (flatworms). It inhabits the liver and the mesenteric veins near the intestines. In its life cycle, it first enters a snail, where it reproduces asexually. The snail is called the intermediate host. It leaves the snail to enter a human, boring through the skin, where two flukes of opposite sexes will pair for life, reproducing sexually; this makes the

human the definitive host. The flukes cause the disease schistosomiasis, which, next to malaria, is the most widespread disease caused by animal parasites.

African sleeping sickness, which differs from ordinary sleeping sickness (encephalitis, caused by a virus), is produced in man by a flagellated protozoan, **Trypanosoma gambiense.** The disease is usually fatal; the nervous system is attacked, and lethargy is produced before death. The vector is the tsetse fly, *Glossina* sp.

Entamoeba histolytica causes amoebic dysentery. While dysentery is also a symptom of schistosomiasis, *E. histolytica* rarely leads to more severe problems. The parasite is a member of class Sarcodina, phylum Protozoa; it inhabits the gut, and is transmitted directly from contaminated food or water to man; there is no intermediate host.

131. **(E)**
132. **(C)**
133. **(B)**
134. **(D)**
135. **(B)**

Glyoxysomes, found only in plant cells that can convert fatty acids to sugar, are organelles adapted to perform the glyoxylate cycle. The overall reaction of that cycle is:

$$2 \text{ Acetyl CoA} \rightarrow \text{ succinate} + 2H + 2CoA$$

Microbodies (peroxisomes) are small membrane-bounded vesicles containing amino acid oxidases; they are relatively primitive oxidative organelles. They are also responsible for photorespiration, in which excess reducing power generated by photosynthesis is dissipated by plants.

Lysosomes are, like peroxisomes, single-membrane organelles, but instead contain hydrolytic enzymes such as phosphatase, ribonuclease, and cathepsin. Their general function is to assimilate (degrade) nutrient molecules of large size that have been absorbed by phagocytosis or pinocytosis.

The **cisternae** are the chambers formed by the infoldings of the endoplasmic reticulum. They interconnect to form channels which aid the transport of proteins synthesized on ribosomes attached to the endoplasmic reticulum to peripheral parts of the cell.

The **cristae** are the folds of the inner membrane of mitochondria. They contain respiratory assemblies, which are functional clusters of the electron-transport enzymes and cytochromes.

136. **(C)**
137. **(D)**
138. **(A)**
139. **(E)**
140. **(B)**

The phylum **Mesozoa** contains about 50 species of parasitic animals that live inside of such invertebrates as squids and octupi. Each organism contains about 25 cells surrounding one or a few reproductive cells. No separate tissues or organs are present.

Coelenterata, a phylum comprising jellyfish, sea anemones, corals, and hydras, is a primitive group. Symmetry is radial throughout the life cycle. Cell specialization is limited; primitive nervous systems, nerve nets, are present. Although a middle germ layer (mesoglea) is present, it is not highly developed; the outer epidermis and inner gastrodermis (ectoderm and endoderm) perform most functions.

Arthopoda, a phylum including insects, crustaceans, and other classes, is a protostome phylum. The Protostomia includes organisms whose embryonic blastopore develops into the adult's mouth, with an anus forming separately. The coelenterate's blastopore develops into a combined anus and mouth (gastrovascular cavity).

Echinoderms and **Chordates** belong to the Deuterostomia, their blastopore becomes the adult's anus, and the mouth forms separately. Echinoderms (starfishes, sea urchins, sea cucumbers) are radially symmetrical as adults, but bilaterally symmetrical as larvae. Chordates (vertebrates, other subphyla) are bilaterally symmetrical in all stages of the life cycle past cleavage.

141. **(B)**
142. **(B)**
143. **(C)**
144. **(E)**
145. **(A)**

After an animal zygote is formed, it divides into smaller cells, producing a small grapelike cluster, a morula, which is the same size as the original ovum. The **blastula** then forms from the morula; it is a spherical body, the center of which is the hollow blastocoel. The blastula gives way to the **gastrula,** in which the spherical shape is lost, the blastopore and archenteron form, and the primary germ layers form. Organogenesis, the process of forming organs, occurs in the next stage, the neurula.

The primary germ layers are the endoderm and ectoderm (inner and outer layers of the gastrula), and the mesoderm, the middle germ layer that begins to form in the gastrula. Each germ layer gives rise to specific organs. In vertebrates, the fates of each primordial germ layer may be summarized as follows:

Endoderm: lungs and respiratory passages, liver, pancreas, bladder, thyroid, digestive tract and its epithelial lining.
Mesoderm: bone, muscle, circulatory system.
Ectoderm: Skin, nervous system, hair, nails, eye lens, many glands, epithelial lining of the mouth, nose, and anus.

146. **(E)**
147. **(A)**
148. **(C)**
149. **(B)**
150. **(D)**

All choices refer to excretory systems. They are discussed in a phylogenetic order.

Contractile vacuoles, found in many protozoans and some sponges, are organelles which gradually absorb water, swelling until they release the water into the external medium; they excrete few waste products. Because fresh-water organisms have a special problem of absorbing too much water from the hypotonic environment, contractile vacuoles are much more common in fresh-water protozoa than in marine forms.

Flame cell systems mark the beginning of a tubular excretory system. They are found in flatworms (turbellarians, flukes, tapeworms). Basically, they consist of paired branching tubes, off of which are bulb-like vesicles (protonephridia). Each bulb contains cilia that sweep the collected water and wastes into the main tubes. Because the beating of the cilia resemble the flickering of a flame, each cell containing them is called a flame cell.

In the earthworm, unlike the flatworm, a circulatory system is present; the earthworm's excretory system, the **nephridium,** is intimately associated with it. Each nephridium, of which there are two per body segment, consists of an open ciliated nephrostome, a coiled tubule running from it into a bladder, and a nephridiopore which releases wastes. Wastes are absorbed from the body fluids and from the surrounding capillaries. Probably, reabsorption from the tubule into the capillaries occurs.

Malpighian tubules are the excretory organs of insects. They are blind sacs located at the intersection of the midgut and the hindgut. Blood from the open circulatory system flows in, and is gradually passed toward the rectum; nitrogenous wastes are turned into uric acid, and almost all water and salts are reabsorbed.

In higher vertebrates such as man, the permanent adult kidney is known as and derives from the metanephros. In embryological development, the pronephros forms and is replaced by the mesonephros, which is finally replaced by the **metanephros.** Briefly described, the kidney works as follows. Each nephron, the functional unit, is composed of a glomerulus which forces blood minus proteins into a collecting capsule (Bowman's capsule). Blood then flows through a convoluted tubule where sodium, glucose, water, etc., are reabsorbed. The remaining fluid is urine.

151. **(D)**
152. **(E)**
153. **(C)**
154. **(A)**
155. **(B)**

Monoecious organisms are those in which each individual contains both male and female organs; the term is usually applied to plants, in which separate flowers of each individual are either staminate or pistillate. Monoecious organisms can breed by themselves in most cases, although some species can only outcross. (Hermaphroditic plants contain stamen and ovary within the *same* flower.)

Dioecious plants contain only male or only female flowers per individual. They are therefore obligate outcrossers, and cannot self-pollinate.

The class Angiospermae (flowering plants) is divided into the subclasses Dicotyledoneae and Monocotyledoneae. **Dicot** embryos contain two cotyledons; **monocot** embryos contain one cotyledon. The vascular bundles in young dicots' stems are arranged in a tubular cylinder, while those of monocots are more scattered. Dicots usually have cambium and secondary growth, leaves with net venation, and flower parts in fours or fives or multiples of those numbers; monocots usually lack cambium and thus secondary growth, have parallel venation in the leaves, and have flower parts that occur in threes or multiples thereof (e.g., three each of stamens, pistils, petals). Some dicots are birches, oaks, roses, and beans; some monocots are grasses, corn, wheat, and palms.

Monotremes are mammals, but also resemble reptiles. Though they have the mammalian traits of lactation and thermoregulation, they lay eggs. The only surviving monotremes are the duck-billed platypus and the spiny anteater, each found in Australia and New Zealand.

156. **(D)**
157. **(B)**
158. **(C)**
159. **(A)**
160. **(E)**

Sympatric species occupy the same geographical area. Sympatric speciation refers to the formation of two species from a pre-existing one without geographical barriers preventing interbreeding; here, ecological and behavioral forces allow speciation.

Allopatry simply means that two groups, usually populations, occur in different places. Allopatric speciation, believed to be responsible for almost all speciation, refers to the introduction of geographical barriers to different members of a species, causing them to form divergent strains which eventually lose the capability of interbreeding; at that point, new species have been formed.

Protandry is the situation in which an organism, in the course of development, changes its sex. It is most common to see changes from male to female, as in fishes which produce more eggs as they get bigger; once a male reaches a certain size, he finds it more reproductively advantageous to become a female. Examples of female-to-male changes are known.

Polyandry and **polygyny** are the two subsets of polygamy. In the former, a female has more than one male mate at a time; in the latter, a male has more than one female mate at a time. Most polygamy is polygyny: among humans, earlier Mormons and Australian aborigines illustrate this. At least one species of a bird, the phalarope, has a polyandrous system; in it, females assume territorial defense duties and males brood the eggs.

161. **(A)**
162. **(D)**
163. **(E)**
164. **(C)**
165. **(E)**

Chiasmata (sing., chiasma) are regions of apparent contact between non-sister chromatids in a bivalent during prophase I of meiosis. The sites of chiasma formation are believed to be the sites at which crossing-over takes place, in which linked alleles become unlinked. Chiasmata are formed in a later stage of prophase I than the

stage during which synapsis occurs. **Synapsis** refers to the precise, point-for-point alignment between homologous pairs of sister chromatids. It is this alignment between homologous, non-sister chromatids that allows chiasmata to form, and is thus necessary for crossing-over.

The **chi-square** test is a statistical procedure most often used in biology to test the significance of deviations of observed frequencies from their expected frequencies. One common application is in experiments in which Mendelian inheritance makes the expected ratios of different genotypes (and thus phenotypes) easy to predict. The statistic used in the test is chi-square, χ^2.

At the end of meiosis (i.e., after telophase II), four haploid gametes, collectively called a **tetrad,** have been formed from each original diploid cell.

A **translocation** may be at least two distinct events in biology. In protein synthesis, translocation is the step in which a new tRNA-aminoacyl complex attaches to the ribosomal-mRNA, displacing a previous tRNA-aminoacyl complex and in which the reading frame of the mRNA is shifted one codon along the ribosome. Translocation, in meiosis, is the attachment of a piece of DNA to a nonhomologous chromosome. This is different than crossing-over, in which homologous chromatids in prophase I exchange genetic material. (Translocation may also mean the transport of solutes within plants.)

166. **(E)**
167. **(A)**
168. **(C)**
169. **(D)**
170. **(D)**

A **vitamin** is an organic trace substance necessary for normal growth, health, or reproduction. It cannot be synthesized endogenously and therefore must be obtained preformed. Vitamins whose biochemical functions are known generally function as coenzymes, small molecules needed for an enzyme to function.

A **nucleic acid,** either DNA or RNA, is a long-chain polymer consisting of nucleotides (DNA) or ribonucleotides (RNA). DNA is the repository of genetic information; RNA carries out its instructions, except for some viruses, in which RNA is the basic carrier of the genetic code.

A **carbohydrate** is a molecule of the form $(CH_2O)_n$. Though less energy-rich than lipids, carbohydrates, through the glycolytic pathway, Krebs cycle, and oxidative phosphorylation are the primary energy source for most, if not all, organisms. It has been estimated that the polysaccharide cellulose, the primary component of plant cell walls and a polymer of glucose molecules, accounts for more than half of all organic carbon in the world.

Protein, composed of amino acids linked by peptide bonds, is the functional expression of DNA. It is a macromolecule composed of 20 major, and some minor, amino acids, such as tyrosine and tryptophan. Proteins are by far the most versatile bilogical molecules: their functions include catalysis, storage, transport, and muscular contraction.

Lipids are water-insoluble organic substances extractable from cells by nonpolar solvents such as chloroform, benzene, and ethyl ether. Lipids function as hormones (including the sex hormones), some vitamins, membrane components, fuel reserves, and protective components of cell walls. The characteristic of saponifiable lipids, but not of terpenes and steroids, is the presence of fatty acids, either free or esterified to a molecule similar to glycerol. A fatty acid is a long hydrocarbon chain with a carboxylic acid group at one end. The chain may contain double or triple bonds.

171. (C) Insolation is the amount of sunlight received over a given area. During the Arctic summer, there is perpetual sunlight for six months of the year.

172. (A) It is during the Southern Hemisphere's summer and the Northern Hemisphere's winter that the earth comes closest to the sun.

173. (A) The calories of insolation that would reach an area of one square foot in a single day can be calculated by the following formula: total area × calories × insolation gain/square inches. The total area whose insolation is to be determined is one square foot. Keeping all measurements constant, there are 144 square inches in one square foot. The chart denotes 800 calories at the equator on June 22, the location and date given in the problem. Insolation given (1.0 − 0.4 = 0.6) is simply determined by subtracting given insolation loss from standard 1.0. The denominator of square inches is arrived at by simply squaring the given measurement of one square inch.

174. (E) May 1st at −40° latitude exhibits an atmospheric absorption rate above 500, the warmest temperature of any of the choices listed.

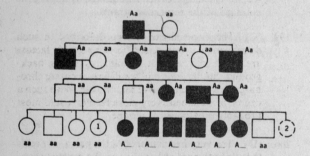

175. (A) The trait is autosomal and dominant. Proof that it is not recessive is shown by the mating producing the F_{3B} generation. Both parents are affected by the trait, but an offspring is not; if the trait were recessive, both parents would be homozygous, and would produce exclusively homozygous offspring. The complete lack of a third phenotype may be taken as proof that the trait is completely dominant, not incompletely dominant. Now that the trait is known to be dominant, the question of sex linkage can be attacked. Consider the P_1 and F_1 generations. If the trait were sex-

linked, the father in P_1 would have an X-chromosome coding for the trait, and an inactive Y-chromosome. All females in F_1 would then carry that X-chromosome, and, since the trait is dominant, would exhibit the trait. Since not all females in F_1 exhibit the trait, the hypothesis of sex linkage leads to a contradiction, indicating that the trait is carried on an autosome.

176. (A) Since neither parent of individual 1 exhibits the trait, each is homozygous recessive (aa). Barring mutation, the cross of two homozygotes yields only homozygotes; therefore, there is no chance of any offspring of these parents exhibiting the trait.

177. (C) One of the parents in the F_1 generation does not exhibit the trait, and is thus double recessive. The other parent exhibits the trait. All offspring must bear a recessive allele from the mother, and thus the affected offspring bear the dominant allele from the father. The parents of individual 2, then, are heterozygous, Aa. The cross, Aa × Aa, should yield ¼ AA, ½ Aa, and ¼ aa. Phenotypically, ¾ are therefore expected to show the trait.

178. (E) Heterosis, also known as hybrid vigor, is the increase in fecundity, health, growth rate, etc., in hybrids as compared to the parents. No hybridization or increased vigor of offspring is indicated here. Linkage involves more than one gene assorting non-independently; only one gene is involved here. Inbreeding, however, which is defined as mating between closely related individuals, such as between siblings, is represented several times in the pedigree.

179. (E) Hemophilia is transmitted as a sex linked recessive trait. Albinism and Tay-Sachs disease are transmitted as autosomal recessive traits. Sickle-cell anemia is transmitted as an autosomal recessive trait in which the heterozygotes have characteristics of each allele. Brachydactyly, in which the fingers are very short, is inherited through an autosome; it is dominant.

180. (E) With small sample sizes, deviations from expectation must be great in order to be significant. In the F_1, out of a sample of 6 offspring, 3 would be expected to bear the trait (50 percent). The only possible results which would be considered statistically significant would be for all offspring to bear the trait, or for all to not bear it. The situation for the F_2 is the same as that for the F_1. In the F_{3A}, the results are exactly as expected. In the F_{3B}, ¾ affected are expected. Of a sample of 7, this corresponds to 5.25 expected to carry the trait. The observed number that do so, 6, is clearly not significantly different from 5.25.

181. (D) The chart shows an array of different radiations that are emitted from radioactive elements.

Some half-lives are very short, others are very long. There seems to be some correlation between the kind of radiation emitted and the duration of half-life.

182. **(C)** It is an established fact that seven half-lives are necessary for a radioactive element to lose approximately 99 percent of its total radioactivity (see next answer). $^{63}/_{64}$ is 95 percent of an atom's total emissions. If, at the end of seven half-lives, 56 days have elapsed ($8 \times 7 = 56$), we can easily calculate that 95 percent of this is 53.2 days. Iron-59 on the chart is the closest isotope to this figure, having a half-life of 45 days.

183. **(C)** If we start with a 100-gram sample of uranium, at the end of the first half-life, 50 grams will be left; at the end of the second half-life, 25 grams will remain; third, 12.5; fourth, 6; fifth, 3; sixth, 1.5; and finally seventh, 0.75 (less than 1 percent will remain).

184. **(B)** The first sentence of the passage states that each judge had to evaluate the sweetness of five compounds by paired comparisons. Therefore, there are five possible pairs for each compound.

185. **(A)** Compound A scored a total of 25 points; B: 23 points; C: 24 points; D: 8 points; and E: 20 points. Simply add the horizontal row of numbers to get the total score.

186. **(D)** With reference to the above scores, compound D achieved the lowest grade of 8 points.

187. **(D)** Compound D is quite isolated from the other four chemicals (as far as score is concerned). The other chemicals are quite close to one another, so the judges had trouble distinguishing among them.

188. **(E)** The judges were split down the middle, giving five points to A and five points to B. All other compound comparisons were rather easily distinguishable.

189. **(A)** There would be no true dominant trait to appear phenotypically, resulting in incomplete dominance or blending, with mulatto as the phenotypic color.

190. **(B)** The first sentence of the third paragraph states that two pairs of alleles are involved (A and a, B and b); each capital letter allele gives one unit of color. Therefore, alleles are genes causing contrasting or different characteristics.

191. **(E)** Adding up the numerator numbers in the fractions displayed in the data chart gives a total of 16. 16 genotypes are given: 1-AABB; 2-AABb; 2-AaBB; 1-AAbb; 4-AaBb; 2-Aabb; 1-aaBB; 2-aaBb; 1-aabb.

192. **(C)** In all cases, figures on both charts show a higher incidence of positive infection among female chickens than among male chickens.

193. **(A)** Table 1 reveals that endothelial invasion of female chickens was quite high after just six days. After eleven days, 90 percent of the female chicks were infected.

194. **(E)** Table 2 reveals a significant difference between male and female chicks with respect to quinine treatment. Among the females, over double the number and percentage of chicks showed a parasite count of 30 percent and above, when compared with the male group.

195. **(A)** The very first sentence shows a comparison of percentages, as do both tables. The explanation of the ratio of the observed difference to its Standard Error with explanation of its significance is given under Table 1.

196. **(C)** The null hypothesis was proved untenable in this instance, because significant results were attained that could be directly attributable to injections of quinine.

197. **(E)** The experiment is concerned with the carotene content of corn. The only reference made to yield per acre occurs in the second sentence of the third paragraph, and the reference is of a vague nature. Much more data is needed to answer the question posed.

198. **(C)** Nebraska 6 scored highest among the choices given, namely 10.17. Illinois A scored second = 9.28; Ohio 28 = 7.64; Ohio 51A = 7.57; Iowa I 205 = 5.52. These figures are determined by adding the columns of the respective strains.

199. **(C)** The experimental design described in such detail herein is very scientific. All possible factors are taken into account — namely, genetic background, similar soils and fertilizers, accurate chromogenic and quantitative factors, etc. With such a degree of exactness, very close results would most probably be attained if redone.

200. **(D)** The very first sentence of the passage reveals that the influence of heredity on the carotene content of corn is a prime factor. The variation in values shown in the data chart bears this out.

201. **(B)** The corn employed herein was subject to exact and complex techniques for storage as described in the second paragraph. Nevertheless, the data chart displays wide variations attained through the performance of several genetic crosses, clearly suggesting the importance of certain genetic factors in relation to carotene production.

202. **(A)** Of the range given, β-lactoglobulin is least soluble at low NaCl concentrations. Its solubility

at 1 mM (0.001 M) is less than that at the other concentrations.

203. **(B)** Increasing interionic distance implies decreasing salt concentration. Decreased salt concentration correlates with decreased solubility.

204. **(C)** From the table, an NaCl concentration of 1 millimole (0.001 M) implies an interionic distance of 94 Å. An angstrom is 10^{-10} meters, or 10^{-4} microns. The interionic distance of 94 Å is equal to $94 \times 10^{-4} = 9.4 \times 10^{-3}$ microns.

205. **(A)** At a salt concentration of 10 mM, the protein has a point of minimum solubility of pH 5.2-5.3. Solubility increases as rapidly (perhaps slightly more rapidly) as pH decreases compared to a pH increase. Since pH 4.7 is 0.5-0.6 pH units from the point of minimum solubility, while pH 5.5 is only 0.2-0.3 pH units from that point, solubility may be predicted to be greatest at the pH 4.7.

206. **(D)** Salting-in is the term used to describe the increase in a protein's solubility due to a small amount of salt. Addition of large amounts of salt often results in the protein's loss of solubility, a phenomenon known as salting-out.

207. **(D)** Almost all globular proteins are least soluble at their isoelectric pH. The isoelectric pH is that pH at which the protein bears no net charge; at that pH, the protein molecules thus possess no electrical repulsion, and tend to clump together, coming out of solution.

208. **(B)** The leaves of the soybean evidently served to inhibit flowering when exposed to a long day, because the plant on the right flowered when its leaves were removed and it was exposed to a long day, whereas no flowering occurred under long-day conditions with the leaves intact. Plate G showed no inhibition taking place in total darkness; the plant flowered in darkness.

209. **(C)** The great majority of researchers feel that a hypothetical hormone, florigen, induces flowering. The cocklebur results are consistent with the concept of a diffusible substance causing flowering.

210. **(C)** The data presented show clearly that the critical day length is a maximum value for short-day plants; above a certain amount of light (long day), flowering did not occur in the soybean until part of the plant was removed. Analogously, long-day plants flower only when they receive more than a certain minimum amount of light.